AF633662

Rare Diseases of the Immune System

Series Editors
Lorenzo Emmi
Domenico Prisco

Editorial Board:
Systemic Vasculitis
L. Emmi
C. Salvarani
R.A. Sinico

Autoimmune Disease
P.L. Meroni
D. Roccatello
M. Matucci Cerinic
L. Emmi

Autoinflammatory Syndromes
M. Gattorno
F. De Benedetti
R. Cimaz

Primary Immunodeficiency
A. Plebani
C.T. Baldari
M.M. D'Elios

Systemic Fibroinflammatory Disorders
A. Vaglio

For further volumes
http://www.springer.com/series/11643

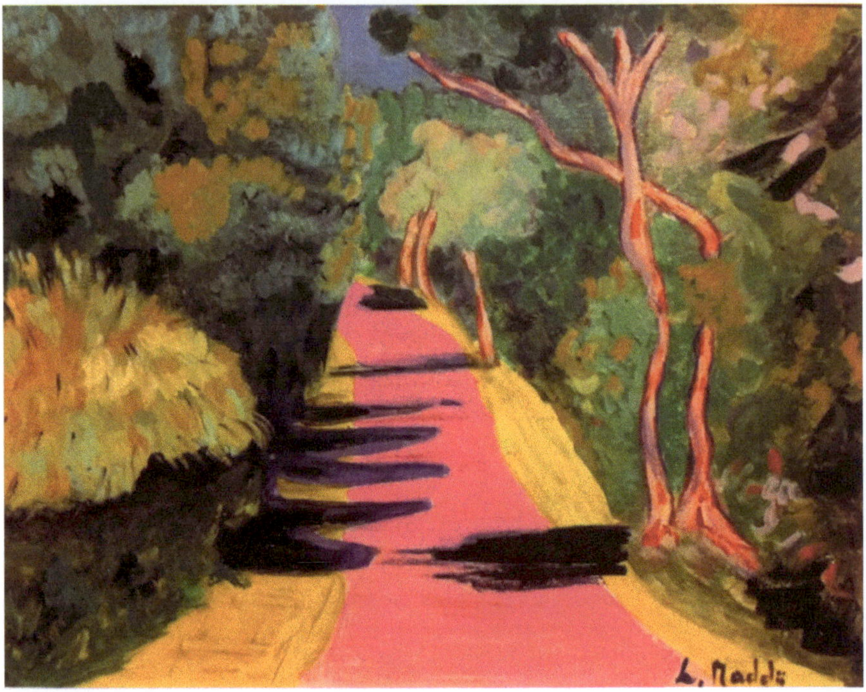

Sentiero Rosa
Laura Maddii Emmi
(private collection)

Pier Luigi Meroni
Editor

Antiphospholipid Antibody Syndrome

From Bench to Bedside

Springer

Editor
Pier Luigi Meroni
Department of Rheumatology
Gaetano Pini Institute
Milan
Italy

ISBN 978-3-319-11043-1 ISBN 978-3-319-11044-8 (eBook)
DOI 10.1007/978-3-319-11044-8
Springer Cham Heidelberg New York Dordrecht London

Library of Congress Control Number: 2014956675

© Springer International Publishing Switzerland 2015
This work is subject to copyright. All rights are reserved by the Publisher, whether the whole or part of the material is concerned, specifically the rights of translation, reprinting, reuse of illustrations, recitation, broadcasting, reproduction on microfilms or in any other physical way, and transmission or information storage and retrieval, electronic adaptation, computer software, or by similar or dissimilar methodology now known or hereafter developed. Exempted from this legal reservation are brief excerpts in connection with reviews or scholarly analysis or material supplied specifically for the purpose of being entered and executed on a computer system, for exclusive use by the purchaser of the work. Duplication of this publication or parts thereof is permitted only under the provisions of the Copyright Law of the Publisher's location, in its current version, and permission for use must always be obtained from Springer. Permissions for use may be obtained through RightsLink at the Copyright Clearance Center. Violations are liable to prosecution under the respective Copyright Law.
The use of general descriptive names, registered names, trademarks, service marks, etc. in this publication does not imply, even in the absence of a specific statement, that such names are exempt from the relevant protective laws and regulations and therefore free for general use.
While the advice and information in this book are believed to be true and accurate at the date of publication, neither the authors nor the editors nor the publisher can accept any legal responsibility for any errors or omissions that may be made. The publisher makes no warranty, express or implied, with respect to the material contained herein.

Printed on acid-free paper

Springer is part of Springer Science+Business Media (www.springer.com)

In spite of the great achievements in APS knowledge, the story is not over and we have to look at the future. So, as the Editor of this book, I would like to dedicate the text and the contents to who is now the future of my family: my grandson Leonardo born on April 28, 2014.

Preface

It is commonly thought that the antiphospholipid syndrome (APS) is a new disorder, but this actually is not correct. The paradox of the association of thrombotic events with the prolongation of blood clotting – the so-called lupus anticoagulant (LAC) phenomenon – has been known since the beginning of the 1950s. Such an association was originally described in a few patients suffering from systemic lupus erythematosus but was then found also in subjects without any other autoimmune condition.

What was thought to represent just an "esoteric" phenomenon was later structured as a condition characterized by the association between LAC and recurrent thrombotic vascular events and/or miscarriages by several groups between 1954 and 1963. However, the milestone in the APS story is represented by the publication in *Lancet* at the end of 1983 by Graham Hughes's group which clearly identified patients with APS for the first time.

In spite of the initial skepticism, APS has grown in the last years as an independent autoimmune disease and generated a large interest in both clinicians and researchers. So, the knowledge on the disease improved in an exponential manner, and it justifies the idea to collect new information in a book dedicated to the clinical and the basic aspects of APS – *Antiphospholipid Antibody Syndrome: From Bench to Bedside*.

The book covers the origin of the so-called antiphospholipid antibodies (aPL) which actually are directed against PL-binding proteins that have been recently characterized. The disease fulfills the usual aspects of every autoimmune condition requiring a genetic background and additional environmental triggers to develop. aPL are not only diagnostic markers but also pathogenic autoantibodies. These aspects are discussed in separate chapters in the book, spanning from the description of the laboratory classification criteria, the pathogenic mechanisms responsible for the vascular and the obstetric manifestations of the syndrome, to the LAC paradox.

Thanks to the new diagnostic tools (in particular, the discovery of the beta-2 glycoprotein I (β2GPI)-dependent aPL), it has been possible to better describe the clinical manifestations of the syndrome and to recognize well-defined clinical classification criteria. However, the larger number of the epidemiological studies suggested new clinical variants such as the catastrophic APS or APS nephropathy. At the same time, additional clinical manifestations have been suggested to represent non-classification criteria still a matter of research. All these aspects are covered by dedicated chapters in the book.

APS can be primary or associated to other systemic autoimmune diseases; in such a case, the presence of aPL may affect the course and the prognosis of the underlying disease in a significant way. This is the reason for a special chapter on the issue. The same is also true for asymptomatic aPL-positive carriers that represent a not-so-rare challenging condition for the physicians in real life.

The treatment of APS is another hot issue. Two different chapters cover the therapy for the vascular and the obstetric manifestations of the syndrome, addressing all the aspects, including the conditions in which there are no well-defined therapeutic approaches. Besides old and new anticoagulant and/or antiplatelet drugs, new therapeutic tools are under active investigation and likely to become available soon. This is covered by a specific chapter.

I do hope that the book may offer a real overview of the APS – from bench to bedside – and represent a useful tool for all the people interested in the syndrome.

Milan, Italy Pier Luigi Meroni

Contents

Genetics and Origin of Antiphospholipid Syndrome

1

Alessandra Soriano, Miri Blank, and Yehuda Shoenfeld

1.1 Introduction

Antiphospholipid syndrome (APS) is a multisystemic autoimmune disorder characterized by vascular thrombosis and/or pregnancy morbidity associated with the concomitant detection of antiphospholipid antibodies (aPL), including lupus anticoagulant (LA), anticardiolipin antibodies (aCL), and anti-β2 glycoprotein I (anti-β2GPI) antibodies [1].

Actually, aPL are a heterogenous group of antibodies that react with a myriad of phospholipids (PLs), PL-protein complexes, and PL-binding proteins. The main antigenic target of these antibodies is recognized to be β2GPI, which along with prothrombin accounts for more than 90 % of the antibody-binding activity in APS patients [2–4].

A. Soriano, MD
Zabludowicz Center for Autoimmune Diseases, Chaim Sheba Medical Center – Affiliated to Tel Aviv University, Tel Hashomer 52621, Israel

Department of Clinical Medicine and Rheumatology, Campus Bio-Medico University, Rome 00128, Italy
e-mail: soriano.alessandra@gmail.com

M. Blank, PhD
Zabludowicz Center for Autoimmune Diseases, Chaim Sheba Medical Center – Affiliated to Sackler Faculty of Medicine, Tel Aviv University, Tel Hashomer 52621, Israel
e-mail: Miri.Blank@sheba.health.gov.il

Y. Shoenfeld, MD, FRCP (Hon), MaACR (✉)
Zabludowicz Center for Autoimmune Diseases, Chaim Sheba Medical Center – Affiliated to Tel Aviv University, Tel Hashomer 52621, Israel

Incumbent of the Laura Schwarz-Kipp Chair for Research of Autoimmune Diseases, Sackler Faculty of Medicine, Tel-Aviv University, Tel Hashomer 52621, Israel
e-mail: Yehuda.Shoenfeld@sheba.health.gov.il

© Springer International Publishing Switzerland 2015

P.L. Meroni (ed.), *Antiphospholipid Antibody Syndrome: From Bench to Bedside*, Rare Diseases of the Immune System, DOI 10.1007/978-3-319-11044-8_1

The genetic basis of aPL [5] and APS [6] has been suggested by several authors according to many clinical evidences, family studies, and experimental models, although the underlying genetic factors predisposing to APS have not been clearly established. Future research in this field may help in delineating also the mechanisms for APS [7].

Similarly, the origin of pathogenic aPL remains to be clearly elucidated. Several environmental factors have been studied in the last decades, with most of the evidence regarding a wide spectrum of infectious agents, which could be responsible for the "second hit" in the APS pathophysiological mechanisms. Molecular mimicry, epitope spreading, and bystander activation are some of the proposed mechanisms through which infectious agents may act in an individual with a procoagulant phenotype, the latter defined as the "first hit" [8].

The focus of this chapter is to gather the most recent scientific evidence with regard to genetics and origin of APS.

1.2 Genetics in APS: Family, Population, and Genome-Wide Association Studies

The human leukocyte antigen (HLA) association with aPL and APS has been studied through various animal models, family and population studies, and more recently, through genome-wide association studies (GWAS). It has emerged that both autoantibody production and disease expression may be influenced by major histocompatibility complex (MHC) genes [8]. In addition, prothrombotic genetic markers may modify the disease expression in APS patients especially when associated with acquired factors such as aPL [9].

APL are a heterogeneous group of antibodies with many different antigenic targets. Today we know that only a limited number of aPL are pathogenic, being induced in most of the cases by certain viral or bacterial products and determining a break in tolerance because of sequence similarities with host antigens [10, 11].

Nevertheless, nowadays it is also clear that a favorable genetic background is essential for the subsequent development of APS, similarly to other autoimmune diseases.

In 1966, Harvey and Shulman [12] described the first family with persistent false-positive tests for syphilis detected in their members, in whom a full-blown autoimmune disease developed years later. In the following decades, several studies described families with high incidence of primary APS associated with LA, aCL, and other autoantibodies [6, 13, 14].

A link with HLA haplotypes has been reported in different family studies on APS: the paternal haplotypes A30, Cw3, B60, DR4, DRw53, and DQw3 have been shown in association with aCL in all the members of an English Canadian family, both in asymptomatic individuals and in those affected with APS secondary to systemic lupus erythematosus (SLE) and autoimmune thyroid disease. In addition, the presence of LA has been demonstrated in family members carrying DR4 and DR7 [15, 16].

A dominant or codominant model for inheritance of the disease by segregation analysis was suggested in a 1998 study considering seven families with a high incidence of primary APS, among which 30 out of 101 members met the diagnostic criteria. However, the study failed to find a linkage to HLA nor to other candidate genes including β2-GPI and Fas [17].

Apart from family studies, association of HLA and APS has been demonstrated in cohorts of patients with primary APS, in which DRB1*04, DR7, DQB1*0301/4, DQB1*0604/5/6/7/8/9, DQA1*0102, and DQA1*0301/2 were found with increased frequency [18–20]. The analysis of a large series of European patients with SLE by Galeazzi et al. [21] has found an association of aCL with HLA-DRB1*04, -DRB1*07, DQA1*0201, DQA1*0301, DQB1*0301, DQB1*0302, and DRB3*0301, while anti-β2GPI were positively associated with DQB1*0302.

Furthermore, the detection of anti-β2GPI was strongly associated with DRB1*1302 and DQB1*0604/0605 haplotypes in African American and in white British patients with primary APS [18, 22], while in Caucasian and Mexican Americans, DQB1*0302 was strongly correlated with anti-β2GPI [18, 22, 23].

Prothrombotic genetic factors have been found playing a role in modifying the disease expression in APS, namely, factor V Leiden mutation; antithrombin III, protein C, and protein S deficiencies; and prothrombin mutations [24]. Subjects with APS carrying factor V Leiden mutation showed an increased incidence of thrombosis in comparison to those without the mutation. On the other hand, other studies comparing the rates of thrombosis in APS patients with factor V Leiden mutation and in the general population (in which the frequency of factor V Leiden mutation ranges from 1 to 15 % for Caucasians) failed to detect a strong influence in APS population on the development of the thrombotic event [24–26]. Moreover, there have been reports of increased risk of thrombosis in APS in case of protein C and S deficiency, as well as in case of association with G20210A mutation [27].

Tissue factor pathway inhibitor [28], type I plasminogen activator inhibitor [29], annexin A5 [30], and p-selectin glycoprotein ligand 21 [31] may potentially positively influence the risk of thrombosis in APS patients.

Recently, Pierangeli et al. [32] showed the in vivo pathogenic role of toll-like receptor 4 (TLR-4) in APS by studying the thrombogenic aPL activity in lipopolysaccharide (LPS) non-responsive (LPS –/–) mice and the association between tlr4 gene polymorphisms and APS in patients affected. The authors found significantly smaller thrombi and fewer white blood cells (WBC) count adhering to endothelial cells in LPS –/– mice displaying a tlr4 spontaneous mutation, when immunized with IgG from patient with APS, suggesting a potential role of TLR-4 in the interaction between aPL and endothelial cells in vivo.

Genome-wide association studies (GWAS) are a relatively new search method based on the study of several single nucleotide polymorphisms (SNPs) in order to identify those occurring more frequently in people affected with a certain disease. This type of study is generally used to pinpoint genes that may contribute to a subject's risk of developing the disease.

Before the GWAS approach, SNPs analyses had been performed to investigate the genetic association between primary APS and SLE, given their clinical and serological similarities.

In 2009, 10 SNPs previously shown to be associated with SLE have been genotyped in a cohort of Italian APS patients [53]. The rationale of the study was to investigate whether the analysis of SLE susceptibility genes could partially provide an explanation for the small percentage of primary APS patients developing a full-blown SLE over the years, despite the similarities between the two conditions.

The study showed a very strong association with *STAT4* and *BLK* SNPs; conversely, no association was detected with *BANK1* [53]. These results were further confirmed when the authors extended their investigation through an additional group of APS patients [54].

Interestingly, in this further study a stronger association with one SNP of *IRF5* (rs2070197), which is a tag for risk haplotype in SLE, was found in the additional group [54]. On the other hand, the lack of association with rs2004640, the strongest *IRF5* SNP associated with SLE, was also confirmed. These last findings underlined that the differences in the genetic effects of *IRF5* between APS and SLE may also account for some of their different clinical expressions.

A genome-wide association study recently performed in an effort to detect loci/genes for aCL, anti-β2GPI, and LA in a cohort of women of European ancestry affected with SLE and carriers of aPL identified a number of suggestive novel loci for aPL, including genes not located near or at the MHC locus [7].

Although the study did not identify loci meeting the conservative threshold of genome-wide significance, it has suggested the potential role in APS of other genes involved in the immune response, like *SESTD1* and *TANK*, which play a role in binding PL species and in type I interferon production, respectively [7]. Undoubtedly, GWAS will contribute to open the way through new directions in the comprehension of APS genetics in the next future.

1.2.1 Genetic Animal Studies

Despite the fact that the first animal models on APS date back to 1980s [33, 34] – before the definition of APS – after three decades animal studies assessing the genetic basis for the development of this syndrome remain few.

The role of certain class of haplotypes in the production of pathogenic aPL came first from a study of Papalardo et al. [35] who elegantly showed the influence of MHC-II and the expression of DQ6, DQ8, and DR4 on the production of pathogenic aPL in mice. MHC-II deficient (−/−), DQ6, DQ8, and DR4 mice, MHC-II-deficient-transgenic mice, or their corresponding wild type (WT) were immunized with human β2GPI or with control protein ovalbumin. WT mice immunized with β2GPI produced significantly higher titers of aCL and anti-β2GPI when compared to controls, and this finding correlated with enhanced thrombus formation and tissue factor activity. MHC (−/−) mice immunized with β2GPI did not produce aCL or anti-β2GPI; mean thrombus sizes and tissue factor activities were significantly diminished, when compared to WT animals. Finally, the pathogenicity of aPL was fully reestablished in MHC (−/−) mice expressing DR4 and DQ8 haplotypes and partially restored in those expressing human DQ6 [35].

In 1992, Hashimoto et al. [36] in their model of APS demonstrated the spontaneous production of IgG aCL antibodies exhibiting the β2GPI-dependent binding to cardiolipin in NZW x BXSB F1 (W/B F1) male mice. Subsequent studies showed a preferential usage of certain VH and VK genes for the production of pathogenic aCL, while random V gene combinations were used for the production of nonpathogenic aCL, suggesting the possible antigen-driven mechanisms.

The search for triggering antigens was proved only in 1992, when Gharavi et al. [37] immunized NIH/Swiss mice with heterologous β2GPI rather than pure PLs, obtaining high-titer production of pathogenic aPL. These results were pivotal to orient research through the concept that the formation of immunogenic complexes against which aPL may be produced may occur when foreign PL-binding proteins with structures similar to β2-GPI bind to self PLs in vivo [8].

Several efforts have then been made in inducing high-titer production of pathogenic aPL in animal models, mainly through the immunization with peptides from microorganisms with functional and sequence similarity to that of the PL-binding site of β2GPI. These studies also contributed to elucidate the origin of pathogenic aPL, as resumed in the following paragraph.

1.3 Infections and Innate Immunity Mechanisms

Apart from the complex aspects of the genetics of APS, the ontogeny itself of the pathogenic aPL remains poorly understood.

As underlined in the introduction to this chapter, despite the presence of an induced procoagulant phenotype which may be genetically determined and finally defines the so-called first hit, an additional inciting factor, namely, "second hit," is necessary for the clinical manifestations of the disease [8].

Currently, infections are considered one of the most relevant environmental factors responsible for both aPL production and APS development.

The first infection recognized to be linked to aPL production was syphilis, although it was first hypothesized that syphilis-linked aPL were nonpathogenic [38–40].

In the following decades, several reports then showed a link between different types of infections and the development of aPL, as well as clinical manifestations of APS. Namely, human immunodeficiency virus (HIV), human T-cell lymphoma/leukemia virus (HTLV), hepatitis B and C virus, varicella-zoster virus (VZV), parvovirus B19, and cytomegalovirus (CMV) have been associated with the production of aPL and the development of clinical manifestations of APS.

Later on, it was clearly postulated that incidental exposure of genetically susceptible individuals to certain infectious agents that bear β2GPI-like structures can induce a break in tolerance to this antigen, thus facilitating the production of pathogenic aPL [8]. In this regard, molecular mimicry has been proposed as one of the pivotal mechanisms for the production of pathogenic aPL, because of the breakdown in the normal mechanisms of peripheral tolerance.

Great part of the efforts in inducing high-titer production of pathogenic aPL in animal models have been made through the immunization with peptides from microorganisms with functional and sequence similarity to that of the PL-binding site of β2GPI [41].

Greater degrees of PL-binding were shown by the peptides TADL from adenovirus (AdV), TIFI and VITT from cytomegalovirus (CMV), and SGDF from Bacillus subtilis, all of them inducing both high-titer aPL and anti-β2GPI production in mice. The pathogenicity of the antibodies induced in TIFI-immunized mice was then confirmed in subsequent experiments in vitro and in vivo [41–43].

Blank et al. [44, 45] added further evidence for a plausible role of molecular mimicry for the infectious origin of aPL: a β2GPI-related hexapeptide, TLRVYK, was identified by anti-β2GPI monoclonal antibodies originated from a patient with recurrent fetal loss on APS peptide background and peptide phage-displayed library. High titers of aCL β2GPI-dependent antibodies were produced through naïve mice immunization with 7 pathogens out of 24 showing high homology to TLRVYK. When purified anti-TLRVYK antibodies were passively transferred to naïve female mice, clinical manifestations of experimental APS were caused only by the autoantibodies originated from Haemophilus influenzae, Neisseria gonorrhoeae, or tetanus toxoid immunized mice, with high affinity to β2GPI.

The use of three synthetic peptides (namely, "A," NTLKTPRVGGC; "B," KDKATFGCHDGC; "C," CATLRVYKGG) derived from a peptide phage-displayed library and reacting specifically with the anti-β2GPI monoclonal antibodies (mAbs) ILA-1, ILA-3, and H-3 has been shown to neutralize the pathogenic functional activity of anti-β2GPI mAbs in vitro [44]. In vivo infusion of each of the anti-β2GPI mAbs into BALB/c mice, followed by administration of the corresponding specific peptides, was able to prevent the peptide-treated mice from developing experimental APS [44].

Moreover, the synthetic peptide named peptide "A" NTLKTPRVGGC that shares similarity with common bacterial antigens prevented induction of thrombosis ex vivo in an aPL-mediated thrombosis [46]. Peptide "A" is also found in region I/II of β2GPI. A scrambled form of peptide "A" (scGTKGCPNVRLT) was used as a control and had no effect.

Evidence that LPS primes the endothelium of rat mesenteric vessels has been provided for anti-β2GPI-mediated thrombosis [55].

Additionally, treatment of mice with intraperitoneal injection of LPS following the injection of cyanine 5.5-labeled β2GPI has been shown to promote protein localization on gut and brain endothelial cells associated with IgG, C1q, and C9 deposition in immunized mice [56].

In this regard, a critical role for complement in inducing aPL-mediated blood clots and fetal resorption has been found first by using aPL of undefined specificity [55] and, afterward, by using specific antibodies to β2GPI [56]. Agostinis et al. [57] recently proposed a novel therapeutic approach based on the use of a high-affinity human monoclonal antibody to β2GPI that competes with the APS patients' antibodies for binding to β2GPI and inhibits their ability to induce blood clots and fetal loss by determining the failure of complement activation [57].

As concerns the intracellular molecular pathways involved in β2GPI-dependent aPL-mediated endothelial cells activation and leading to procoagulating state of the cells, Meroni et al. [47] showed the role of TLR-4 as a co-receptor for MyD88 upregulation with the subsequent NFκB activation. This molecular pathway is specific for LPS-triggered innate immunity. In addition, as previously underlined, Pierangeli et al. [32] studied in vivo the pathogenic role of TLR-4 through evaluating the aPL activity in LPS non-responsive (LPS –/–) mice. It was shown that smaller thrombi developed in LPS –/– mice in comparison to LPS +/+ mice.

Three main plausible mechanisms have been proposed in order to explain the enhanced aPL production in the presence of LPS: (1) the interaction of T cells with antigen-presenting cells (APC) due to overexpression of co-stimulatory molecules induced by LPS, (2) the activation of APC and the subsequent production of TNF-α, and (3) the bystander activation of B cells [48, 49].

Recently, the role of LPS in the in vitro interaction of β2GPI with endothelial TLR-4 has been investigated by Raschi et al. [58]. In their model, the authors demonstrated a threshold effect for the action of LPS on endothelial cells, different from what was observed on monocyte/macrophages cultures.

Indeed, LPS has been found to enhance anti-β2GPI antibody endothelial cells binding only at cell-activating concentrations, shown to increase TLR-4 expression. Thereby, it has been speculated that LPS may act as an inflammatory stimulus upregulating TLR-4 expression and at the same time favoring the formation of β2GPI/LPS complexes. The interaction of β2GPI with TLR-4 – directly or complexed with LPS – can finally increase the presence of β2GPI on the endothelial cell surface, eventually allowing antibody binding, complement fixation, and clotting.

A similar cascade of events could explain the in vivo LPS effect in animal models [56] and can be hypothesized in vivo in APS patients who experienced some types of infectious processes that may represent trigger hits for clotting [58, 59].

Moreover, infectious agents could potentially induce autoimmune response through the selection (or destruction) of specific lymphocyte subsets, by releasing specific subsets of chemokines and cytokines, or by the exposure of cryptic autoantigens that can follow the cell necrosis and apoptosis.

The concept that cell damage could be one of the origins of aPL was first formulated by Piroux et al. [50] in 1997, who provided evidence about the peculiar recognition of surface epitopes – including β2GPI and anionic phospholipid complexes like phosphatidylserine (PS) – that are exposed following the cell apoptosis.

The binding of β2GPI to the surface of apoptotic cells was shown to generate an epitope recognized by aPL in patients affected with primary APS and SLE by Levine et al. [51].

Long-lasting circulating apoptotic cells presenting PS on the apoptotic blebs may lead to presentation of hidden epitopes or neo-epitopes of β2GPI once the complex PS/β2GPI has been constituted, finally triggering the immune response to self and inducing the production of aPL, including anti-β2GPI antibodies.

Similarly, it has been recently investigated the role of bacterial proteins in determining β2GPI conformational changes with following exposure of cryptic epitopes.

In particular, conformational changes in β2GPI have been hypothesized to trigger the formation of antibodies against a cryptic epitope in domain I of β2GPI, after its exposure on the outside of the molecule. Autoantibodies against the domain I of β2GPI have been found to be strongly associated with thrombotic events in APS patients and still represent a matter of extensive investigations [60].

Starting from these assumptions and given the previous evidence that β2GPI interacts with Streptococcus pyogenes [61], van Os et al. [62] recently injected mice with Streptococcus pyogenes-derived surface proteins, including M1 protein, protein H, streptococcal collagen-like protein A [SclA], and streptococcal collagen-like protein B [SclB].

They showed that the interaction of streptococcal protein H with plasma-derived β2GPI resulted in a conformational change in β2GPI, namely, from the plasmatic circular conformation through the fishhook shape, the latter being adopted after binding to phospholipids [62]. Anti-murine β2GPI IgM and IgG were detected only in mice challenged with multiple boosts of protein H (and not with boosts of the three other streptococcal proteins) and were mainly directed against domain I of β2GPI.

In their model, the authors hypothesized that during a long-lasting infection and probably following repetitive interactions between β2GPI and streptococcal protein H, the fishhook conformation of β2GPI triggers the immune system, resulting in the development of antibodies against the cryptic epitope in domain I of β2GPI. They finally speculated that proteins present on other microorganism may also bind to β2GPI and induce such a conformational change [62].

1.4 Other Potential Environmental Triggers Inducing the Production of aPL

Among other potential environmental triggers involved in the production of aPL, both solid and hematological malignancies have been reported in association with aPL and secondary APS, although the mechanisms remain to be elucidated. High levels of VEGF in patients affected with malignancies might contribute to tissue factor generation and procoagulant status in APS patients. The inflammatory network induced by the tumor cells, together with the pharmacological effects of chemotherapeutic drugs, could result in an increased amount of apoptotic cells which, as discussed above, are a further source of aPL and contribute to the development of thrombosis and also of catastrophic form of APS.

Several drugs including antiepileptic agents, antiarrhythmic drugs (procainamide), antipsychotic drugs such as chlorpromazine, antibiotics such as amoxicillin, and oral contraceptive drugs have been linked to increased titers of aPL, although data about prevalence of drug-induced aPL in APS are still lacking.

Furthermore, the exposure to acrylamide has been associated with the development of high levels of aCL and anti-β2GPI.

Finally, postvaccination-induced aPL following tetanus toxoid vaccine, hepatitis B vaccine, and influenza vaccine have been described in rare cases in association with APS clinical manifestations, but the pathophysiological mechanisms remain to be clarified [52].

References

1. Meroni PL, Borghi MO, Raschi E et al (2011) Pathogenesis of antiphospholipid syndrome: understanding the antibodies. Nat Rev Rheumatol 7:330–339
2. McNeil HP, Simpson RJ, Chesterman CN et al (1990) Antiphospholipid antibodies are directed against a complex antigen that includes lipid binding inhibitor of coagulation: β2 glycoprotein I (apolipoprotein H). Proc Natl Acad Sci U S A 87:4120–4124
3. Galli M, Comfurius P, Maassen C et al (1990) Anticardiolipin antibodies (ACA) directed not to cardiolipin but to a plasma protein cofactor. Lancet 335:1544–1547
4. Amengual O, Atsumi T, Koike T (2004) Antiprothrombin antibodies and the diagnosis of antiphospholipid syndrome. Clin Immunol 112:144–149
5. Mackworth-Young C, Chan J, Harris N (1987) High incidence of anticardiolipin antibodies in relatives of patients with systemic lupus erythematosus. J Rheumatol 14:723–726
6. Matthey F, Walshe K, Mackie IJ et al (1989) Familial occurrence of the antiphospholipid syndrome. J Clin Pathol 42:495–497
7. Ilyas Kamboh M, Wang X, Kao HA et al (2013) Genome wide association study for antiphospholipid antibodies. Autoimmune Dis 2013:761046
8. Willis R, Nigel Harris E, Pierangeli SS (2012) Pathogenesis of the antiphospholipid syndrome. Semin Thromb Hemost 38:305–321
9. Castro-Marrero J, Balada E, Vilardell-Tarrés M et al (2009) Genetic risk factors of thrombosis in the antiphospholipid syndrome. Br J Haematol 147:289–296
10. Gharavi AE, Pierangeli SS, Harris EN (2001) Origin of antiphospholipid antibodies. Rheum Dis Clin North Am 27:551–563
11. Gharavi AE, Pierangeli SS, Harris EN (2003) Viral origin of antiphospholipid antibodies: endothelial cell activation and thrombus enhancement by CMV peptide-induced APL antibodies. Immunobiology 207:37–42
12. Harvey AM, Shulman LE (1966) Connective tissue disease and the chronic biologic false-positive test for syphilis (BFP reaction). Med Clin North Am 50:1271–1279
13. Exner T, Barber S, Kronenberg H et al (1980) Familial association of the lupus anticoagulant. Br J Haematol 45:89–96
14. Jolidon RM, Knecht H, Humair L et al (1991) Different clinical presentations of a lupus anticoagulant in the same family. Klin Wochenschr 69:340–344
15. Rouget JP, Goudemand J, Montreuil G et al (1982) Lupus anticoagulant: a familial observation. Lancet 2(8289):105
16. Mackie IJ, Colaco CB, Machin SJ (1987) Familial lupus anticoagulants. Br J Haematol 67:359–363
17. Goel N, Ortel TL, Bali D et al (1999) Familial antiphospholipid antibody syndrome: criteria for disease and evidence for autosomal dominant inheritance. Arthritis Rheum 42:318–327
18. Caliz R, Atsumi T, Kondeatis E et al (2001) HLA class II gene polymorphisms in antiphospholipid syndrome: haplotype analysis in 83 Caucasoid patients. Rheumatology (Oxford) 40:31–36
19. Bertolaccini ML, Atsumi T, Caliz AR et al (2000) Association of antiphosphatidylserine/prothrombin autoantibodies with HLA class II genes. Arthritis Rheum 43:683–688

20. Vargas-Alarcon G, Granados J, Bekker C et al (1995) Association of HLA-DR5 (possibly DRB1*1201) with the primary antiphospholipid syndrome in Mexican patients. Arthritis Rheum 38:1340–1341
21. Galeazzi M, Sebastiani GD, Tincani A et al (2000) HLA class II alleles associations of anticardiolipin and anti-beta2GPI antibodies in a large series of European patients with systemic lupus erythematosus. Lupus 9:47–55
22. Arnett FC, Thiagarajan P, Ahn C et al (1999) Associations of anti-beta2-glycoprotein I autoantibodies with HLA class II alleles in three ethnic groups. Arthritis Rheum 42:268–274
23. Reverter JC, Tassies MD (2009) Genetic aspects of the antiphospholipid syndrome: associations with clinical manifestations. In: Handbook of systemic autoimmune diseases. Antiphospholipid syndrome in systemic autoimmune diseases. (Ed. by R. Cervera, J.C. Reverter and M. Khamashta). 10:91–103.
24. Schütt M, Klüter H, Hagedorn-Greiwe M et al (1998) Familial coexistence of primary antiphospholipid syndrome and factor V Leiden. Lupus 7:176–182
25. Brenner B, Vulfsons SL, Lanir N et al (1996) Coexistence of familial antiphospholipid syndrome and factor V Leiden: impact on thrombotic diathesis. Br J Haematol 94:166–167
26. Chopra N, Koren S, Greer WL et al (2002) Factor V Leiden, prothrombin gene mutation, and thrombosis risk in patients with antiphospholipid antibodies. J Rheumatol 29:1683–1688
27. Ames PR, Margaglione M, Tommasino C et al (2001) Impact of plasma homocysteine and prothrombin G20210 A on primary antiphospholipid syndrome. Blood Coagul Fibrinolysis 12:699–704
28. Lincz LF, Adams MJ, Scorgie FE et al (2007) Polymorphisms of the tissue factor pathway inhibitor gene are associated with venous thromboembolism in the antiphospholipid syndrome and carriers of factor V Leiden. Blood Coagul Fibrinolysis 18:559–564
29. Yasuda S, Tsutsumi A, Atsumi T et al (2002) Gene polymorphisms of tissue plasminogen activator and plasminogen activator inhibitor-1 in patients with antiphospholipid antibodies. J Rheumatol 29:1192–1197
30. de Laat B, Derksen RH, Mackie IJ et al (2006) Annexin A5 polymorphism (−1C-->T) and the presence of anti-annexin A5 antibodies in the antiphospholipid syndrome. Ann Rheum Dis 65:1468–1472
31. Bugert P, Pabinger I, Stamer K et al (2007) The risk of thromboembolic disease in lupus anticoagulant patients due to pathways involving P-selectin and CD154. Thromb Haemost 97:573–580
32. Pierangeli SS, Vega-Ostertag ME, Raschi E et al (2007) Toll-like receptor and antiphospholipid mediated thrombosis: in vivo studies. Ann Rheum Dis 66:1327–1333
33. Hang LM, Izui S, Dixon FJ (1981) (NZW x BXSB)F1 hybrid. A model of acute lupus and coronary vascular disease with myocardial infarction. J Exp Med 154:216–221
34. Oyaizu N, Yasumizu R, Miyama-Inaba M et al (1988) (NZW x BXSB) F1 mouse. A new animal model of idiopathic thrombocytopenic purpura. J Exp Med 167:2017–2022
35. Papalardo E, Romay-Penabad Z, Christadoss P et al (2010) Induction of pathogenic antiphospholipid antibodies in vivo are dependent on expression of MCH-II genes. Lupus 19:496
36. Hashimoto Y, Kawamura M, Ichikawa K et al (1992) Anticardiolipin antibodies in NZW x BXSB F1 mice. A model of antiphospholipid syndrome. J Immunol 149:1063–1068
37. Gharavi AE, Sammaritano LR, Wen J et al (1992) Induction of antiphospholipid antibodies by immunization with beta 2 glycoprotein I (apolipoprotein H). J Clin Invest 90:1105–1109
38. Wasserman A (1907) Über Entwicklung und den Gegenwartingen Stand der Serodiagnostic gegenüber Syphilis. Berl Klin Wochenschr 44:1599–1634
39. Harris EN, Gharavi AE, Boey ML et al (1983) Anticardiolipin antibodies: detection by radioimmunoassay and association with thrombosis in systemic lupus erythematosus. Lancet 2:1211–1214
40. Levy Y, Almog O, Gorshtein A et al (2006) The environment and antiphospholipid syndrome. Lupus 15:784–790

41. Gharavi EE, Chaimovich H, Cucurull E et al (1999) Induction of antiphospholipid antibodies by immunization with synthetic viral and bacterial peptides. Lupus 8:449–455
42. Gharavi AE, Pierangeli SS, Espinola RG et al (2002) Antiphospholipid antibodies induced in mice by immunization with a cytomegalovirus-derived peptide cause thrombosis and activation of endothelial cells in vivo. Arthritis Rheum 46:545–552
43. Gharavi AE, Vega-Ostertag M, Espinola RG et al (2004) Intrauterine fetal death in mice caused by cytomegalovirus-derived peptide induced aPL antibodies. Lupus 13:17–23
44. Blank M, Shoenfeld Y, Cabilly S et al (1999) Prevention of experimental antiphospholipid syndrome and endothelial cell activation by synthetic peptides. Proc Natl Acad Sci 96:5164–5168
45. Blank M, Krause I, Fridkin M, Keller N, Kopolovic J, Goldberg I, Tobar A, Shoenfeld Y (2002) Bacterial induction of autoantibodies to beta2-glycoprotein-I accounts for the infectious etiology of antiphospholipid syndrome. J Clin Invest 109:797–804
46. Pierangeli SS, Blank M, Liu X, Espinola R, Fridkin M, Ostertag MV, Roye-Green K, Harris EN, Shoenfeld Y (2004) A peptide that shares similarity with bacterial antigens reverses thrombogenic properties of antiphospholipid antibodies in vivo. J Autoimmun 22: 217–225
47. Meroni PL, Raschi E, Testoni C, Parisio A, Borghi MO (2004) Innate immunity in the antiphospholipid syndrome: role of toll-like receptors in endothelial cell activation by antiphospholipid antibodies. Autoimmun Rev 3:510–515
48. Benson MJ, Elgueta R, Schpero W et al (2009) Distinction of the memory B cell response to cognate antigen versus bystander inflammatory signals. J Exp Med 206:2013–2025
49. Khoruts A, Mondino A, Pape KA et al (1998) A natural immunological adjuvant enhances T cell clonal expansion through a CD28-dependent, interleukin (IL)-2-independent mechanism. J Exp Med 187:225–236
50. Piroux V, Eschwege V, Freyssinet JM (1997) Cell damage at the origin of antiphospholipid antibodies and their pathogenic potential in recurrent pregnancy loss. Infect Dis Obstet Gynecol 5:176–180
51. Levine JS, Koh JS, Subang R et al (1999) Apoptotic cells as immunogen and antigen in the antiphospholipid syndrome. Exp Mol Pathol 66:82–98
52. Blank M, Israeli E, Shoenfeld Y (2012) When APS (Hughes syndrome) met the autoimmune/inflammatory syndrome induced by adjuvants. Lupus 21:711–714
53. Yin H, Borghi MO, Delgado-Vega AM, Tincani A, Meroni PL, Alarcon-Riquelme ME (2009) Association of STAT4 and BLK, but not BANK1 or IRF5, with primary antiphospholipid syndrome. Arthritis Rheum 60:2468–2471
54. Fredi M, Tincani A, Yin H, Delgado-Vega AM, Borghi MO, Meroni PL, Alarcon-Riquelme ME (2010) IRF5 is associated with antiphospholipid syndrome but is not a major risk factor. Arthritis Rheum 62:1201–1202
55. Fischetti F, Durigutto P, Pellis V, Debeus A, Macor P, Bulla R, Bossi F, Ziller F, Sblattero D, Meroni PL, Tedesco F (2005) Thrombus formation induced by antibodies to β2-glycoprotein I is complement dependent and requires a priming factor. Blood 106:2340–2346
56. Agostinis C, Biffi S, Garrovo C, Durigutto P, Lorenzon A, Bek A, Bulla R, Grossi C, Borghi MO, Meroni PL, Tedesco F (2011) In vivo distribution of β2-glycoprotein I under various pathophysiologic conditions. Blood 118:4231–4238
57. Agostinis C, Durigutto P, Sblattero D, Borghi MO, Grossi C, Giuda F, Bulla R, Macor P, Pregnolato F, Meroni PL, Tedesco F (2014) A non-complement fixing antibody to β2-glycoprotein I as a novel therapy for antiphospholipid syndrome. Blood 123:3478–3487
58. Raschi E, Chighizola C, Grossi C, Ronda N, Gatti R, Meroni PL, Borghi MO (2014) β2-glycoprotein I, lipopolysaccharide and endothelial TLR4: three players in the two hit theory for anti-phospholipid-mediated thrombosis. J Autoimmun Mar 27 [Epub ahead of print]
59. Shoenfeld Y, Blank M, Cervera R, Font J, Raschi E, Meroni PL (2006) Infectious origin of the antiphospholipid syndrome. Ann Rheum Dis 65:2–6

60. de Laat B, van Berkel M, Urbanus RT, Siregar B, de Groot PG, Gebbink MF, Maas C (2011) Immune responses against domain I of β2-glycoprotein I are driven by conformational changes. Arthritis Rheum 63:3960–3968
61. Nilsson M, Wasylik S, Morgelin M, Olin AI, Meijers JC, Derksen RH, de Groot PG, Herwald H (2008) The antibacterial activity of peptides derived from human β2-glycoprotein I is inhibited by protein H and M1 protein from Streptococcus pyogenes. Mol Microbiol 67:482–492
62. van Os GM, Meijers JC, Agar C, Seron MV, Marquart JA, Akesson P, Urbanus RT, Derksen RH, Herwald H, Morgelin M, de Groot PG (2011) Induction of anti β2-glycoprotein I autoantibodies in mice by protein H of Streptococcus pyogenes. J Thromb Haemost 9:2447–2456

2 The Paradox of Lupus Anticoagulant

Alessandra Banzato and Vittorio Pengo

2.1 History

In the 1940s a report from the University of California Medical School described a young man with a fatal condition manifesting as moderate thrombocytopenia and prolonged whole blood clotting time with a hemorrhagic diathesis and intracranial and peripheral venous thrombosis [1]. Even if the prolonged clotting time was attributed to "hypothromboplastinemia" and the crude tests available did not demonstrate a coagulation inhibitor, it may be speculated whether this was the first description of a lupus inhibitor. Afterward, Ley et al. [2] reported on a young man with a fatal disease with abnormal bleeding, arthralgias, and leg vein thrombosis, with prolonged blood clotting time and prothrombin time attributed to hypoprothrombinemia. At examination, as well as tissue bleeds, there were renal changes indicative of SLE and cerebral infarcts.

In the 1950s it was progressively more acknowledged that some patients with systemic lupus erythematosus (SLE) have a circulating anticoagulant factor. Conley [3], of Johns Hopkins, wrote a brief report about two patients with lupus and a "peculiar hemorrhagic disorder" with prolonged blood clotting and prothrombin times, and clear evidence of an anticoagulant in plasma mixing studies. Especially, both patients had biological false-positive tests for syphilis.

These observations were complemented by Frick and Weimer in the 1955s, who reported three patients with convincing evidence of coagulation inhibitors, including in one subject with confirmed lupus. In each case there were positive serological tests for syphilis, and in only one of the three was there a definite hemorrhagic

A. Banzato • V. Pengo (✉)
Department of Cardiologic Thoracic and Vascular Sciences, Padua University Hospital, Via Giustiniani, 2, Padua 35121, Italy
e-mail: alessandra.banzato@unipd.it; vittorio.pengo@unipd.it

© Springer International Publishing Switzerland 2015
P.L. Meroni (ed.), *Antiphospholipid Antibody Syndrome: From Bench to Bedside*, Rare Diseases of the Immune System, DOI 10.1007/978-3-319-11044-8_2

diathesis. Furthermore, they provided evidence for transplacental transfer of the anticoagulant in one subject and postulated an "immunologic" pathogenesis [4]. The picture of lupus anticoagulant was slowly emerging, with evidence of its immunoglobulin association, and, in retrospect, the link to anticardiolipin was present, identified through the biological false-positive tests for syphilis in these patients. Subsequent case reports demonstrated that on serum electrophoresis the Wasserman reagent and the anticoagulant localized to the same region of gamma globulins [5]. The hypothesis of Frick [4] that the mechanism of action was "directed against thromboplastin" was reasonable at the time and not all that far from the truth.

In the 1960s it was increasingly recognized that the in vitro anticoagulant phenomenon in SLE could be associated with a thrombotic rather than a hemorrhagic diathesis: Bowie et al. [6] reported on the presence of circulating anticoagulant in eight of 11 patients with SLE of whom three suffered from deep vein thrombosis and one from ischemic leg ulcers and livedo reticularis.

The term "lupus anticoagulant" (LAC) was coined only later [7], in 1972, to designate an inhibitor of coagulation that impairs prothrombinase activation of prothrombin (PT), which was recognized in the plasma of patients with systemic SLE. Some arguments favored the hypothesis that the inhibitor was directed against phospholipids (PL) since preincubation with PL reduced its activity and the inhibitory effect was more pronounced when PL were diluted. It seems likely that the excess of descriptions of a hemorrhagic diathesis in the early case reports with what came to be known in the 1970s as lupus coagulation inhibitor [8], and soon after lupus anticoagulant, was simply due to the presentation with bleeding as the principal symptom in these unusual cases and the lack of any reason to explore coagulation in SLE patients without such a history of bleeding. Subsequent case reports highlighted that the lupus anticoagulant-associated prothrombotic condition can arise in the absence of SLE or other connective tissue disorders [9]. A significant diagnostic breakthrough occurred with the development of assays for anticardiolipin (aCL) that were considerably more sensitive than other assays. Harris et al. in 1983 [10] demonstrated that almost two-thirds of serum samples from a cohort of 65 patients with SLE had high levels of anticardiolipin.

Furthermore, over 90 % of those with LAC had raised anticardiolipin antibody levels, confirming the relationship previously suggested by cases with both LAC and biological false-positive tests for syphilis. Finally, there was a correlation between raised aCL titer and history of thrombosis within this patient cohort with SLE [10]. In the '80s, observations in four women, only one of whom had SLE, led to the postulation of a possible correlation between LAC and pregnancy morbidity [11]. This postulation was later confirmed [12]. Further case reports around this time suggested additional disease associations, for example, chorea gravidarum [13]. It was in the 1980s that the nomenclature "antiphospholipid antibody syndrome" (APS) began to be generally used [14], abbreviated to "antiphospholipid syndrome" afterward. The term primary antiphospholipid syndrome was introduced to describe those cases in which there was no background disease [15, 16]. There were also reports of cases with unusually acute and severe multiorgan vasoocclusive episodes associated with positive tests for antiphospholipid antibodies (aPL) [17, 18]. In 1992 Ronald Asherson of Cape Town, South Africa, coined the term catastrophic antiphospholipid syndrome (CAPS) [19]. It became clear that CAPS is a rare form of microangiopathic thrombosis that has shared features with thrombotic thrombocytopenic purpura, disseminated intravascular coagulation, and systemic inflammatory response syndrome (SIRS) as seen in sepsis. Because of these similarities, there is the possibility of both under- and over-diagnosis, especially in view of the lack of specificity of aPL. Multiorgan involvement is typical with a predilection for the lung, brain, and kidney. It may complicate previously diagnosed more typical APS or be the presenting manifestation, and there is often a trigger for the acute episode, such as infection or anti-coagulant withdrawal.

LAC is now considered the most important acquired risk factor for thrombosis and fetal loss. The current definition of LAC is autoantibodies that in vitro inhibit PL-dependent coagulation reactions in the absence of specific coagulation factor inhibition.

2.2 Autoantigen

Individuals with LAC have circulating autoantibodies that inhibit blood coagulation. The autoantibodies are of the IgG or IgM isotype and are mainly directed against two phospholipid (PL)-binding plasma proteins, β_2GPI and PT [20]. The presence of such inhibitors represents a well-recognized risk factor for venous and arterial thromboembolism, as well as pregnancy loss. These two proteins are mainly involved in the LAC phenomenon. β_2GPI is a 326-amino-acid PL-binding protein with a molecular weight of 50 kDa belonging to the complement control protein superfamily.

Its plasma concentration is approximately 200 μg/ml, and as 40 % is bound to lipoproteins, it is also termed "apolipoprotein H." Composed of five homologous "sushi" domains of approximately 60 amino acids and binding to anionic PL (aPL) with its fifth positively charged domain, it may have a role in the elimination of apoptotic cells from circulation.

Prothrombin (PT), a 579-amino-acid-long vitamin K-dependent glycoprotein with a molecular weight of 72 kDa, has central role in blood coagulation. Its plasma concentration is approximately 1.5 μmol/l. PT binds to PL through N-terminal γ-carboxyglutamic acid domain in the presence of calcium ions and is activated to thrombin by the prothrombinase complex (activated factor X, factor V, calcium ions, and negatively charged PL).

Both proteins can be purified from human plasma. Human β_2GPI is purified from normal plasma by means of perchloric acid precipitation and affinity chromatography on heparin–sepharose followed by cation-exchange chromatography. β_2GPI is a very conserved protein among species, and bovine and human β_2GPI cannot be distinguished from an antigenic point of view.

PT is purified from normal plasma by precipitation with barium chloride, which is then removed by ammonium sulfate. The supernatant is then applied to an anion-exchange column, and PT is eluted with a gradient of sodium chloride. Human and bovine PT differ as bovine PT may not be recognized by some LACs.

2.3 Autoantibody

The LAC phenomenon is related to the presence of autoantibodies of IgG or IgM isotypes directed against β_2GPI, PT, or both. This has been demonstrated by testing the anticoagulant properties of affinity-purified aβ_2GPI antibodies on normal plasma. By prolonging PL-dependent coagulation tests (in particular diluted Russell viper venom time (dRVVT)), the action of these antibodies is inhibited by an excess of PL. It has been proposed that the molecular mimicry mechanism between infectious agents and the β_2GPI molecule may generate anti-β_2GPI antibodies [21].

Moreover, a strong homology exists between β_2GPI-related peptides (target epitopes for anti-β_2GPI antibodies) and different common pathogens. Furthermore, β_2GPI polymorphism (in particular the Val 247 allele) has recently been associated with both a high frequency of anti-β_2GPI antibodies and a stronger antibody reactivity than the Leu247 β_2GPI allele. It is possible that this type of polymorphism may favor the occurrence of molecular mimicry. With regard to antiprothrombin antibodies, LAC activity was first demonstrated in the purified system consisting of human PT, factor Xa, factor Va, and calcium. The same properties have been shown by murine monoclonal antibodies against human β_2GPI and PT. How these immunoglobulins determine thromboembolic events or obstetric complications is still unknown as many theories have been put forward but none are considered totally resounding. One possibility is that antibodies responsible for LAC in vitro also interfere with the in vivo function of PL-dependent anticoagulant pathways. In fact, PL-dependent inactivation of factors Va/VIIIa by the thrombomodulin–protein C–protein S system or by PL-dependent tissue factor (TF) inhibition by tissue factor pathway inhibitor (TFPI) may be impaired in the presence of LAC [22].

Alternatively, β_2GPI (or annexin V, another putative autoantigen for LAC) may exert an anticoagulant effect in vivo, whereas autoantibodies to β_2GPI (or annexin V) may damage it. Thrombus formation may thus take place on the surface of activated monocytes, platelets, or endothelial cells. While original, these theories are controverted by the fact that congenital β_2GPI deficiency is not a risk factor for thrombosis.

Many autoimmune diseases are associated with genes in the major histocompatibility complex (MHC) region. MHC class II alleles (HLA-DR and DQ) may be involved in the genetic predisposition to develop LAC. HLA-DQw7 (DQB1*0301), linked to HLA-DR5 and -DR4 haplotypes, was significantly increased in LAC-positive patients as compared to race-matched normal controls. Moreover, the HLADQB1*0302 (DQ8) allele, typically carried on HLA-DR4 haplotypes, was associated with anti-β_2GPI, but there are variations in HLA associations in different ethnic groups. The HLA-DPB1 locus may also contribute to the genetic predisposition to develop anti-β_2GPI and clinical manifestations of APS in patients with SLE, but this association is unclear.

Previous criteria for the diagnosis of LAC were those proposed by Brandt in 1995 [23]: prolongation in at least one PL-dependent coagulation test out of two or more screening assays (activated partial thromboplastin time (aPTT), kaolin clotting time (KCT), dRVVT, diluted PT time (dPT)).

2.4 LAC Detection

According to the Brandt guidelines, in our laboratory dRVVT was determined essentially [24, 25], by using a single batch of reagents and an automatic coagulation analyzer. The screening test was considered positive when a 1:1 mixture of test plasma and normal plasma yielded a clotting time exceeding 42″. This cutoff value was usually calculated by using the 95th percentile of coagulation times obtained in frozen plasma samples from healthy subjects and corresponded to a ratio to normal plasma of 1.19. Results were confirmed in patient plasmas by test normalizing clotting time (confirming test), which has been reported to be diagnostic also in patients on oral anticoagulant treatment [26, 27]. KCT was determined using 2 % kaolin in distilled water [25] and was considered positive when a 1:1 mixture of normal and patient plasma yielded a coagulation time greater than 159″. This meant a ratio to pooled normal plasma of 1.31 (the cutoff value is calculated as for dRVVT). To exclude factor deficiency, test plasma was mixed with pooled plasma at a ratio of 1:1. A confirmatory test using an excess of PL or activated platelets (platelet neutralization procedure) or exagonal PL will neutralize the anticoagulant effect, demonstrating that the inhibitor is actually sensitive to PL. In any case, the presence of other inhibitors or heparin, which interferes with most LAC assays, should be excluded (Fig. 2.1).

Numerous variables affect screening tests for LAC detection. The low content of PL renders the test more sensitive, and KCT can be considered the most sensitive as no external PL is added to the assay, with the only available PL being those present

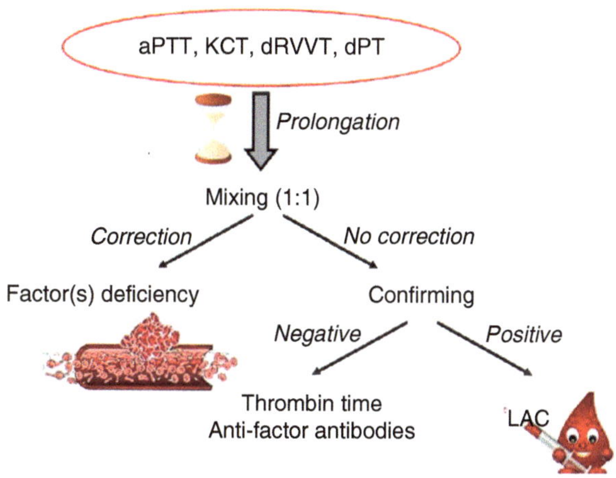

Fig. 2.1 Flow chart for diagnosis of LAC

in the plasma tested. Unfortunately, KCT is hard to automate, as most photo-optical devices cannot be used in the presence of the kaolin reagent, which tends to scatter light. The presence of platelets in this and in other assays greatly affects the results, particularly when plasma is frozen before testing. Centrifuging fresh plasma twice or using a double filter (through a 0.2-μm filter) may get around this problem. aPTT is a general coagulation screening test, KCT and dPT are used less frequently, and dRVVT has become the most commonly used screening assay for detection of LAC. We have modified the original test by diluting both the venom and the PL, thereby greatly increasing its sensitivity. Because Russell viper venom activates factor X directly, the test is normal in patients with some factor deficiency and in those with an inhibitor to factor VIII, the most common coagulation inhibitor associated with a bleeding tendency.

The performance of laboratories across the world to detect LA is a matter of concern. Misclassification of positive or negative LA plasma sample is commonly encountered in external surveys. Recently, in a survey of centralized LA diagnosis, we reported that about 33 % of plasma samples collected by thrombosis centers and labeled locally as LA positive were reported as LA negative in a central laboratory [28].

The poor laboratory performance is due to the lack of standardized tests and/or inappropriate application of the diagnostic criteria. Recently, the Brandt guidelines were updated [29]. Particular emphasis was given to several aspects discussed in this official communication. A new paragraph was dedicated to the patient selection. Testing for LAC should be limited to patients who have a significant probability of having the antiphospholipid syndrome (APS). Appropriateness to search for LAC can be graded according to clinical characteristics into low, moderate, and high.

- High: unprovoked venous thromboembolism (VTE) and (unexplained) arterial thromboembolism (ATE) in young patients (<50 years of age), thrombosis at unusual sites, late pregnancy loss, any thrombosis, or pregnancy morbidity in patients with autoimmune diseases (systemic lupus erythematosus, rheumatoid arthritis, autoimmune thrombocytopenia, autoimmune hemolytic anemia)
- Moderate: accidentally found prolonged aPTT in asymptomatic subjects, recurrent spontaneous early pregnancy loss, and provoked VTE in young patients
- Low: VTE or ATE in elderly patients

Modalities for blood collection and processing are fully delineated, and the choice of tests is limited to dRVVT and a sensitive aPTT. Calculation of cutoff values for each diagnostic step are clearly stated. To avoid misinterpretation, it is recommended to perform laboratory procedures 1–2 weeks after discontinuation of treatment or when the INR is less than 1.5. Bridging VKA discontinuation with LMWH is recommended with the last dose of LMWH administered more than 12 h before the blood is drawn for LAC testing. LAC result should always be considered in the context of a full laboratory aPL profile comprising aCL and aβ2GPI antibodies ELISAs. The presence of medium- to high-titer aCL and aβ2GPI of the same isotype (most often IgG) is in agreement with a positive LAC and identifies patients at high risk for thrombosis and fetal losses [30]. Diagnostic steps are confirmed to be those of previous guidelines: (a) screening step, (b) mixing test, and (c) confirmatory test.

Results of screening tests are potentially suggestive of LA when their clotting times are longer than the local cutoff value. Results should be expressed as follows:

$$\text{dRVVT Screen Ratio} = \frac{\text{Patient dRVVT Screen results (in seconds)}}{\text{PNP dRVVT Screen (in seconds)}}$$

Perform testing on patient plasmas mixed with the pooled normal plasma (PNP) at 1:1 proportion and express results as follows:

$$\text{dRVVT mixing Ratio} = \frac{\text{Patient dRVVT mixing (1:1)}}{\text{PNP dRVVT (in seconds)}}$$

Confirmatory Test: Results are confirmatory of LA if the % correction of patient's plasma at low (screen) and high (confirm) phospholipid concentration is above the local cutoff value.

Sensitive aPTT: same procedure as dRVVT should be used.

2.5 Significance of Positive LAC

LAC is an important test in vascular medicine, since its detection on two occasions 12 weeks apart in a patient with venous or arterial thromboembolism allows us to suspect the antiphospholipid syndrome (APS), and this in turn determines a different approach to secondary prevention and treatment. As thrombosis is a common event, laboratory diagnosis of LAC becomes crucial in identifying patients with APS.

When medium- to high-titer beta-2 glycoprotein I-dependent anticardiolipin antibodies and LAC are both present in the same patient's plasma, a complete positive antiphospholipid profile may render physicians more confident with the diagnosis of APS. However, APS diagnosis becomes problematic, due to the abovementioned laboratory pitfalls, when LAC is the only positive test among those used to study antiphospholipid antibodies. Moreover, if antihuman prothrombin antibodies are responsible for LAC, they are poorly associated with thromboembolic events [31]. Therefore, the development of simple coagulation tests improving the clinical significance of positive LA is important [32].

Among the so-called antiphospholipid antibodies, the presence of LAC is strongly associated with thrombosis and obstetric complications. Thromboembolic complications, venous thromboembolism (deep vein thrombosis and/or pulmonary embolism), and cerebral ischemia (transient ischemic attack (TIA) or stroke) are the most frequent. In a systematic review of the literature, LAC has been shown to be statistically associated with both venous and arterial thromboembolism with an odds ratio ranging from 4.09 to 16.2. Obstetric complications include fetal death, preeclampsia or eclampsia, and multiple abortions. The association of other antiphospholipid antibodies such as anticardiolipin antibodies (aCL) and aβ_2GPI with the clinical manifestations described above is less striking. The contemporaneous positivity in coagulation (LAC) and solid-phase assays (aCL and aβ_2GPI antibodies) is due to the presence of a common pathogenic group of aβ_2GPI antibodies.

As LAC is less sensitive with respect to solid-phase assays, triple positivity suggests that the aβ_2GPI antibodies present in plasma are able to express LAC activity. In the absence of standardization and reference material for testing, an antiphospholipid laboratory profile could help to better classify these patients [33]. With this in mind we examined the results of all the three tests obtained in 618 consecutive subjects and compared subjects with previously documented thrombosis-related events with those without, for the most part, normal subjects. When antiphospholipid antibody profiles, instead of individual test positivity, were considered in a multivariate analysis taking into account age, gender, the presence of SLE or other autoimmune diseases, and established risk factors for venous and arterial thromboembolism, triple positivity was found to be a strong independent risk factor (odds ratio 33.3, confidence interval 7.0–157.6). Significance was maintained when an association with venous or arterial thromboembolism was considered. Double positivity with negative LAC was a highly significant risk factor for obstetric complications only (odds ratio 10.8, confidence interval 2.9–40.8). Other combinations were not statistically significant. The analysis of a complete antiphospholipid antibody profile, as compared to a single testing, can thus better identify patients at risk. In fact, it is a common experience that some isolated and often transient episodes of LAC positivity, such as those not infrequently found in children or young adults during a coagulation screening before surgery, are benign and not associated with thromboembolism. In the same way, isolated aCL positivity can easily be found in infectious diseases where no association with thrombosis has been reported. It is important to underline that only some antibodies to a specific domain of β_2GPI express LAC activity and correlate strongly with thromboembolic events [34]. Other autoantibodies to β_2GPI may not be pathogenic, and this may explain why studies on aβ_2GPI antibody detection in solid-phase assays do not produce uniform results as IgG aβ_2GPI is associated with thrombosis in only a subset of patients. In those cases (from 2 to 10 %) in which aβ_2GPI is the sole antibody detected in patients with clinical manifestations of APS, it may not be pathogenic. In conclusion, a complete pattern of aPL antibodies comprising LAC, aCL, and aβ_2GPI is important for identifying pathogenic aβ_2GPI antibodies and the associated risk of clinical manifestations.

The prevalence of LAC in the normal population is reported to be 3.6 % according to screening using the KCT, but it may be much less. The prevalence of LAC in the SLE population has been reported to be between 10 and 50 %, depending on the test used [35].

The lupus anticoagulant is detected according to a set of diagnostic criteria recommended by the Scientific and Standardization Committee of the International Society of Thrombosis and Haemostasis. The sensitivity and specificity of these procedures vary, depending on the type of test, reagents, instrumentation, cutoff values, and the expression of results utilized. Many surveys have been carried out to evaluate the performance of clinical laboratories in LAC diagnosis. A recent survey was carried out within the framework of activities of the Italian Federation of Anticoagulation Clinics using affinity-purified lyophilized IgG aβ_2GPI from a single patient. Overall, 69, 68, and 59 out of 70 participants were able to detect LAC in plasma with high, intermediate, and low potency (sensitivity 99, 97, and 84 %).

Conversely, 69, 50, and 53 out of 70 were able to rule out LAC when examining normal, heparinized, and deficient plasma (specificity, 99, 71, and 76 %). This survey showed that sensitivity is satisfactory, whereas specificity should be improved.

We have recently demonstrated that LAC with associated aCL and aβ_2GPI antibody positivity (triple positivity) is a risk factor for thromboembolic recurrence. Moreover, LAC in these patients constantly remains positive with time. Thromboembolic events may occur anywhere without provocation. It is the experience of authors that appropriate oral anticoagulant treatment is essential as recurrence is more frequent at the subtherapeutic international normalized ratio (i.e., INR <2.0). A first distinction in methods to detect LAC in relation to clinical manifestation of APS considered LAC to be clinically relevant when detected by means of dRVVT. In fact, the dRVVT rather than the KCT profile may better identify β_2GPI-dependent LAC and is associated with thrombosis in LAC-positive patients. Coagulation tests assessing LAC can be improved by making them very sensitive to the presence of aβ_2GPI antibodies. The mechanism underlying LAC activity of aβ_2GPI antibodies is related to their ability to enhance binding of β_2GPI to PL, thus impeding binding/activation of clotting factors. Since β_2GPI binding to aPL as well as its enhanced binding to PL in the presence of specific autoantibodies might be influenced by calcium and ionic strength, we evaluated the effect of various calcium concentrations in common tests assessing the presence of LAC in patients with functionally active aβ_2GPI antibodies. We were thus able to distinguish plasmas from patients with clinically relevant antihuman β_2GPI LAC. A reduction in the final calcium concentration (from 10 to 5 mM) increased coagulation times in both dRVVT and dilute dPT when plasmas of patients with aβ_2GPI antibodies were used. Instead, all LAC-positive antiβ_2GPI antibody-negative patients showed decreased coagulation times. These results were confirmed by running dRVVT of normal plasma spiked with affinity-purified IgG anti-aβ_2GPI antibodies. Thus when a PL-dependent coagulation test is run twice at different final calcium concentrations, aβ_2GPI LAC can be identified. Another test system to discriminate between LAC caused by anti-β_2GPI from those due to antiprothrombin antibodies has recently been described [32]. In an aPTT-based test, the addition of cardiolipin vesicles shortened or prolonged coagulation time in the presence of aβ_2GPI or antiprothrombin LAC, respectively.

References

1. Aggeler PM, Lindsay S, Lucia SP (1946) Studies on the coagulation defect in a case of thrombocytopenic purpura complicated by thrombosis. Am J Pathol 22:1181–1203
2. Ley AB, Reader GG, Sorenson CW, Overman RS (1951) Idiopathic hypoprothrombinemia associated with hemorrhagic diathesis, and the effect of vitamin K. Blood 6:740–755
3. Conley CL (1952) Disorders of the blood in disseminated lupus erythematosus. Am J Med 13:1–2
4. Frick PG (1955) Acquired circulating anticoagulants in systemic collagen disease; autoimmune thromboplastin deficiency. Blood 10:691–706
5. Laurell AB, Nilsson IM (1957) Hypergammaglobulinemia, circulating anticoagulant, and biologic false positive Wassermann reaction; a study in two cases. J Lab Clin Med 49:694–707
6. Bowie EJ, Thompson JH, Pascuzzi CA Jr, Owen CA Jr (1963) Thrombosis in systemic lupus erythematosus despite circulating anticoagulants. J Lab Clin Med 62:416–430
7. Jayakody Arachchillage D, Greaves M (2014) The chequered history of the antiphospholipid syndrome. Br J Haematol 165:609–617
8. Exner T, Rickard KA, Kronenberg H (1975) Studies on phospholipids in the action of a lupus coagulation inhibitor. Pathology 7:319–328
9. Manoharan A, Gibson L, Rush B, Feery BJ (1977) Recurrent venous thrombosis with a "lupus" coagulation inhibitor in the absence of systemic lupus. Aust N Z J Med 7:422–426
10. Harris EN, Gharavi AE, Boey ML et al (1983) Anticardiolipin antibodies: detection by radioimmunoassay and association with thrombosis in systemic lupus erythematosus. Lancet 2:1211–1214
11. Firkin BG, Howard MA, Radford N (1980) Possible relationship between lupus inhibitor and recurrent abortion in young women. Lancet 2:366
12. Boey ML, Colaco CB, Gharavi AE, Elkon KB, Loizou S, Hughes GR (1983) Thrombosis in systemic lupus erythematosus: striking association with the presence of circulating lupus anticoagulant. Br Med J (Clin Res Ed) 287:1021–1023
13. Lubbe WF, Walker EB (1983) Chorea gravidarum associated with circulating lupus anticoagulant: successful outcome of pregnancy with prednisone and aspirin therapy. Case report. Br J Obstet Gynaecol 90:487–490
14. Bingley PJ, Hoffbrand BI (1987) Antiphospholipid antibody syndrome: a review. J R Soc Med 80:445–448
15. Asherson RA (1988) A "primary" antiphospholipid syndrome? J Rheumatol 15:1742–1746
16. Alarcon-Segovia D, Sanchez-Guerrero J (1989) Primary antiphospholipid syndrome. J Rheumatol 16:482–488
17. Bird AG, Lendrum R, Asherson RA, Hughes GR (1987) Disseminated intravascular coagulation, antiphospholipid antibodies, and ischaemic necrosis of extremities. Ann Rheum Dis 46:251–255
18. Ingram SB, Goodnight SH Jr, Bennett RM (1987) An unusual syndrome of a devastating noninflammatory vasculopathy associated with anticardiolipin antibodies: report of two cases. Arthritis Rheum 30:1167–1172
19. Asherson RA (1992) The catastrophic antiphospholipid syndrome. J Rheumatol 19:508–512
20. Roubey RA (1994) Autoantibodies to phospholipid-binding plasma proteins: a new view of lupus anticoagulants and other "antiphospholipid" autoantibodies. Blood 84:2854–2867
21. Shoenfeld Y, Krause I, Kvapil F et al (2003) Prevalence and clinical correlations of antibodies against six beta2-glycoprotein-I-related peptides in the antiphospholipid syndrome. J Clin Immunol 23:377–383
22. McIntyre JA, Wagenknecht DR, Faulk WP (2003) Antiphospholipid antibodies: discovery, definitions, detection and disease. Prog Lipid Res 42:176–237
23. Brandt JT, Triplett DA, Alving B, Scharrer I (1995) Criteria for the diagnosis of lupus anticoagulants: an update. On behalf of the Subcommittee on Lupus Anticoagulant/Antiphospholipid

Antibody of the Scientific and Standardisation Committee of the ISTH. Thromb Haemost 74:1185–1190

24. Thiagarajan P, Pengo V, Shapiro SS (1986) The use of the dilute Russell viper venom time for the diagnosis of lupus anticoagulants. Blood 68:869–874
25. Pengo V, Biasiolo A, Rampazzo P, Brocco T (1999) dRVVT is more sensitive than KCT or TTI for detecting lupus anticoagulant activity of anti-beta2-glycoprotein I autoantibodies. Thromb Haemost 81:256–258
26. Lawrie AS, Purdy G, Mackie IJ, Machin SJ (1997) Monitoring of oral anticoagulant therapy in lupus anticoagulant positive patients with the anti-phospholipid syndrome. Br J Haematol 98:887–892
27. Tripodi A, Chantarangkul V, Clerici M, Mannucci PM (2002) Laboratory diagnosis of lupus anticoagulants for patients on oral anticoagulant treatment. Performance of dilute Russell viper venom test and silica clotting time in comparison with Staclot LA. Thromb Haemost 88:583–586
28. Pengo V, Biasiolo A, Gresele P et al; Participating Centres of Italian Federation of Thrombosis Centres (FCSA) (2007) Survey of lupus anticoagulant diagnosis by central evaluation of positive plasma samples. J Thromb Haemost 5:925–930
29. Pengo V, Tripodi A, Reber G, Rand JH, Ortel TL, Galli M, de Groot PG (2009) Update of the guidelines for lupus anticoagulant detection. J Thromb Haemost 7:1737–1740
30. Pengo V, Ruffatti A, Legnani C, Gresele P, Barcellona D, Erba N et al (2010) Clinical course of high-risk patients diagnosed with antiphospholipid syndrome. J Thromb Haemost 8:237–242
31. Galli M, Barbui T (1999) Antiprothrombin antibodies: detection and clinical significance in the antiphospholipid syndrome. Blood 93:2149–2157
32. Simmelink MJ, Derksen RH, Arnout J, De Groot PG (2003) A simple method to discriminate between beta2-glycoprotein I- and prothrombin-dependent lupus anticoagulants. J Thromb Haemost 1:740–747
33. Pengo V, Biasiolo A, Pegoraro C, Iliceto S (2004) A two-step coagulation test to identify antibeta-glycoprotein I lupus anticoagulants. J Thromb Haemost 2:702–707
34. de Laat B, Derksen RH, Urbanus RT, de Groot PG (2005) IgG antibodies that recognize epitope Gly40-Arg43 in domain I of beta 2-glycoprotein I cause LAC, and their presence correlates strongly with thrombosis. Blood 105:1540–1545
35. Thiagarajan P, Shapiro SS (1998) Lupus anticoagulants and antiphospholipid antibodies. Hematol Oncol Clin North Am 12:1167–1192

Antiphospholipid Antibody Mechanisms of Thrombosis

3

Pier Luigi Meroni, Chiara Crotti, and Cecilia Chighizola

3.1 Introduction

Arterial and/or venous thrombosis in association with the persistent presence of antiphospholipid antibodies (aPL) is the hallmark of the antiphospholipid antibody syndrome (APS).

aPL can be detected by solid-phase assays (anticardiolipin [aCL] and/or anti-β2 glycoprotein I [β2GPI]) and/or by a functional assay (lupus anticoagulant [LA]) [1]. Besides their diagnostic value, aPL are also pathogenic autoantibodies that mediate the vascular manifestations in association with an additional second hit (*two hits theory*) [2].

3.2 Pathogenic aPL

aPL are mainly directed against two PL-binding proteins: β2GPI and prothrombin (PT). β2GPI-dependent aPL can be detected by both aCL and anti-β2GPI assay and are responsible for most of the LA positivities. There is a general agreement that

P.L. Meroni, MD (✉)
Department of Clinical Sciences and Community Health, University of Milan, Milan, Italy

Istituto G. Pini and IRCCS Istituto Auxologico Italiano, Milan, Italy

Division of Rheumatology, Istituto G. Pini, Pzza. C. Ferrari, 1, Milan 20122, Italy
e-mail: pierluigi.meroni@unimi.it

C. Crotti • C. Chighizola
Department of Clinical Sciences and Community Health, University of Milan, Milan, Italy

Istituto G. Pini and IRCCS Istituto Auxologico Italiano, Milan, Italy
e-mail: chiara.crotti@unimi.it; cecilia.chighizola@unimi.it

© Springer International Publishing Switzerland 2015

P.L. Meroni (ed.), *Antiphospholipid Antibody Syndrome: From Bench to Bedside*,
Rare Diseases of the Immune System, DOI 10.1007/978-3-319-11044-8_3

β2GPI-dependent aPL are more predictive for the vascular (and the obstetric) manifestations of the syndrome [2, 3].

aPL reacting with human β2GPI and cross-reacting with the animal molecule were shown to be pathogenic in all the in vivo experimental models. More importantly, the thrombogenic effect was reproduced by affinity-purified anti-β2GPI IgG and inhibited by specific absorption of the anti-β2GPI activity [2]. Accordingly, β2GPI-dependent aPL are generally thought to represent the main pathogenic antibody subpopulation for the APS thrombotic manifestations.

β2GPI is a large molecule belonging to the complement control protein (CCP) family and consists of 326 amino acid residues arranged in 5 CCP repeat domains, termed "sushi" domains. Hence, it is not surprising that autoantibodies can recognize several epitopes in the molecule. However, there is growing evidence that a cryptic epitope (Gly40-Arg43) of domain I (DI) may represent the immunodominant epitope that is recognized by most of the APS sera and closely related to the clinical manifestations of the syndrome [3, 4].

We recently demonstrated that a human monoclonal antibody (moAb) specific for DI is pathogenic in a murine model of vascular thrombosis further supporting the hypothesis that such a subpopulation of anti-β2GPI may play a pathogenic role [5].

aPL are also known to react with other PL-binding proteins and in particular with PT. Although in vitro studies suggested that anti-PT may perturb endothelial cells (EC) by reacting with the molecule on the cell surface, still there is no clear evidence for anti-PT pathogenic activity in animal models and their possible pathogenic role is only supported by the epidemiological association with thrombosis [2, 3]. The best association was reported for antibodies detected by the PS-PT assay, suggesting that the pathogenic antibodies may react with a conformational epitope(s) expressed by PT when complexed with anionic PL in the presence of calcium ions [6].

3.3 Why We Break the Tolerance Against Beta2GPI?

The mechanism(s) through which the tolerance towards β2GPI is lost is still matter of research, and several hypotheses have been suggested.

There is sound evidence that aPL can be detectable in the course of viral, bacterial, and parasitic infections as a transient phenomenon [7, 8]. This is also true for anti-β2GPI antibodies suggesting a possible link between the production of β_2GPI-dependent aPL antibodies and infectious processes or even an active immunization [9].

Infectious agents may induce conformational changes in antigens, exposing hidden epitopes and leading to autoantibodies production. Accordingly, it has been suggested that the contact of β2GPI with an infectious agent or with endotoxin may favor the exposure of immunogenic epitopes. Beta2GPI is a plasma protein that may act as a scavenger molecule for lipopolysaccharide (LPS) through its C-terminal part [10]. Circulating plasma β_2GPI exists in a circular form that, upon binding to suitable anionic surfaces as CL and other PL or to LPS, opens up to a J-shaped fish-hook configuration [11]. Such a conformational change exposes DI that has been suggested to be the main antigenic target for anti-β_2GPI antibodies [12, 13]. In particular, it has been recently demonstrated that the antibodies recognize the sequence of arginine 39-arginine 43, aspartic acid 8-aspartic acid 9, and possibly the inter-linker region between DI and DII, with R39 being the most important residue [14, 15]. This epitope was reported to be a cryptic and conformation-dependent structure. In the β_2GPI circular conformation, DI interacts with DV and the critical epitope is thus hidden. Conversely, upon opening to a J-configuration, the critical epitope arginine 39-glycine 43 is exposed, thus becoming available for antibody binding [16]. It has been suggested that upon the binding to LPS (or after the contact with an infectious agent) β_2GPI may circulate in the open form, offering the DI immunodominant epitope to the afferent limb of the immune system and eventually triggering antibody production in susceptible individuals [17].

Besides exposing hidden epitopes, infections could also increase the immunogenicity of the molecule β2GPI by changing its redox potential. It has been reported, in fact, that the majority of circulating β2GPI exists in a reduced form and that oxidation increases immunogenicity. Accordingly, the generation of reactive oxidative and nitroxidative species by certain infectious agents may favor the generation of oxidized β2GPI and foster autoantibodies production [18].

Molecular mimicry is another suggested mechanism: nonself molecules (frequently infectious agents) may share similar amino acid sequences with β2GPI and may trigger the production of antibodies against the infectious antigen(s) cross-reacting with the β2GPI itself [19].

3.4 Pathogenesis of the Vascular Manifestations: Introduction

Traditionally, the clotting cascade is depicted as consisting of an intrinsic and extrinsic pathway (Fig. 3.1). The intrinsic pathway is initiated by the exposure of blood to a negatively charged surface. The extrinsic pathway is activated by tissue factor (TF) exposed at the site of injury or by TF-like material. Both pathways converge on the activation of factor X which, as a component of prothrombinase, converts prothrombin to thrombin, the final enzyme of the clotting cascade. Thrombin converts fibrinogen from a soluble plasma protein into an insoluble fibrin clot.

Fluid-phase coagulation components are involved in propagation of the clotting process, in termination of clotting by antithrombotic control mechanisms, and in the removal of the clot by fibrinolysis. At the same time, endothelium and peripheral blood monocytes play a main role in expressing TF and supporting clot formation, while platelets are pivotal in the initiation and formation of the plug.

aPL procoagulant mechanism(s) has been initially related to the antibody's binding to β2GPI or PT and the consequent interference with the natural anticoagulant

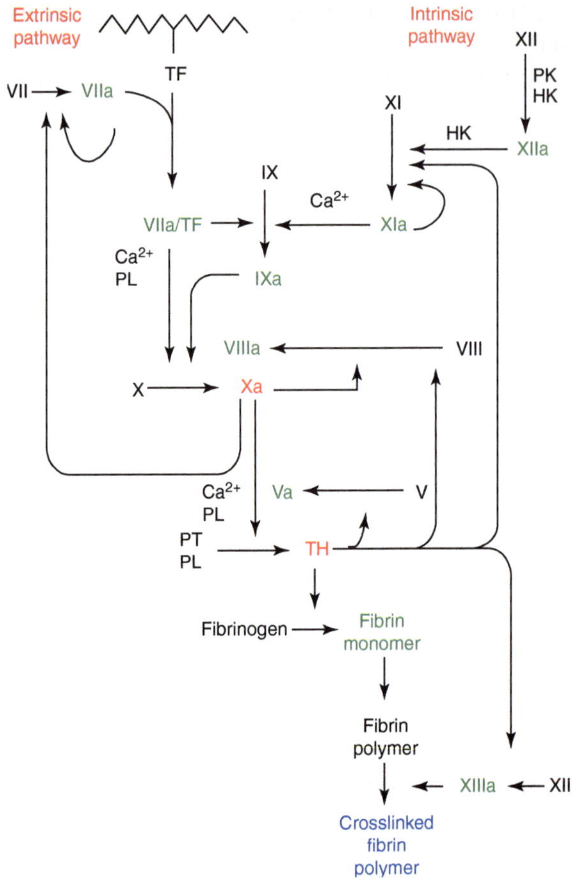

Fig. 3.1 Schematic representation of the coagulation cascade. *HK* high-molecular-weight kininogen, *PK* prekallikrein, *PL* phospholipid, *PT* prothrombin, *TH* thrombin coagulation cascade

system of protein C and with the reduction of fibrinolysis. However, two main reasons supported the search for additional pathogenic mechanisms:

(a) Vascular events in APS patients are affecting both arterial and venous vessels, while abnormal protein C and fibrinolysis may account mainly for venous events.
(b) It is still not clear whether aPL react in a significant manner with the PL-binding proteins (β2GPI and PT) in fluid phase. In fact, all aPL are low-avidity antibodies suggesting that complex formation in the fluid phase requires stechiometric antigen-antibody ratios that are uncommon in patients [20].

As a consequence, a lot of investigations have been focused on aPL ability to react with PL-binding proteins expressed on the cell membrane of the cells involved in the coagulation cascade.

In this regard, β2GPI is expressed on the cell membranes at high antigenic density and so more easily recognized by low-avidity autoantibodies. In addition, it has

Table 3.1 Antiphospholipid antibody-mediated pathogenic mechanisms for thrombosis

Interference with fluid-phase coagulation components:
Inhibition of natural anticoagulants
Inhibition of protein C activation[a]
Disruption of the annexin V shield[a]
Inhibition of fibrinolysis
Interference with cells of the coagulation cascade:
Endothelial cell perturbation[a]
Monocyte activation (TF expression)[a]
Platelet activation[a]
Complement activation[a]

[a]β2GPI/anti-β2GPI antibody involvement

been reported that circulating β2GPI is usually present in the circular-closed form, while it is opened only after binding to negative PL or after complexing with LPS. Since the autoantibodies were reported to react mainly with the opened form (i.e., reacting with the exposed cryptic epitope of DI), this finding may further explain the reason of the limited reactivity with the circulating form.

Most of the pathogenic mechanisms potentially responsible for thrombus formation have been demonstrated using in vitro models. However, three different in vivo models of thrombosis induced respectively by mechanical, chemical, or photochemical trauma have confirmed the pathogenic effect of aPL [2]. Two of these experimental models showed an increase of the thrombus size already triggered respectively by the mechanical or the chemical stimulus and a delayed dissolution. On the other hand, the third model showed that the passive infusion of human aPL IgG together with a small amount of LPS is able by itself to start clotting in the rat mesenteric arterial microcirculation [21].

Table 3.1 and Fig. 3.2 summarize the main pathogenic mechanisms that have been reported in the literature [2, 22].

Still open is the question why some aPL-positive patients develop both arterial and venous events and why others can display arterial or venous thrombosis only.

3.5 Interference of aPL with Fluid-Phase Coagulation Cascade

The evidence of aPL interference with fluid-phase components of coagulation has been provided mostly by in vitro models [2, 22].

aPL can bind some members of the serine protease (SP) family, which enlists proteins involved in hemostasis (procoagulant factors such as thrombin, PT, FVIIa, FIXa, and FXa and natural anticoagulants as protein C) and in fibrinolysis (plasmin and tissue plasminogen activator (tPA)). The fact that β2GPI and SP enzymatic domain share conformational epitopes was suggested to be the reason for the cross-reactivity.

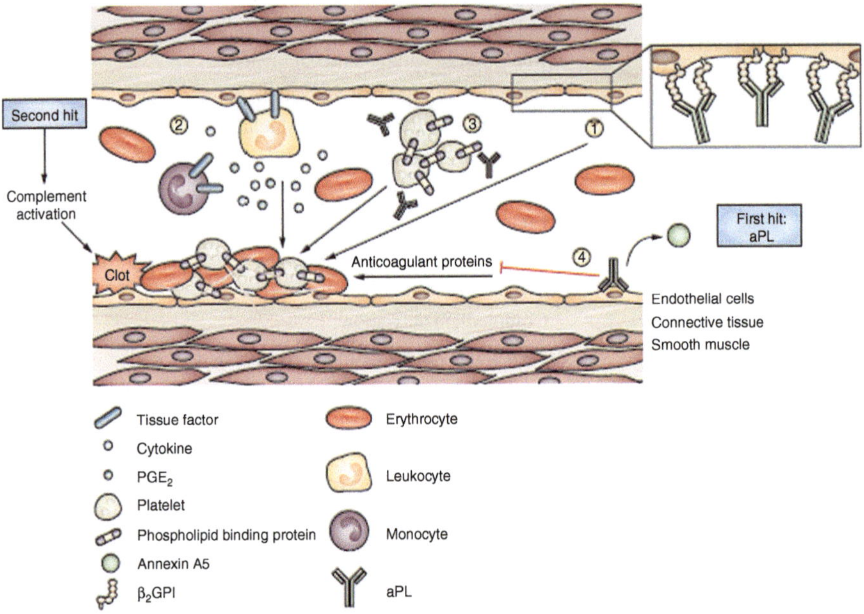

Fig. 3.2 Pathogenic clotting mechanisms mediated by aPL. aPL actions favor clot formation through several routes. *1* aPL interact with endothelial cells, primarily through binding of β2GPI on the cell surface, and induce a procoagulant and proinflammatory endothelial phenotype. *2* aPL upregulate tissue factor expression on endothelial cells and blood monocytes, and promote endothelial leukocyte adhesion, cytokine secretion, and PGE2synthesis. *3* aPL recognize phospholipid-binding proteins expressed on platelets—aPL binding potentiates platelet aggregation induced by another agonist. *4* aPL interfere with plasma components of the coagulation cascade, by inhibiting anticoagulant activity, by affecting fibrinolysis, and by displacing the binding of the natural anticoagulant annexin A5 to anionic structures. These mechanisms all contribute to a procoagulant state that is necessary but not sufficient for clotting. Clot formation seems to require two steps: the presence of aPL provides the 'first hit', which produces clotting when accompanied by another procoagulant condition, a 'second hit'. Complement activation seems to be necessary for clot formation in vivo. Abbreviations: aPL anti-phospholipid autoantibodies, β2GPI β2 glycoprotein I, PGE2 prostaglandin E2 (Permission from Meroni et al [2])

aPL interact with thrombin and FXa, interfering with the formation of thrombin-antithrombin (AT) and FXa-AT complexes, thus affecting the AT inactivation of thrombin and FXa. Moreover, aPL are reported to decrease activated protein C (APC) activity by competing with APC for PL binding. Accordingly, an increased APC resistance has been reported in APS. Several groups have also found decreased levels of both proteins C and S and aPL with affinity for either protein S or C. In addition, some aPL were shown to inhibit plasmin-mediated fibrinolysis, eventually leading to an impairment of fibrin dissolution by plasmin. Some aPL subpopulations were also found to bind to tPA, inhibiting tPA-mediated conversion of plasminogen to plasmin. Anti-tPA antibodies were shown to inversely correlate with plasma tPA activity in APS.

Besides the inhibitory effects on the natural anticoagulant systems, aPL may also increase the enzymatic activity of procoagulants. In fact some aPL subpopulations were shown to induce a gain of function of PT leading to increased fibrin production. In addition, aPL have been reported to disrupt the crystallization of annexin A5 on EC monolayer. The "shield" of annexin A5 is thought to represent a potent anticoagulant barrier that prevents PL bioavailability for coagulation enzymes [2, 22].

3.6 Interference of aPL with Cells Involved in the Coagulation Cascade

More recently, research has focused on aPL interaction with cells involved in the hemostatic balance as platelets, monocytes, and EC [2].

3.6.1 Platelet Involvement

The occurrence of mild thrombocytopenia is a frequent clinical finding among APS patients and strongly suggested the possible interaction between platelets and aPL.

aPL reactivity with platelets has been shown only after their pre-activation by agonists such as thrombin or collagen. The reason for this was thought to be related to the exposure of phosphatidylserine (PS) on the cell outer membrane after platelet activation and the consequent binding of the cationic β2GPI. However, β2GPI can also bind two surface receptors on platelets. Apolipoprotein E receptor 2' (ApoER2') is a member of low-density lipoprotein (LDL) receptor family expressed by platelets; its LDL-binding domain I recognizes the PL-binding site of β2GPI domain V. Lastly β2GPI has been shown to bind directly GPIba, a subunit of the GPIb-IX-V platelet receptor [23] and to platelet factor 4 [24].

Altogether these findings suggest that the main antigenic target on platelets is the β2GPI itself which can be recognized by specific antibodies.

There is evidence that such interaction may be responsible for several biological effects. In general, the binding of the antibodies with their own antigenic target can trigger platelet activation. In addition, aPL have been shown to neutralize β2GPI interaction with von Willebrand factor (vWF). β2GPI acts as a biologically relevant inhibitor of vWF function, thus interfering with vWF-dependent platelet adhesion. This action could be hampered by aPL so favoring thrombosis and may explain the consumptive thrombocytopenia frequently observed in aPL carriers. Once bound, aPL have been shown to enhance the expression of platelet membrane glycoproteins (GPs) IIb/IIIa and IIIa. GPs are fibrinogen receptors that mediate platelet aggregation, whose role in APS pathogenesis is further supported by in vivo findings [25]. In fact, aPL did not affect thrombus formation in GPIIb/IIIa-deficient mice and pretreatment with a monoclonal anti-GPIIb/IIIa antibody inhibited aPL-mediated reduced thrombus formation. In vivo evidence of platelet activation by aPL has been gained in other models: (i) aPL produced a platelet-rich thrombus in rats, after treatment with low concentration of adenosine diphosphate (ADP), and (ii) platelet involvement was reported in the thrombus formation by photochemical injury in the rat. Platelet activation by aPL has been supported by ex vivo studies since elevated levels of thromboxane (TX, the major eicosanoid metabolic breakdown product) have been found in the urine of APS patients [26].

3.6.2 Involvement of Monocytes

aPL upregulate TF expression on peripheral blood monocytes. In particular, monocyte TF expression is increased in patients with APS and correlates with the expression of β2GPI. Accordingly, cell-surface TF on monocytes is higher in APS patients than in subjects without thrombotic events. Interestingly, vascular endothelial growth factor (VEGF) stimulates TF expression in monocytes through its tyrosine-kinase receptor Flt-1, and expression of both VEGF and Flt-1 is increased in monocytes from APS patients [27]. On monocytes, aPL have been suggested to interact with β2GPI in association with annexin A2 [28] and toll-like receptor (TLR) 4 within lipid rafts [29]. Other authors provided indirect evidence of TLR2 involvement in mediating aPL-induced monocyte activation [2].

3.6.3 Involvement of Endothelial Cells

Endothelium has been suggested to represent a cell type deeply involved in APS pathogenesis since the earliest pathogenic studies. The milestone was the demonstration that aPL could react with EC mainly recognizing β2GPI present on the cell membrane [30, 31]. Once bound the β2GPI-dependent aPL can trigger EC perturbation with the induction of a proinflammatory and procoagulant cell phenotype [2, 22, 26].

The majority of the studies have been performed in vitro showing an upregulation of endothelial cellular adhesion molecules (such as ICAM-1, VCAM-1, and E-selectin) and the synthesis of proinflammatory cytokines (as interleukin (IL)-1β, IL-6, and IL-8). Accordingly, in vivo studies have shown that passive infusion of aPL induced an increase in the rate of leukocytes adhering to the endothelium. Lastly, aPL may modulate the vascular tone by inhibiting endothelial nitric oxide synthase and altering prostaglandin metabolism [2, 26].

Ex vivo studies in APS subjects reported raised levels of soluble cellular adhesion molecules such as s-ICAM-1, VCAM-1, and P-selectin although with contrasting results among the different groups. More importantly, APS patients were found to display endothelial perturbation, as suggested by the impaired brachial artery flow-mediated vasodilation responses and the significant increase in the numbers of circulating ECs and in tPA and vWF titers [32].

aPL reactivity with EC is mainly mediated by autoantibodies to β2GPI expressed on the endothelial cell membrane. Since endothelial synthesis of the molecule has not been confirmed, it has been suggested that β2GPI is adhering to EC membrane. The adhesion is apparently mediated by several different receptors. Annexin A2, a receptor for tPA and plasminogen, has been demonstrated to directly bind β2GPI. As annexin A2 lacks an intracytoplasmic tail, a coreceptor is required to trigger signaling cascade. TLRs 2 and 4, heparan sulfate, and ApoER2' have all been indirectly shown to bind β2GPI on endothelial surface. TLRs 2 and 4 have been found to mediate also intracellular aPL signaling in ECs; to note, TLR2 is expressed by ECs only upon cell activation, while TLR4 is constitutively expressed [2]. A direct interaction between β2GPI and TLR4 has been recently reported [33]. More recently, it has been suggested that a multiprotein complex including TLR4 and annexin A2 is involved in aPL-induced EC activation [34].

Annexin A2, TLR4, and ApoER2' have also been investigated in in vivo models. Animals deficient in any one of these molecules are only partially protected against aPL thrombogenic effects, suggesting redundancy in the receptor function and signaling cascade [2].

There is general agreement that nuclear factor κ B (NFκB) and p38 mitogen-activated protein kinase (MAPK) are the main downstream signaling pathways engaged by aPL in EC and monocyte activation [2].

3.7 The "Two-Hit Hypothesis"

To explain the clinical observation that the thrombotic events occur only occasionally in spite of the persistent presence of aPL a *two-hit hypothesis* has been suggested [2].

The antibody (*first hit*) induces a thrombophilic condition, but clotting takes place in the presence of another thrombophilic condition (*second hit*). Accordingly, the administration of small amount of LPS was required for human β2GPI-specific aPL IgG to display their thrombogenic effect in the mesenteric microcirculation [5, 21]. Such animal models fits very well with the clinical observation that infectious processes may frequently precede the full-blown picture of the syndrome and may be the initiator of the catastrophic subtype [35]. To explain the relationship between infections and APS the potential involvement of pattern recognition receptors (i.e., TLRs) in sensing microbes and triggering an inflammatory response was suggested. Since TLRs 2 and 4 have been reported to contribute to EC and/or monocyte activation by β2GPI-dependent aPL, it has been suggested that the infection plus TLR perturbation mediated by the autoantibodies overcomes the threshold for triggering thrombosis [2]. Alternatively, infection/inflammation may increase the expression of the target antigen for aPL or the expression of antigenic epitopes that are hidden in resting conditions as shown in murine tissues after LPS injection [36].

Additional second hits have been reported in two other different models: (i) mechanical trauma on the mouse femoral vein [37] and (ii) a photochemical injury [38].

3.8 Complement Activation

APS animal models showed that complement activation is a necessary requirement since animals deficient in complement components or complement receptors or treated with inhibitors of complement activation were protected from the aPL thrombogenic effects [2, 5].

On the other hand, sera from the majority of APS patients were found to fix complement in vitro.

However, a clear complement consumption has not been described in patients, with only two studies reporting mild hypocomplementemia in primary APS [2]. So, if definite conclusions about the involvement of complement in APS-associated thrombosis cannot currently be drawn, the potential role of complement in aPL-mediated thrombosis should not be neglected.

References

1. Miyakis S et al (2006) International consensus statement on an update of the classification criteria for definite antiphospholipid syndrome (APS). J Thromb Haemost 4:295–306
2. Meroni PL et al (2011) Pathogenesis of antiphospholipid syndrome: understanding the antibodies. Nat Rev Rheumatol 7:330–339
3. Meroni PL, Chighizola C, Rovelli F, Gerosa M (2014) Antiphospholipid syndrome 2013: more than autoantibodies only. Arthr Res Ther 16:209
4. Chighizola CB et al (2014) New tests to detect antiphospholipid antibodies: anti-domain I beta-2-glycoprotein-I antibodies. Curr Rheumatol Rep 16:402–407
5. Agostinis C et al (2014) A non-complement-fixing antibody to β2 glycoprotein I as a novel therapy for antiphospholipid syndrome. Blood 123:3478–3487
6. Sciascia S et al (2014) New tests to detect antiphospholipid antibodies: antiprothrombin (aPT) and anti-phosphatidylserine/prothrombin (aPS/PT) antibodies. Curr Rheumatol Rep 16:415
7. S'ene D et al (2009) Antiphospholipid antibodies, antiphospholipid syndrome and viral infections. Rev Med Interne 30:135–141
8. Ben-Chetrit E et al (2013) Antiphospholipid antibodies during infectious mononucleosis and their long term clinical significance. J Clin Virol 56:312–315
9. Cruz-Tapias P et al (2012) Infections and vaccines in the etiology of antiphospholipid syndrome. Curr Opin Rheumatol 24:389–393
10. Agar C et al (2011) Beta2-glycoprotein I: a novel component of innate immunity. Blood 117:6939–6947
11. De Laat B et al (2011) Autoantibodies directed against domain I of beta2-glycoprotein I. Curr Rheumatol Rep 13:70–76
12. Iverson GM et al (1998) Anti-β2 glycoprotein I (β2GPI) autoantibodies recognize an epitope on the first domain of β 2GPI. Proc Natl Acad Sci U S A 95:15542–15546
13. McNeely PA et al (2001) β 2-glycoprotein I-dependent anticardiolipin antibodies preferentially bind the amino terminal domain of β 2-glycoprotein I. Thromb Haemost 86:590–595
14. Iverson GM et al (2002) Use of single point mutations in domain I of β_2-glycoprotein I to determine fine antibody specificity of antiphospholipid autoantibodies. J Immunol 169: 7097–7103
15. Ioannou Y et al (2007) Binding of antiphospholipid antibodies to discontinuous epitopes on domain I of human beta(2)-glycoprotein I: mutation studies including residues R39 to R43. Arthritis Rheum 56:280–290
16. De Laat B et al (2006) Pathogenic anti-beta2 glycoprotein I antibodies recognize domain I of beta-2 glycoprotein I only after a conformational change. Blood 107:1916–1924

17. De Laat B et al (2011) Immune responses against domain I of β2-glycoprotein I are driven by conformational changes: domain I of β2-glycoprotein I harbors a cryptic immunogenic epitope. Arthritis Rheum 63:3960–3968
18. Passam FH et al (2011) Molecular pathophysiology of the antiphospholipid syndrome: the role of oxidative post-translational modification of beta 2 glycoprotein I. J Thromb Haemost 9(Suppl 1):275–282
19. Blank M et al (2002) Bacterial induction of autoantibodies to beta2-glycoprotein-I accounts for the infectious etiology of antiphospholipid syndrome. J Clin Invest 109:797–804
20. Tincani A et al (1996) The anti-beta2-glycoprotein I activity in human anti-phospholipid syndrome sera is due to monoreactive low-affinity autoantibodies directed to epitopes located on native beta2-glycoprotein I and preserved during species' evolution. J Immunol 157: 5732–5738
21. Fischetti F et al (2005) Thrombus formation induced by antibodies to beta2-glycoprotein I is complement dependent and requires a priming factor. Blood 106:2340–2346
22. Giannakopoulos B et al (2013) The pathogenesis of the antiphospholipid syndrome. N Engl J Med 368:1033–1044
23. Pennings MT et al (2006) Interaction of beta2-glycoprotein I with members of the low density lipoprotein receptor family. J Thromb Haemost 4:1680–1690
24. Sikara MP et al (2010) {beta}2 Glycoprotein I ({beta}2GPI) binds platelet factor 4 (PF4): implications for the pathogenesis of antiphospholipid syndrome. Blood 115(3):713–723
25. Shi T et al (2006) Anti-beta2-glycoprotein I antibodies in complex with beta2-glycoprotein I can activate platelets in a dysregulated manner via glycoprotein Ib-IX-V. Arthritis Rheum 54:2558–2567
26. Pierangeli SS et al (2008) Antiphospholipid antibodies and the antiphospholipid syndrome: pathogenic mechanisms. Semin Thromb Hemost 34:236–250
27. Boles J et al (2010) Role of tissue factor in thrombosis in antiphospholipid antibody syndrome. Lupus 19:370–378
28. Zhang J et al (2005) Annexin A2 mediates endothelial cell activation by antiphospholipid/anti-beta2 glycoprotein I antibodies. Blood 105:1964–1969
29. Sorice M et al (2007) Anti-beta2-glycoprotein I antibodies induce monocyte release of tumor necrosis factor alpha and tissue factor by signal transduction pathways involving lipid rafts. Arthritis Rheum 56:2687–2697
30. Vismara A et al (1988) Relationship between anti-cardiolipin and anti-endothelial cell antibodies in systemic lupus erythematosus. Clin Exp Immunol 74:247–253
31. Del Papa N et al (1995) Relationship between anti-phospholipid and anti-endothelial cell antibodies III: beta 2 glycoprotein I mediates the antibody binding to endothelial membranes and induces the expression of adhesion molecules. Clin Exp Rheumatol 13:179–185
32. Cugno M et al (2010) Patients with antiphospholipid syndrome display endothelial perturbation. J Autoimmun 34:105–110
33. Raschi E et al. (2014) β2-glycoprotein I, lipopolysaccharide and endothelial TLR4: three players in the two hit theory for anti-phospholipid-mediated thrombosis. J Autoimmun 1–9. doi: 10.1016/j.jaut.2014.03.001
34. Allen KL et al (2012) A novel pathway for human endothelial cell activation by antiphospholipid/anti-β2 glycoprotein I antibodies. Blood 119:884–893
35. Shoenfeld Y et al (2006) Infectious origin of the antiphospholipid syndrome. Ann Rheum Dis 65:2–6
36. Agostinis C et al (2011) In vivo distribution of β2 glycoprotein I under various pathophysiologic conditions. Blood 118:4231–4238
37. Pierangeli SS et al (1996) Thrombogenic properties of murine anti-cardiolipin antibodies induced by beta 2 glycoprotein 1 and human immunoglobulin G antiphospholipid antibodies. Circulation 94:1746–1751
38. Jankowski M et al (2003) Thrombogenicity of beta 2-glycoprotein I-dependent antiphospholipid antibodies in a photochemically induced thrombosis model in the hamster. Blood 101:157–162

4 The Pathogenic Mechanisms for Antiphospholipid Antibodies (aPL)-Mediated Pregnancy Loss

Nicoletta Di Simone and Silvia D'Ippolito

4.1 Introduction

The revised Sapporo criteria established that pregnancy morbidity in antiphospholipid syndrome (APS) encloses ≥3 consecutive and spontaneous early miscarriages before 10 weeks of gestation, at least one unexplained fetal death after the 10th week of gestation of a morphologically normal fetus, and a premature birth before the 34th week of gestation of a normal neonate due to eclampsia or severe preeclampsia or placental insufficiency [1].

During the years several researchers tried to find an etiopathogenic explanation for pregnancy morbidity in APS. The results underlined the heterogeneity of the pathogenic mechanisms involved in antiphospholipid antibody (aPL)-mediated fetal loss, all taking place within the placenta [1–5]. Actually, intraplacental thrombotic phenomena, a direct aPL-mediated placental damage, and inflammatory processes involving the complement cascade are considered the most important mechanisms underlying miscarriages in APS [3–5]. It is now well accepted that these mechanisms are not mutually exclusive and may play a role together or in different combination at different times of the pregnancy. Such a variety in the aPL-mediated action fits well with the heterogeneity of the clinical manifestations of the obstetric APS, spanning from early to late miscarriages or preeclampsia [6].

N. Di Simone (✉) • S. D'Ippolito
Department of Obstetrics and Gynecology, Università Cattolica del Sacro Cuore Rome, Largo Agostino Gemelli 8, Rome 00168, Italy
e-mail: nicolettadisimone@rm.unicatt.it; silviadippolito@yahoo.it

© Springer International Publishing Switzerland 2015
P.L. Meroni (ed.), *Antiphospholipid Antibody Syndrome: From Bench to Bedside*, Rare Diseases of the Immune System, DOI 10.1007/978-3-319-11044-8_4

4.2 The Human Implantation and Placentation

Human implantation and placentation represent a complex process based on subsequent steps. In particular, trophoblast cells play a key role in placental development. After implantation, they differentiate into villous and extravillous trophoblast cells (VTC and EVTC, respectively) [6]. VTC support the maternal-fetal exchange of nutrients and the endocrine functions of the placenta. EVTC invade the maternal endometrium and, through the formation of cellular plugs, gradually erode local spiral arteries to provide access to the maternal blood. The invasive nature of EVTC is dependent on the activity of matrix metalloproteases (MMPs) [7, 8], proteolytic enzyme degrading the extracellular matrix (ECM), and on the secretion of a number of molecules such as heparin-binding epidermal growth factor (HB-EGF), a strong mitogenic molecule expressed in VTC and EVTC, able to stimulate trophoblast differentiation, invasive phenotype, and motility [9–12].

During the early phase of pregnancy, also the endometrium of the uterus undergoes profound changes and transforms into decidua, a newly formed tissue that plays a critical role for successful embryo implantation and regular fetal growth. The decidua provides a physical anchorage for the implanted embryo tightly attached to the maternal tissue through anchoring villi which float in the intervillous space, surrounded by an outer layer of trophoblast cells. An important feature of the decidual tissue in the early phase of pregnancy is represented by the active angiogenic differentiation of endometrial endothelial cells (HEECs) and the vascular remodeling of the spiral arteries [13]. In particular decidualizing endometrial cells produce critical angiogenic molecules, such as vascular endothelial growth factor (VEGF) able to promote the angiogenic differentiation of HEECs [14–16]. These changes facilitate a regular supply of maternal blood to the developing placenta at an optimal flow rate necessary for the adequate delivery of nutrients to the developing embryo [13–16]. Noteworthy, VTC exposed to maternal blood circulating in the intervillous space and EVTC present in human decidua, being of fetal origin, represent a real challenge for the maternal immune system. As a result, a vigorous response may be mounted against paternal antigens expressed on trophoblasts leading to potential deleterious effects on fetal survival [17]. Trophoblast invasion of decidua results in recruitment and activation of leukocytes and precursors of endothelial cells and in the release of various cytokines, chemokines, and growth factors that promote tissue remodeling [3, 17, 18]. There is evidence for a dynamic balance between proinflammatory and anti-inflammatory mediators in normal pregnancy [3, 17–20].

Embryo implantation is, therefore, strictly based on trophoblast invasion and endometrial decidualization both associated with an inflammatory process and a highly regulated maternal immune response which rather than having deleterious effects help to promote fetal survival and allow normal progression of pregnancy [3, 17–19].

4.3 aPL and Intraplacental Thrombotic Phenomena

In line with the thrombogenic effect of aPL, intraplacental thrombotic phenomena and the subsequent impaired maternal-fetal blood exchange were initially suggested as the main pathogenic mechanism underlying the poor obstetric outcome [21, 22].

Accordingly placental thrombosis and infarction were reported. It was suggested that such an effect might be due to the in vitro ability of aPL, mainly anti-ß2 glycoprotein 1 antibodies (anti-ß2GP1), to induce a procoagulant state via disruption of annexin A5 shield on trophoblast and endothelial cell monolayers. These findings were supported by the observation of reduced annexin A5 expression in placentas from aPL-positive women compared to those lacking the autoantibodies [23, 24]. However further histological studies revealed that neither thrombosis nor infarction is common in the placentas of patients with APS [25, 26]. Specifically, the prevalence of intervillous thrombosis in women with aPL was similar to that found in aPL-negative pregnancies. Moreover, due to the presence of trophoblast plugs in the uterine spiral arteries, significant maternal blood flow does not occur in the intervillous space until the end of the first trimester, suggesting that placental thrombosis and infarction are unlikely causes of embryonic or early fetal loss in APS patients.

4.4 aPL and Direct Placental Damage

Besides thrombosis, several evidence indicated that alternative aPL-mediated pathogenic mechanisms directly affect placental tissue. The observation of β2GPI reactivity with trophoblast cell membranes, human stromal decidual cells, and HEECs suggested the placental tropism of anti-β2GPI antibodies [15, 27, 28]. β2GPI has been shown to bind to target cells through the phospholipid-binding site in the fifth domain of the molecule [4, 19, 28]. Accordingly polyclonal IgG antibodies from APS patients and human IgM monoclonal antibodies with anti-β2GPI activity can react in vitro with β2GPI both at the fetal side of human placenta (i.e., on trophoblast cells) and at the maternal one (i.e., on stromal decidual cells and HEECs) [15, 27, 28]. Subsequent studies demonstrated that, after reacting with target cells, aPL are able to:

- Inhibit trophoblast differentiation, as shown by the reduced secretion of human chorionic gonadotrophin (hCG) [28, 29].
- Impair EVTC invasiveness in an in vitro Matrigel assay. This effect is well correlated with a significant inhibition of expression/activity of MMPs [28, 29] and of HB-EGF production [30].
- Induce trophoblast injury and apoptosis [31].
- Be endocytosed into the human syncytiotrophoblast in a ß2GPI-dependent process, disrupting the normal apoptotic turnover and to induce the extrusion of necrotic trophoblast debris which are able to activate the maternal endothelium [32].
- Induce a proinflammatory phenotype in stromal decidual cells [27].
- Block endometrial angiogenesis both in vitro and in vivo, by inhibiting the HEECs angiogenic differentiation and the production of specific factors upregulated during angiogenesis, such as VEGF [15].

As a whole, all of these aPL-mediated effects might contribute to a final functional cellular damage resulting in a defective placentation and eventually in the poor obstetric outcome. Furthermore these findings suggest that APS-associated pregnancy complications can be mediated by several distinct pathogenic events not necessarily related to the procoagulant action of aPL [3, 4, 19].

The above results suggest β2GPI-dependent aPL as the main pathogenic autoantibodies in obstetric APS. Accordingly, it has been hypothesized that most of these potentially pathogenic autoantibodies should be absorbed at the placental level (where β2GPI is expressed) and should not be transferred to the fetus. This mechanism would explain why thrombotic events are rarely reported in babies born to aPL-positive mothers, in spite of the high thrombophilic profile of neonates.

4.5 aPL and Inflammation-Mediated Damage

Acute inflammatory events can be responsible for a negative pregnancy outcome via the activity of proinflammatory mediators, such as complement, tumor necrosis factor-α [TNF-α], and chemokines that have been shown to have a role in animal models of aPL-induced fetal loss [3, 4, 19, 20]. Evidence from experimental animal models confirmed the ability of human IgG with aPL activity, passively infused after implantation (10 mg/mouse per injection), to induce fetal resorption and growth retardation. The decidual immunohistochemical and histological demonstration of human IgG and mouse complement deposition, neutrophil infiltration, and local TNF-α secretion suggested a placental inflammatory damage [33–35]. The involvement of the complement system, in particular the cleaved product C5a, was supported by the observation that complement-deficient animal models are protected from pregnancy complications [20, 36–39]. In another experimental model of fetal loss, mice deficient in chemokine-binding protein D6, a placental scavenger receptor which controls local inflammation by degrading the majority of inflammatory chemokines, are more susceptible to fetal loss when passively infused with a small amount of human aPL IgG than wild-type mice or mice infused with normal IgG [40]. Further in vitro studies reported the ability of aPL to directly induce human first trimester trophoblasts to generate a potent proinflammatory and potentially damaging cytokine, interleukin-1ß (IL-1ß). This is possible via the aPL-mediated activation of the uric acid response which in turn activates the inflammasome, a protein complex containing the Nod-like receptor and the apoptosis-associated speck-like protein (Nalp3/ASC) able to facilitate pro-IL-1ß processing in the trophoblast [41].

Altogether, these findings suggest that a local acute inflammatory response might have a role in experimental aPL-mediated fetal loss.

In spite of the experimental results, the role of inflammation in determining APS pregnancy complications still remains a debated issue. In APS placentas a strong infiltration of complement components, as well as histopathological findings of deciduitis and villous infiltration, has been found more frequently compared to normal controls [42–45]. On the contrary, further ex vivo examinations of APS placentas and subsequent in vivo studies, using another model of fetal resorption and growth retardation, injected with small amount of human aPL IgG (10–50 μg/mouse) before implantation, failed to show any sign of acute placental inflammatory events and complement deposition [46]. These discrepancies in the results might be due to the different experimental models used and to the fact that experimental observations are often restricted to a given period of the pregnancy, that is, when the investigation is performed or at the time of autoantibody passive infusion. For the same reason, histological examination of human term placentae may show only the resulting damage without providing any insight on the events taking place at the beginning of the aPL-mediated insult.

4.6 Conclusions and Implications from a Practical Point of View

Taken together, the above reported findings suggest that numerous, heterogeneous and complex events underlie pregnancy complications in APS patients. However several aspects with regard to the events that break out the aPL activity and precipitate the different clinical manifestations of obstetric APS are still debated and need further investigation. Nevertheless, it is nowadays well established the ability of aPL to directly target both the invading trophoblasts and the maternal decidua/endometrial endothelial cells in the human placenta and, then, to induce a negative effect on placentation not necessarily related to prothrombotic or inflammatory events.

From a practical point of view, the knowledge of the aPL-mediated placental action has allowed important therapeutical implications. In clinical practice, several strategies have been proposed to improve the pregnancy outcome, including combinations of aspirin and unfractionated (UFH) or low molecular weight (LMWH) heparin [47–49]. Treatment with heparin is mainly based on the initial assumption that thrombotic events played the major role in APS pregnancy morbidity [46, 47]. However the evidence of alternative mechanisms of aPL-induced placental damage and the success of treatment with heparin on the pregnancy outcome suggested additional mechanisms of action for the drug [50, 51]. Actually it has been demonstrated the ability of LMWH to prevent the aPLs binding to trophoblast cells and to restore in vitro placental invasiveness and differentiation [49]. Accordingly, heparin has been shown to prevent the binding of β2GPI to negatively charged phospholipids (PL), which in turn prevents the deposition of the anti-β2GPI in tissues. Subsequent studies reported the ability of heparin to block the aPL-mediated inhibition of HEEC angiogenic differentiation [52]. As a whole, these results suggest that heparin, by interfering with the aPL binding, is able to prevent the aPL pathogenic action not only on the fetal side of the placenta (trophoblast cells) but also on the maternal one (HEECs).

In addition, other researchers, in line with the aPL/complement-mediated pathogenic action, demonstrated that the protective effect of heparin in the mouse model is linked to its anticomplement activity [50].

The likelihood of a good pregnancy outcome in women with APS is around 75–80 % under correct management. Unfortunately, a significant proportion of women, about 20–21 %, does not respond to the standard treatment and still suffer from miscarriages and adverse pregnancy events [53, 54]. The role of glucocorticoids remains still worthy of further assessment. The addition of 40–60 mg of prednisolone to aspirin alone or associated to heparin during gestation has shown no clear benefits in APS pregnant women in spite of important side effects, such as preterm delivery because of premature rupture of membranes or preeclampsia [55–57]. By contrast, a recent study by Brahman et al. seems to suggest that the addition of low-dose prednisolone (10 mg) from the time of positive pregnancy test up to 14 weeks of gestation may be effective in increasing live birth rate [58]. The addition of intravenous immunoglobulin (IVIg) has not been shown to be superior to heparin and aspirin in unselected patients, while it seems to be efficacious in obstetric APS patients selected for poor prognosis or autoimmune phenomena [59].

A possible explanation for the high proportion of refractory APS might be that not all the mechanisms underlying aPL-mediated pregnancy complications have been clarified. Novel alternative therapies are urgently needed [60]. Given the evidence that β2GPI and the related autoantibodies play a central role in aPL-mediated obstetric manifestations, new molecules able to interfere with β2GPI expression at the placental level have been recently investigated. This is the case of a synthetic peptide, TIFI, sharing structural similarity with the PL-binding site of β2GPI. Through this similarity, TIFI can compete with the β2GPI PL-binding site and displace the molecule from the cell surface, ultimately inhibiting the aPL reaction with the target tissues [61]. Accordingly, this peptide is able to prevent aPL-mediated thrombosis in vivo and to inhibit the in vitro binding of β2GPI to human endothelial cells, murine monocytes, trophoblast cells, and HEECs [46, 61, 62]. Furthermore, when passively infused in naïve pregnant mice, TIFI prevents the aPL-mediated fetal loss [46]. As a whole, these results show how molecules, possibly disrupting the β2GPI placental expression, can inhibit the binding of β2GPI-dependent aPL and, in turn, the aPL-mediated placental damage. At the same time, these results lead to investigate a further and more specific therapeutical approach able to abrogate the aPL pathogenic effects. Indeed, the observation that mice lacking β2GPI show a compromised early pregnancy suggested that functional β2GPI is necessary for optimal implantation and placental morphogenesis [63]. This has led researchers to conceive novel and promising biological therapies useful for refractory APS patients and based on the use of immunomodulatory drugs [64] or a monoclonal antibody which are able to prevent the aPL-mediated activation of the complement and the procoagulant and pro-abortive effects, without interfering with the expression of the placental β2GPI [65, 66].

References

1. Miyakis S, Lockshin MD, Atsumi T et al (2006) International classification consensus statement on an update of the classification criteria for definite antiphospholipid syndrome (APS). J Thromb Haemost 4:295–306
2. Gómez-Puerta JA, Cervera R (2014) Diagnosis and classification of the antiphospholipid syndrome. J Autoimmun 48:20–25

3. Meroni PL, Borghi MO, Raschi E et al (2011) Pathogenesis of antiphospholipid syndrome: understanding the antibodies. Nat Rev Rheumatol 7:330–339
4. Pierangeli SS, Chen PP, Raschi E et al (2008) Antiphospholipid antibodies and the antiphospholipid syndrome: pathogenic mechanisms. Semin Thromb Hemost 34:236–250
5. Meroni PL, Raschi E, Grossi C et al (2012) Obstetric and vascular APS: same autoantibodies but different diseases? Lupus 21:708–710
6. D'Ippolito S, Meroni PL, Koike T et al (2014) Obstetric antiphospholipid syndrome: a recent classification for an old defined disorder. Autoimmunity Reviews 13:901–908
7. Chen JZ, Sheehan PM, Brennecke SP et al (2012) Vessel remodelling, pregnancy hormones and extravillous trophoblast function. Mol Cell Endocrinol 349:138–144
8. Cohen M, Meisser A, Bischof P (2006) Metalloproteinases and human placental invasiveness. Placenta 27:783–793
9. Ferretti C, Bruni L, Dangles-Marie V et al (2007) Molecular circuits shared by placental and cancer cells, and their implications in the proliferative, invasive and migratory capacities of trophoblasts. Hum Reprod Update 13:121–141
10. Raab G, Klagsbrun M (1997) Heparin binding EGF growth factor. Biochim Biophys Acta 1333:F179–F199
11. Jessmon P, Leach RE, Randal Armant D (2009) Diverse functions of HBEGF during pregnancy. Mol Reprod Dev 76:1116–1127
12. Chen Y, Xiao-Xia W, Tan J et al (2012) Effect of low molecular weight heparin and heparin-binding epidermal growth factor on human trophoblast in first trimester. Fertil Steril 97:764–770
13. Lyall F, Bulmer JN, Duffie E et al (2001) Human trophoblast invasion and spiral artery transformation: the role of PECAM- 1 in normal pregnancy, preeclampsia, and fetal growth restriction. Am J Pathol 158:1713–1721
14. Yagel S (2011) Angiogenesis in gestational vascular complications. Thromb Res 127: S64–S66
15. Di Simone N, Di Nicuolo F, D'Ippolito S et al (2010) Antiphospholipid antibodies affect human endometrial angiogenesis. Biol Reprod 83:212–219
16. Pijnenborg R, Vercruysse L, Hanssens M (2006) The uterine spiral arteries in human pregnancy: facts and controversies. Placenta 27:939–958
17. Bulla R, Bossi F, Tedesco F (2012) The complement system at the embryo implantation site: friend or foe. Front Immunol 3:55
18. Chaouat G (2007) The Th1/Th2 paradigm: still important in pregnancy? Semin Immunopathol 29:95–113
19. Meroni PL, Tedesco F, Locati M et al (2010) Antiphospholipid antibody mediated fetal loss: still an open question from a pathogenic point of view. Lupus 19:453–456
20. Girardi G, Yarilin D, Thurman JM et al (2006) Complement activation induces dysregulation of angiogenic factors and causes fetal rejection and growth restriction. J Exp Med 203: 2165–2175
21. De Wolf F, Carreras FO, Moernan P et al (1982) Decidual vasculopathy and extensive placental infarction in a patient with repeated thromboembolic accidents, recurrent fetal loss, and a lupus anticoagulant. Am J Obstet Gynecol 142:829–834
22. Out HJ, Kooijman CD, Bruinse HW (1991) Histopathological finding from patient with intrauterine fetal death and antiphospholipid antibodies. Eur J Obstet Gynecol Reprod Biol 41:179–186
23. Rand JH, Wu XX, Quinn AS et al (2010) The annexin A5-mediated pathogenic mechanism in the antiphospholipid syndrome: role in pregnancy losses and thrombosis. Lupus 19:460–469
24. Rand JH, Wu XX, Guller S et al (1994) Reduction of annexin-V (placental anticoagulant protein-I) on placental villi of women with antiphospholipid antibodies and recurrent spontaneous abortion. Am J Obstet Gynecol 171:1566–1572
25. Sebire NJ, Fox H, Backos M et al (2002) Defective endovascular trophoblast invasion in primary antiphospholipid antibody syndrome-associated early 1078 pregnancy failure. Hum Reprod 17:1067–1071

26. Salafia CM, Cowchock FS (1997) Placental pathology and antiphospholipid antibodies: a descriptive study. Am J Perinatol 14:435–441
27. Borghi MO, Meroni PL, Raschi E et al (2009) Antiphospholipid antibodies reactivity with human decidual cells: an additional mechanism of pregnancy complications in APS and a potential target for innovative therapeutic intervention. Ann Rheum Dis [abstract OP-0119] 68(Suppl 3):109
28. Di Simone N, Raschi E, Testoni C et al (2005) Pathogenic role of anti-β2-glycoprotein I antibodies in antiphospholipid-associated fetal loss: characterisation of β2-glycoprotein I binding to trophoblast cells and functional effects of anti-β2-glycoprotein I antibodies *in vitro*. Ann Rheum Dis 64:462–467
29. Di Simone N, Meroni PL, del Papa N et al (2000) Antiphospholipid antibodies affect trophoblast gonadotropin secretion and invasiveness by binding directly and through adhered beta2-glycoprotein I. Arthritis Rheum 43:140–150
30. Di Simone N, Marana R, Castellani R et al (2010) Decreased expression of heparin-binding epidermal growth factor-like growth factor as a newly identified pathogenic mechanism of antiphospholipid-mediated defective placentation. Arthritis Rheum 62:1504–1512
31. Di Simone N, Castellani R, Raschi E et al (2006) Anti-beta-2 glycoprotein I antibodies affect Bcl-2 and Bax trophoblast expression without evidence of apoptosis. Ann N Y Acad Sci 1069:364–376
32. Viall CA, Chen Q, Liu B et al (2013) Antiphospholipid antibodies internalised by human syncytiotrophoblast cause aberrant cell death and the release of necrotic trophoblast debris. J Autoimmun 47:45–57
33. Holers VM, Girardi G, Mo L et al (2002) Complement C3 activation is required for antiphospholipid antibody-induced fetal loss. J Exp Med 195:211–220
34. Girardi G, Berman J, Redecha P et al (2003) Complement C5a receptors and neutrophils mediate fetal injury in the antiphospholipid syndrome. J Clin Invest 112:1644–1654
35. Berman J, Girardi G, Salmon JE (2005) TNF-α is a critical effector and a target for therapy in antiphospholipid antibody-induced pregnancy loss. J Immunol 174:485–490
36. Thurman JM, Kraus DM, Girardi G et al (2005) A novel inhibitor of the alternative complement pathway prevents antiphospholipid antibody-induced pregnancy loss in mice. Mol Immunol 42:87–97
37. Redecha P, Tilley R, Rencati M et al (2007) Tissue factor: a link between C5a and neutrophil activation in antiphospholipid antibody induced fetal injury. Blood 110:2423–2431
38. Redecha P, Franzke CW, Ruf W et al (2008) Neutrophil activation by the tissue factor/Factor VIIa/PAR2 axis mediates fetal death in a mouse model of antiphospholipid syndrome. J Clin Invest 118:3453–3461
39. Seshan SV, Franzke CW, Redecha P et al (2009) Role of tissue factor in a mouse model of thrombotic microangiopathy induced by antiphospholipid antibodies. Blood 114:1675–1683
40. Martinez de la Torre Y, Buracchi C, Borroni EM et al (2007) Protection against inflammation- and autoantibody-caused fetal loss by the chemokine decoy receptor D6. Proc Natl Acad Sci U S A 104:2319–2324
41. Mulla MJ, Salmon JE, Chamley LW et al (2013) A role for uric acid and the Nalp3 inflammasome in antiphospholipid antibody-induced IL-1β production by human first trimester trophoblast. PLoS One 8:e65237
42. Park AL (2006) Chapter 28. Placental pathology in antiphospholipid syndrome. In: Khamashta MA (ed) Hughes' syndrome. Springer, London, pp 362–374
43. Shamonki JM, Salmon JE, Hyjek E et al (2007) Excessive complement activation is associated with placental injury in patients with antiphospholipid antibodies. Am J Obstet Gynecol 196:e1–e5
44. Cavazzana I, Nebuloni M, Cetin I et al (2007) Complement activation in anti-phospholipid syndrome: a clue for an inflammatory process? J Autoimmun 28:160–164

45. Meroni PL, Tincani A, Alarcón-Riquelme ME et al (2009) European Forum on Antiphospholipid Antibodies: research in progress. Lupus 18:924–929
46. Martinez de la Torre Y, Pregnolato F, D'Amelio F et al (2012) Anti-phospholipid induced murine fetal loss: novel protective effect of a peptide targeting the β2 glycoprotein I phospholipid-binding site. Implications for human fetal loss. J Autoimmun 38:J209–J215
47. Arnaud L, Mathian A, Ruffatti A et al (2014) Efficacy of aspirin for the primary prevention of thrombosis in patients with antiphospholipid antibodies: an international and collaborative meta-analysis. Autoimmun Rev 13:281–291
48. Branch W, Obstetric Task Force (2011) Report of the Obstetric APS Task Force: 13th International Congress on Antiphospholipid Antibodies, 13th April 2010. Lupus 20: 158–164
49. Hoppe B, Burmester GR, Dörner T (2011) Heparin or aspirin or both in the treatment of recurrent abortions in women with antiphospholipid antibody syndrome. Curr Opin Rheumatol 23:299–304
50. Girardi G, Redecha P, Salmon JE (2004) Heparin prevents antiphospholipid antibody induced fetal loss by inhibiting complement activation. Nat Med 10:1222–1226
51. Di Simone N, Caliandro D, Castellani R (1999) Low molecular weight heparin restores *in vitro* trophoblast invasiveness and differentiation in presence of immunoglobulin G fractions obtained from patients with antiphospholipid syndrome. Hum Reprod 14:489–495
52. D'Ippolito S, Marana R, Di Nicuolo F et al (2012) Effect of Low molecular weight heparins (LMWHs) on antiphospholipid antibodies (aPL)—mediated inhibition of endometrial angiogenesis. PLoS One 7:e29660
53. Ziakas PD, Pavlou M, Voulgarelis M (2010) Heparin treatment in antiphospholipid syndrome with recurrent pregnancy loss: a systematic review and meta-analysis. Obstet Gynecol 115:1256–1262
54. Ruffatti A, Tonello M, Visentin MS et al (2011) Risk factors for pregnancy failure in patients with anti-phospholipid syndrome treated with conventional therapies: a multicentre, case–control study. Rheumatology 50:1684–1689
55. Lockshin MD, Drunzin M, Qamar T (1989) Prednisone does not prevent recurrent fetal death in women with antiphospholipid antibody. Am J Obstet Gynecol 160:439–443
56. Silver RK, MacGregor SN (1993) Comparative trial of prednisone plus aspirin versus aspirin alone in the treatment of anticardiolipin antibody-positive obstetric patients. Am J Obstet Gynecol 169:1411–1417
57. Cowchock FS, Reece EA, Balaban D (1992) Repeated fetal losses associated with antiphospholipid antibodies: a collaborative randomized trial comparing prednisone with low-dose heparin. Am J Obstet Gynecol 166:1318–1323
58. Bramham K, Thomas M, Nelson-Piercy C et al (2011) First-trimester low-dose prednisolone in refractory antiphospholipid antibody-related pregnancy loss. Blood 117:6948–6951
59. Carp HJ, Sapir T, Shoenfeld Y (2005) Intravenous immunoglobulin and recurrent pregnancy loss. Clin Rev Allergy Immunol 29:327–332
60. Erkan D, Aguiar CL, Andrade D et al (2014) 14th International Congress on Antiphospholipid Antibodies: task force report on antiphospholipid syndrome treatment trends. Autoimmun Rev 13:685–696
61. Ostertag MV, Liu X, Henderson V, Pierangeli SS (2006) A peptide that mimics the Vth region of beta-2-glycoprotein I reverses antiphospholipid-mediated thrombosis in mice. Lupus 15:358–365
62. Di Simone N, D'Ippolito S, Marana R et al (2013) Antiphospholipid antibodies affect human endometrial angiogenesis: protective effect of a synthetic peptide (TIFI) mimicking the phospholipid binding site of β2 glycoprotein I. Am J Reprod Immunol 70:299–308
63. Miyakis S, Robertson SA, Krilis SA (2004) Beta-2 glycoprotein I and its role in antiphospholipid syndrome-lessons from knockout mice. Clin Immunol 112:136–143

64. Comarmond C, Cacoub P (2013) Antiphospholipid syndrome: from pathogenesis to novel immunomodulatory therapies. Autoimmun Rev 12:752–757
65. Berman H, Rodríguez-Pintó I, Cervera R et al (2013) Catastrophic Antiphospholipid Syndrome (CAPS) Registry Project Group (European Forum on Antiphospholipid Antibodies). Rituximab use in the catastrophic antiphospholipid syndrome: descriptive analysis of the CAPS registry patients receiving rituximab. Autoimmun Rev 12:1085–1090
66. Agostinis C, Durigutto P, Sblattero D et al (2014) A non complement-fixing antibody to β2 glycoprotein I as a novel therapy to control abortions and thrombosis in antiphospholipid syndrome. Blood 123:3478–3487

5 Classification Criteria for the Antiphospholipid Syndrome

Ronald H.W.M. Derksen and Ruth Fritsch-Stork

5.1 Introduction

The history of antiphospholipid antibodies (aPL) dates back to 1952, when both the phenomenon of "biological false-positive serological tests for syphilis" (BFP-STS), which is the presence of antibodies that are reactive with extracts from bovine heart as detected with the Wassermann or the VDRL tests, with negative results with more specific syphilis tests [49], and a peculiar inhibitor of coagulation in patients with systemic lupus erythematosus (SLE) [10] were described. The latter was shown to be caused by antibodies and appeared phospholipid dependent [39]. It was termed lupus anticoagulant (LAC) in 1972 [19]. Recognition that BFP-STS associate with LAC [38] and that the phospholipid cardiolipin is the major antigen in serological screening tests for syphilis resulted in development of solid phase assays to detect anticardiolipin antibodies (aCL) [23, 29, 43]. Major interest in aPL arose worldwide when clinical studies showed that both presence of LAC [6] and aCL [29] characterize a subset of SLE patients with thrombosis and/or fetal loss [14, 40] and associate with thrombocytopenia [6, 27, 30]. The presence of LAC or aCL in combination with thrombosis, fetal loss, and/or thrombocytopenia was named antiphospholipid syndrome (APS) in 1985 [31]. Originally, APS was described in patients with SLE, but soon, similar combinations of serological and clinical findings were recognized in otherwise healthy people (primary APS) [2, 3]. Over the years it became clear that LAC and aCL also associate with clinical features like livedo reticularis, heart valve lesions, microangiopathic nephropathy, cognitive

R.H.W.M. Derksen (✉) • R. Fritsch-Stork
Department of Rheumatology and Clinical Immunology, University Medical Centre Utrecht, 85500, Utrecht 3508 GA, The Netherlands
e-mail: r.h.w.m.derksen@umcutrecht.nl; R.Fritsch@umcutrecht.nl

© Springer International Publishing Switzerland 2015
P.L. Meroni (ed.), *Antiphospholipid Antibody Syndrome: From Bench to Bedside*, Rare Diseases of the Immune System, DOI 10.1007/978-3-319-11044-8_5

dysfunction, and chorea [17]. Recognition that autoimmune aCL and LAC require the plasma protein β2-glycoprotein I (β2GPI) as cofactor for binding to anionic phospholipids [20, 46, 47] led to development of solid phase assays to detect anti-β2GPI antibodies. Although by definition a misnomer, LAC, aCL, and anti-β2GPI collectively are indicated by the term aPL. This umbrella comprises overlapping, not necessarily identical antibodies. Clinicians are interested in APS as its recognition influences treatment [13, 16, 24, 36, 44, 61], whereas fundamental researchers unraveled many possible pathogenic pathways [11, 12, 24, 62].

5.2 Classification Criteria

5.2.1 1987: The First Proposal

The risks of therapy that follows a diagnosis of APS, combined with difficulties in standardization of aCL assays, led to the first proposal for APS criteria (Table 5.1) [26]. As low aCL levels are clinically irrelevant, a cutoff was set in GPL and MPL units for both IgG and IgM isotypes, based on association studies and standardization efforts [28, 32]. IgG class aCL antibodies were found more relevant than IgM [28], and the latter were not included as a stand-alone serologic criterion [26]. Definitions of the clinical criteria were not provided. To be "more sure" about the diagnosis, it was advised to have positive serology confirmed with an interval of at least 8 weeks.

5.2.2 1999: Preliminary Classification Criteria for Definite APS

To facilitate studies of treatment and causation and to align the diverse clinical and basic science disciplines involved in APS, consensus criteria were formulated in October 1998 in Sapporo, Japan (Table 5.2) [69]. Clinical criteria included: (1) objectively verified vascular thrombosis of any vessel and (2) pregnancy morbidity defined according to strict definitions [7]. There was consensus that presence of other contributing causes of thrombosis does not preclude a diagnosis of APS.

Table 5.1 Proposed criteria for antiphospholipid antibody syndrome[a] [26]

Clinical	Serology
1. Venous thrombosis	1. IgG anticardiolipin antibody (>20 GPL units)
2. Arterial thrombosis	2. Positive test for lupus anticoagulant
3. Recurrent fetal loss	3. IgM anticardiolipin antibody (>20 GPL units) AND positive test for lupus anticoagulant
4. Thrombocytopenia	

[a]Patients with APS should have at least one clinical and one serological feature at some time in their disease course. An aPL test should be positive on at least two occasions, more than 8 weeks apart

Table 5.2 Preliminary criteria for the classification of APS[a] [69]

Clinical criteria
1. Vascular thrombosis
One or more clinical episodes of arterial, venous, or small vessel thrombosis, in any tissue or organ
Thrombosis must be confirmed by imaging or Doppler studies or histopathology, with the exception of superficial venous thrombosis
For histopathologic confirmation, thrombosis should be present without significant evidence of inflammation in the vessel wall
2. Pregnancy morbidity
(a) One or more unexplained deaths of a morphologically normal fetus at or beyond the 10th week of gestation, with normal fetal morphology documented by ultrasound or by direct examination of the fetus
(b) One or more premature births of a morphologically normal neonate at or before the 34th week of gestation because of severe preeclampsia or eclampsia or severe placental insufficiency
(c) Three or more unexplained consecutive spontaneous abortions before the 10th week of gestation, with maternal anatomic or hormonal abnormalities and paternal and maternal chromosomal causes excluded
In studies of populations of patients who have more than one type of pregnancy morbidity, investigators are strongly encouraged to stratify groups of subjects according to a, b, or c above
Laboratory criteria
1. Anticardiolipin antibody of IgG and/or IgM isotype in blood, present in medium or high titer, on 2 or more occasions, at least 6 weeks apart, measured by a standardized enzyme-linked immunosorbent assay for β2-glycoprotein I-dependent anticardiolipin antibodies
2. Lupus anticoagulant present in plasma, on 2 or more occasions at least 6 weeks apart, detected according to the guidelines of the International Society on Thrombosis and Haemostasis [8], in the following steps:
(a) Prolonged phospholipid-dependent coagulation demonstrated on a screening test, e.g., activated partial thromboplastin time, kaolin clotting time, dilute Russell's viper venom time, dilute prothrombin time, Textarin time
(b) Failure to correct the prolonged coagulation time on the screening test by mixing with normal platelet-poor plasma
(c) Shortening or correction of the prolonged coagulation time on the screening test by the addition of excess phospholipid
(d) Exclusion of other coagulopathies, e.g., factor VIII inhibitor or heparin, as appropriate

[a]APS is considered to be present in a given patient when at least 1 of the clinical criteria and at least 1 of the laboratory criteria are met

For future studies, it was recommended to stratify patients according to presence or absence of additional thrombotic risk factors besides aPL. Also by consensus it was decided not to designate other features of APS (such as thrombocytopenia, transient cerebral ischemia, cardiac valve disease, and livedo reticularis) as criteria, because their associations with aPL were judged not as strongly based on clinical and experimental data as the chosen clinical criteria. Further studies of these additional associated features of APS are encouraged.

The laboratory criteria included aCL and LAC. For aCL it was specified that the assay should be β2GPI dependent [33] and titers medium or high. IgG and IgM isotypes were weighted equally. Guidelines for the detection of LAC were provided [8]. Extension of the laboratory criteria with anti-β2GPI antibodies was discussed but not executed because the assay was insufficiently standardized and it was felt that association studies did not convincingly show that their inclusion would have added value.

The criteria require that positive laboratory tests are confirmed with an interval of at least 6 weeks, reasoning that this will help to exclude aPL positivity that represents an epiphenomenon to clinical events. However, it was explicitly stated that no specific limits are placed on the interval between a clinical event and positive laboratory findings.

Two validation studies have been performed in patients regarded as having APS by their physicians [42, 68]. Because patients with low aCL levels, thrombocytopenia, or livedo reticularis in absence of classical clinical features do not classify for APS according to the criteria, reported sensitivities of 70–80 % are not surprising.

5.2.3 2006: Update of the Classification Criteria for Definite APS

In November 2004 the classification criteria for APS were revised in Sydney, Australia [48] (Table 5.3). The update resulted from a review of literature data in different fields of APS, grading of evidence, and consensus reached by open discussions. The classical clinical criteria were left unchanged, but some clarifications were added. These include (1) a list of coexisting inherited or acquired factors for thrombosis for which patients should be stratified in clinical studies, (2) strict definitions of eclampsia and severe preeclampsia [1], and (3) a list of commonly used clinical definitions for placental insufficiency. Superficial venous thrombosis was omitted as clinical criterion.

The committee advised against subdivision between primary and secondary APS as the clinical consequences of aPL among patients in these two categories are the same (Evidence Level I) but regarded documentation of coexisting SLE (or other disease) as advantageous.

The committee considered adoption of additional clinical features like heart valve disease, livedo reticularis, thrombocytopenia, nephropathy, and neurological manifestations as independent criteria for definite APS. It was decided not to do so, as it was felt that this would decrease the diagnostic specificity, even though association of these features with APS is recognized. Separate recognition of non-criteria features of APS in studies is, however, encouraged, and definitions of these features were provided.

Significant changes were executed in the laboratory criteria. Based on expert opinion the time interval for repeated testing for aPL was extended from 6 (Sapporo criteria) to 12 weeks, to reduce the risk for misclassification by transient presence of epiphenomenal aPL. Also new was the inclusion of a maximum time interval

Table 5.3 Revised classification criteria for APS[a] [48]

Clinical criteria
1. Vascular thrombosis
One or more clinical episodes of arterial, venous, or small vessel thrombosis, in any tissue or organ
Thrombosis must be confirmed by ***objective validated criteria*** (i.e., unequivocal findings of appropriate imaging studies or histopathology)
For histopathologic confirmation, thrombosis should be present without significant evidence of inflammation in the vessel wall
2. Pregnancy morbidity
(a) One or more unexplained deaths of a morphologically normal fetus at or beyond the 10th week of gestation, with normal fetal morphology documented by ultrasound or by direct examination of the fetus
(b) One or more premature births of a morphologically normal neonate before the 34th week of gestation because of: (i) ***eclampsia or severe preeclampsia defined according to standard definitions*** [1], or (ii) ***recognized features of*** placental insufficiency
(c) Three or more unexplained consecutive spontaneous abortions before the 10th week of gestation, with maternal anatomic or hormonal abnormalities and paternal and maternal chromosomal causes excluded
In studies of populations of patients who have more than one type of pregnancy morbidity, investigators are strongly encouraged to stratify groups of subjects according to a, b, or c above
Laboratory criteria
1. Lupus anticoagulant present in plasma, on two or more occasions at least ***12 weeks*** apart, detected according to the guidelines of the International Society on Thrombosis and Haemostasis (Scientific Subcommittee on LAs/phospholipid-dependent antibodies) [8]
2. Anticardiolipin (aCL) antibody of IgG and/or IgM isotype in ***serum or plasma***, present in medium or high titer ***(i.e., >40 GPL or MPL, or >the 99th percentile)***, on two or more occasions, at least ***12 weeks apart***, measured by a ***standardized ELISA***
3. ***Anti-β2GPI antibody of IgG and/or IgM isotype in serum or plasma (in titer >the 99th percentile), present on two or more occasions at least 12 weeks apart, measured by a standardized ELISA, according to recommended procedures*** [56]

Differences between these and the Sapporo criteria are indicated in bold-italics
[a]APS is present if at least 1 of the clinical criteria and at least 1 of the laboratory criteria are met

(5 years) between a clinical manifestation and aPL testing. It was felt that a longer interval may not reflect a causative relationship. Recommendations for LAC testing became more stringent. Use of two or more LAC tests with different assay principles was advised before presence of LAC is excluded, as no single test is 100 % sensitive for LAC. The issue of testing for LAC in patients using vitamin K antagonists was addressed. With an international normalized ratio (INR) >3.5, testing for LAC should not be performed. With less prolonged INRs test samples should be diluted with normal plasma.

There was a strong debate on the difficulties with testing for aCL, which include the still marginal interlaboratory agreement, absence of a standard for the threshold used to distinguish between moderate/high and low aCL levels, and the difficult definition of the level that best corresponds to clinical manifestations. There was, however, no consensus to remove aCL tests completely from the criteria. The committee decided to define new cutoff levels that were felt to be appropriate until an international consensus is reached. These new cutoffs are >40 GPL or MPL or >99th percentile.

The most important revision in the criteria was the inclusion of IgG and IgM isotype anti-β2 GPI antibodies as a stand-alone laboratory criterion for APS, despite recognition of problems with standardization of the anti-β2 GPI assay (results being among others dependent on types of plates and purity, concentration, and source of β2 GPI) and with the definition of appropriate cutoffs (no uniformly accepted calibrators and units). Statements that anti-β2 GPI antibodies are independent risk factors for thrombosis and pregnancy complications were graded with evidence level II and I, respectively. Of note, at least two members voted against inclusion of anti-β2 GPI in the criteria as they considered existing evidence too weak. It was decided to use a threshold of >99th percentile of controls for both IgG and IgM class anti-β2 GPI to define a positive result.

The committee strongly advised to classify APS patients in studies according to their serological profile as follows: (I) more than one laboratory criteria present (any combination), (IIa) LA present alone, (IIb) aCL antibody present alone, and (IIc) anti-β2 GPI antibody present alone.

Not surprisingly, studies that applied both the Sapporo and revised criteria on patients in aPL databases found that 3–9 % more patients classify for APS with the revised criteria, simply because these had anti-β2 GPI antibodies in presence of classical clinical criteria, but negative LAC and aCL assays [15, 35, 55, 63, 64]. This increase in patients classifying for APS due to introduction of anti-β2 assays is counteracted by loss of patients that do not fulfill the revised criteria, when these are applied strictly. One study found that only 58 % of patients that classified APS according to the Sapporo criteria also fulfilled the updated criteria [35]. The patients that did not classify any more had aCL levels below the newly defined cutoff and had an interval greater than 5 years between a clinical event and the first aPL test and/or an interval between test and retest between 6 and 12 weeks.

5.3 Critics on and Shortcomings of Current Classification Criteria

The revisions that the committee made in the clinical and laboratory criteria for APS evoked many comments. A major contributor to the confusion on APS is the unclear border between diagnostic and classification criteria. Although it is acknowledged that classification criteria are intended to serve research, they are uniformly applied for diagnostic purposes and to guide treatment [37, 63]. In APS the situation is complex because thrombosis and pregnancy morbidities are multicausal and relatively common in the general population and the tests included in the laboratory criteria are unspecific and difficult to standardize.

5.3.1 Methodological Issues

Serious shortcomings were noted in an evaluation of the developmental methodology and measurement properties of both sets of classification criteria [4]. Although the revised criteria may have incremental face and content validity over the Sapporo criteria, the complexity of both the criteria and the diagnostic and immunologic tests limits their feasibility. Before a classification criterion can confidently be used in multicenter trials, it is a prerequisite that its reliability is established [34]. However, at present the reliability of individual APS criteria is unknown.

5.3.2 Comments on Clinical Criteria

It has been questioned, whether removal of superficial thrombosis (confirmed by imaging techniques), as clinical criterion and exclusion of APS when vasculitis is simultaneously present is correct [9]. Mondor's disease can be a manifestation of APS [5, 45] and APS can coexist with vasculitis [50, 57]. Lackner et al. argued against joining of primary and secondary APS [37] because the prevalence of APS is low in otherwise healthy persons and high in SLE and test performances always depend strongly on prevalence of disease. Based upon interpretation of reported inconsistent findings on associations between aPL and consecutive spontaneous abortions before the 10th week, and increasing evidence that this clinical problem has other etiologies than late fetal loss or early delivery with placental insufficiency, some advocate withdrawal of the "recurrent spontaneous abortions" criterion from clinical APS criteria [25].

5.3.3 Comments on Laboratory Criteria

Lackner et al. strongly criticized the decision of the committee to include anti-β2 GPI as stand-alone laboratory criterion by showing that they strongly overestimated the power of studies used to justify their decision [37]. The authors stress that clinicians need solid tests with high predictive values for future APS manifestations and prefer tests with high specificity over high sensitivity. They warned that addition of inconclusive laboratory tests without firm evidence to support their use can be harmful [37].

Although specification of time intervals between serologic tests and between serology and clinical manifestations in the revised criteria improves face validity, the value of these time intervals must be tested in clinical studies before these can be useful [4]. Formulation of these time intervals was not based on scientific data. One study found that a wider time interval between serologic tests is unlikely to make a difference [63].

In the revised criteria the cutoff for positive aCL was set at >40 GPL or MPL or >the 99th percentile, suggesting these are similar. This, however, is not the case. The 99th percentile of the geometric mean of 100 normal subjects is always lower than 40 Units and corresponds with 15–26 GPL and 16–27 MPL [22, 58, 59, 64]. Most APS patients with IgG aCL levels between the 99th percentile and 40 GPL have pregnancy morbidity and test negative for LAC and anti-β2 GPI (category IIb of the revised criteria) [58]. Others plead to use different cutoffs for obstetric and thrombotic APS, namely, the 95th and the 99th percentile, respectively [22], as many patients with obstetric APS have, in contrast to those with thrombotic APS IgG class aCL or anti-β2 GPI antibodies between 5 and 20 Units. It was argued that by applying the higher cutoff, such patients will probably be withhold proper treatment [22]. Clinically relevant aPL levels for thrombotic APS are higher than for obstetric APS, but in absence of a generally accepted international definition cutoff level, any arbitrarily chosen value will leave doubts about its validity [64]. However, good arguments to prefer a cutoff for a positive aCL test based on the 99th percentile of the healthy population instead of 40 GPL/MPL include: (1) the 99th percentile is simple, objective (for the given population and laboratory), and uniform; (2) there are no widely accepted and validated calibrators; and (3) the available standard has fluctuations from lot to lot [65].

There is general agreement that aCL and anti-β2-GPI of IgM isotype are of significantly less clinical importance than those of the IgG class [4, 64, 66]. It is to be regretted that the updated criteria do not separate IgG and IgM isotypes in the laboratory subclassification (categories IIb and IIc) [64]. Subclassification of patients based on aPL test results is relevant as multiple positivity (category I of the revised criteria) associates with higher risks. Presence of LAC together with IgG aCL and/or IgG anti-β2 GPI associates with higher risk for clinical complications (notably thrombosis) than presence of LAC alone (category IIa of the revised criteria) [64]. Patients with obstetric APS have significantly more often than those with thrombotic APS an IgG aCL level <40 GPL [58]. Furthermore, there is a progressive increase in IgG aCL level when one compares groups of APS patients that are only aCL positive (category IIb), double positive, or triple positive in that order [58].

In 2008 a group of prominent APS researchers published a provocative paper to evoke a debate on the serological criteria, so that these would identify exclusively patients who suffer from APS with high probability and simultaneously reduce over diagnosis of APS [21]. The group proposed (1) implementation of strict guidelines for performance of LAC assays, (2) exclusion of aCL from the criteria, and (3) limitation of anti β2-GPI antibody measurement to IgG isotype. Several groups responded [51, 65–67]. There was not much discussion on the need for updated guidelines for LAC that should include rules for pre-analytic handling of plasma samples, expression of results of LAC assays, interpretation of the degree of reduction that extra phospholipids must induce to mark the LAC assay as positive, and for the minimal number, type and combination of assays that reach a sufficiently high sensitivity and specificity for proper diagnosis of LAC. An update along these lines, including guidelines for LAC detection in patients on antithrombotic treatment [66], was soon delivered by the subcommittee on lupus anticoagulant/phospholipid-dependent antibodies from the International Society on Thrombosis and Haemostasis (ISTH) [54].

The arguments to remove the aCL test from APS criteria as proposed by Galli et al. [21] were both clinical and technical. The association between a solitary positive aCL test (category IIb of the revised criteria) and thrombosis is poor, and the assay has many technical difficulties and also detects irrelevant antibody reactivity. Respondents of the evoked debate [51, 65, 67] agreed to maintain aCL of medium/high titer as criterion, although they conceded the validity of the issues raised [21]. This also applied for 9/13 international experts in the field who participated in a 2007 survey [51]. Arguments to maintain the aCL test for APS classification included that, in patients with negative LAC assays, a positive result for the same isotype in both aCL and anti-β2-GPI assays reinforces suspicion of APS and that aCL values serve as a control both for the quality of the antibodies tested and performance of the anti-β2-GPI test [51]. Swadzba added that it has not been proven beyond doubt that aCL antibodies directed against proteins other than β2-GPI are completely devoid of prothrombotic properties [65]. Another argument to maintain the aCL test is that positivity in both LAC, aCL, and anti-β2-GPI tests (triple positivity) strongly associates with classical clinical APS events [52, 53, 60]. On a different note, Wahl [67] counters the proposed modifications of the APS criteria by stating that such important decision should not be based on expert opinion, but on new data and appropriate systematic reviews.

The many data showing that IgM class antibodies are not associated with thrombosis and pregnancy morbidity [4, 64, 66] support the proposal made by Galli et al. [21] to remove these as laboratory criterion for APS. Pengo, however, considers the IgM tests still useful in special cases where LAC is not associated with positive IgG aCL or IgG anti-β2-GPI [51].

5.4 Concluding Remarks

There is no doubt that some aPL(-profiles) associate with risks for thrombosis and pregnancy morbidity and that APS exists. Classification criteria aim at provision of homogeneous groups of patients in clinical and laboratory studies. In APS, clinical studies should aim at identification of aPL profiles that distinguish patients at high risk for (recurrent) manifestations from those patients with a low risk, while taking into account the presence or absence of other risk factors for thromboembolic events, cardiovascular disease, and pregnancy complications. In that way, the context can be discovered where the presence of aPL should dictate management and medical treatment of patients. We agree with Wahl that we should leave the concept of a syndrome and regard aPL as risk factors for recurrent clinical events, a policy that is also advocated for hereditary thrombophilia [67]. We strongly feel that laboratory criteria for classification and diagnosis of obstetric APS should not necessarily be the same. The associations linking aPL subtypes and obstetrical morbidities show variable specificities and sensitivities and are different from those with thrombotic APS, although LAC apparently is a strong risk factor for both [25, 41, 58]. Most women presenting with pregnancy failure and aPL do not experience thromboembolic events, and the pathogenetic mechanisms of aPL-mediated thrombosis and pregnancy loss are diverging [24, 62].

Inevitably, classification criteria are used in daily practice for diagnosis and to guide therapy. A decision to reserve adaptations of treatment for (suggested) high-risk aPL profiles (e.g., triple positivity) simultaneously leaves many patients with other profiles (e.g., single positivity for aCL or anti-β2-GPI positivity or IgM) with standard treatment. We see in daily life that clinicians often feel uncomfortable to go for high specificity instead of high sensitivity as they fear that they wrongly withhold adaptation of (suggested) beneficial treatment. Unfortunately, one has to ascertain that decades after the first proposal of APS classification, no unequivocal data on risks for clinical events and treatment are available, because undisputable, large-scale prospective clinical studies have not been performed. This explains why all (suggestions for) adaptations of criteria were mainly based on consensus, using data from imperfect studies.

It is a great step forward that the Antiphospholipid Syndrome Alliance for Clinical Trials and International Networking (APS-ACTION) was recently founded and started international initiatives [18]. Hopefully APS-ACTION succeeds in execution of appropriate trials that are so urgently needed in this field to get answers to at least part of the many uncertainties that surround APS.

References

1. Anonymous (2002) ACOG Committee on Obstetric Practice. Diagnosis and management of preeclampsia and eclampsia. Number 33, January 2002. American College of Obstetricians and Gynecologists. Int J Gynaecol Obstet 77(1):67–75
2. Alarcon-Segovia D, Sanchez-Guerrero J (1989) Primary antiphospholipid syndrome. J Rheumatol 16(4):482–488
3. Asherson RA (1988) A "primary" antiphospholipid syndrome? J Rheumatol 15(12):1742–1746
4. Bobba RS, Johnson SR, Davis AM (2007) A review of the sapporo and revised Sapporo criteria for the classification of antiphospholipid syndrome. Where do the revised sapporo criteria add value? J Rheumatol 34(7):1522–1527
5. Boehlen F, Bader M, de Moerloose P (2004) Superficial thrombophlebitis of the chest wall associated with anticardiolipin antibodies: antiphospholipid syndrome or Mondor's disease? Lupus 13(1):70–71
6. Boey ML, Colaco CB, Gharavi AE, Elkon KB, Loizou S, Hughes GR (1983) Thrombosis in systemic lupus erythematosus: striking association with the presence of circulating lupus anticoagulant. Br Med J (Clin Res Ed) 287(6398):1021–1023
7. Branch DW, Silver RM (1996) Criteria for antiphospholipid syndrome: early pregnancy loss, fetal loss, or recurrent pregnancy loss? Lupus 5(5):409–413
8. Brandt JT, Triplett DA, Alving B, Scharrer I (1995) Criteria for the diagnosis of lupus anticoagulants: an update. On behalf of the Subcommittee on Lupus Anticoagulant/Antiphospholipid Antibody of the Scientific and Standardisation Committee of the ISTH. Thromb Haemost 74(4):1185–1190
9. Carvalho JF (2008) Some concerns about the Sydney criteria for antiphospholipid syndrome. Lupus 17(8):770
10. Conley CL, Hartmann RC (1952) A hemorrhagic disorder caused by circulating anticoagulant in patients with disseminated lupus erythematosus. J Clin Invest 31:621–622

11. De Groot PG, Urbanus RT (2014) Cellular signaling by antiphospholipid antibodies. J Thromb Haemost 12:773–5
12. De Groot PG, Urbanus RT, Derksen RH (2012) Pathophysiology of thrombotic APS: where do we stand? Lupus 21(7):704–707
13. Derksen RH, de Groot PG (2008) The obstetric antiphospholipid syndrome. J Reprod Immunol 77(1):41–50
14. Derue GJ, Englert HJ, Harris EN, Gharavi AE, Morgan SH, Hull RG (1985) Fetal loss in systemic lupus erythematosus: association with anticardiolipin antibodies. J Obstet Gynecol Neonatal Nurs 5:207–209
15. Drijkoningen J, Damoiseaux J, van Pieter P, Tervaert JW (2007) Clinical manifestations of the anti-phospholipid syndrome as defined by the updated Sapporo classification criteria. Ann Rheum Dis 66(10):1407–1408
16. Empson M, Lassere M, Craig JC, Scott JR (2002) Recurrent pregnancy loss with antiphospholipid antibody: a systematic review of therapeutic trials. Obstet Gynecol 99(1):135–144
17. Erkan D, Lockshin MD (2010) Non-criteria manifestations of antiphospholipid syndrome. Lupus 19(4):424–427
18. Erkan D, Lockshin MD (2012) APS ACTION–AntiPhospholipid Syndrome Alliance for Clinical Trials and International Networking. Lupus 21(7):695–698
19. Feinstein DI, Rapaport SI (1972) Acquired inhibitors of blood coagulation. Prog Hemost Thromb 1:75–95
20. Galli M, Comfurius P, Maassen C, Hemker HC, de Baets MH, van Breda-Vriesman PJ, Barbui T, Zwaal RF, Bevers EM (1990) Anticardiolipin antibodies (ACA) directed not to cardiolipin but to a plasma protein cofactor. Lancet 335(8705):1544–1547
21. Galli M, Reber G, de Moerloose P, de Groot PG (2008) Invitation to a debate on the serological criteria that define the antiphospholipid syndrome. J Thromb Haemost 6(2):399–401
22. Gardiner C, Hills J, Machin SJ, Cohen H (2013) Diagnosis of antiphospholipid syndrome in routine clinical practice. Lupus 22(1):18–25
23. Gharavi AE, Harris EN, Asherson RA, Hughes GR (1987) Anticardiolipin antibodies: isotype distribution and phospholipid specificity. Ann Rheum Dis 46(1):1–6
24. Giannakopoulos B, Krilis SA (2013) The pathogenesis of the antiphospholipid syndrome. N Engl J Med 368(11):1033–1044
25. Gris JC, Bouvier S (2013) Antiphospholipid syndrome: looking for a refocusing. Thromb Res 131(Suppl 1):S28–S31
26. Harris EN (1987) Syndrome of the black swan. Br J Rheumatol 26(5):324–326
27. Harris EN, Asherson RA, Gharavi AE, Morgan SH, Derue G, Hughes GR (1985) Thrombocytopenia in SLE and related autoimmune disorders: association with anticardiolipin antibody. Br J Haematol 59(2):227–230
28. Harris EN, Chan JK, Asherson RA, Aber VR, Gharavi AE, Hughes GR (1986) Thrombosis, recurrent fetal loss, and thrombocytopenia. Predictive value of the anticardiolipin antibody test. Arch Intern Med 146(11):2153–2156
29. Harris EN, Gharavi AE, Boey ML, Patel BM, Kworth-Young CG, Loizou S, Hughes GR (1983) Anticardiolipin antibodies: detection by radioimmunoassay and association with thrombosis in systemic lupus erythematosus. Lancet 2(8361):1211–1214
30. Harris EN, Gharavi AE, Hegde U, Derue G, Morgan SH, Englert H, Chan JK, Asherson RA, Hughes GR (1985) Anticardiolipin antibodies in autoimmune thrombocytopenic purpura. Br J Haematol 59(2):231–234
31. Harris EN, Gharavi AE, Hughes GR (1985) Anti-phospholipid antibodies. Clin Rheum Dis 11(3):591–609
32. Harris EN, Gharavi AE, Patel SP, Hughes GR (1987) Evaluation of the anti-cardiolipin antibody test: report of an international workshop held 4 April 1986. Clin Exp Immunol 68(1):215–222
33. Harris EN, Pierangeli SS, Gharavi AE (1998) Diagnosis of the antiphospholipid syndrome: a proposal for use of laboratory tests. Lupus 7(Suppl 2):S144–S148

34. Johnson SR, Goek ON, Singh-Grewal D, Vlad SC, Feldman BM, Felson DT, Hawker GA, Singh JA, Solomon DH (2007) Classification criteria in rheumatic diseases: a review of methodologic properties. Arthritis Rheum 57(7):1119–1133
35. Kaul M, Erkan D, Sammaritano L, Lockshin MD (2007) Assessment of the 2006 revised antiphospholipid syndrome classification criteria. Ann Rheum Dis 66(7):927–930
36. Khamashta MA, Cuadrado MJ, Mujic F, Taub NA, Hunt BJ, Hughes GR (1995) The management of thrombosis in the antiphospholipid-antibody syndrome. N Engl J Med 332(15): 993–997
37. Lackner KJ, Peetz D, Peetz D, von Landenberg P (2006) Revision of the Sapporo criteria for the antiphospholipid syndrome– coming to grips with evidence and Thomas Bayes? Thromb Haemost 95(6):917–919
38. Laurell AB, Nilsson IM (1957) Hypergammaglobulinemia, circulating anticoagulant, and biologic false positive Wassermann reaction; a study in two cases. J Lab Clin Med 49(5): 694–707
39. Lee SL, Sanders M (1955) A disorder of blood coagulation in systemic lupus erythematosus. J Clin Invest 34(12):1814–1822
40. Lockshin MD, Druzin ML, Goei S, Qamar T, Magid MS, Jovanovic L, Ferenc M (1985) Antibody to cardiolipin as a predictor of fetal distress or death in pregnant patients with systemic lupus erythematosus. N Engl J Med 313(3):152–156
41. Lockshin MD, Kim M, Laskin CA, Guerra M, Branch DW, Merrill J, Petri M, Porter TF, Sammaritano L, Stephenson MD, Buyon J, Salmon JE (2012) Prediction of adverse pregnancy outcome by the presence of lupus anticoagulant, but not anticardiolipin antibody, in patients with antiphospholipid antibodies. Arthritis Rheum 64(7):2311–2318
42. Lockshin MD, Sammaritano LR, Schwartzman S (2000) Validation of the Sapporo criteria for antiphospholipid syndrome. Arthritis Rheum 43(2):440–443
43. Loizou S, McCrea JD, Rudge AC, Reynolds R, Boyle CC, Harris EN (1985) Measurement of anti-cardiolipin antibodies by an enzyme-linked immunosorbent assay (ELISA): standardization and quantitation of results. Clin Exp Immunol 62(3):738–745
44. Lubbe WF, Butler WS, Palmer SJ, Liggins GC (1983) Fetal survival after prednisone suppression of maternal lupus-anticoagulant. Lancet 1(8338):1361–1363
45. Magy N, Gil H, Racadot E, Dupond JL (2003) Mondor's thrombophlebitis and antiphospholipid antibodies. Presse Med 32(2):70–71
46. Matsuura E, Igarashi Y, Fujimoto M, Ichikawa K, Koike T (1990) Anticardiolipin cofactor(s) and differential diagnosis of autoimmune disease. Lancet 336(8708):177–178
47. McNeil HP, Simpson RJ, Chesterman CN, Krilis SA (1990) Anti-phospholipid antibodies are directed against a complex antigen that includes a lipid-binding inhibitor of coagulation: beta 2-glycoprotein I (apolipoprotein H). Proc Natl Acad Sci U S A 87(11):4120–4124
48. Miyakis S, Lockshin MD, Atsumi T, Branch DW, Brey RL, Cervera R, Derksen RH, de Groot PG, Koike T, Meroni PL, Reber G, Shoenfeld Y, Tincani A, Vlachoyiannopoulos PG, Krilis SA (2006) International consensus statement on an update of the classification criteria for definite antiphospholipid syndrome (APS). J Thromb Haemost 4(2):295–306
49. Moore JE, Mohr CF (1952) Biologically false positive serologic tests for syphilis; type, incidence, and cause. J Am Med Assoc 150(5):467–473
50. Norden DK, Ostrov BE, Shafritz AB, Von Feldt JM (1995) Vasculitis associated with antiphospholipid syndrome. Semin Arthritis Rheum 24(4):273–281
51. Pengo V (2008) A contribution to the debate on the laboratory criteria that define the antiphospholipid syndrome. J Thromb Haemost 6(6):1048–1049
52. Pengo V, Ruffatti A, Legnani C, Gresele P, Barcellona D, Erba N, Testa S, Marongiu F, Bison E, Denas G, Banzato A, Padayattil JS, Iliceto S (2010) Clinical course of high-risk patients diagnosed with antiphospholipid syndrome. J Thromb Haemost 8(2):237–242
53. Pengo V, Ruffatti A, Legnani C, Testa S, Fierro T, Marongiu F, De Micheli V, Gresele P, Tonello M, Ghirarduzzi A, Bison E, Denas G, Banzato A, Padayattil JS, Iliceto S (2011) Incidence of a first thromboembolic event in asymptomatic carriers of high-risk antiphospholipid antibody profile: a multicenter prospective study. Blood 118(17):4714–4718

54. Pengo V, Tripodi A, Reber G, Rand JH, Ortel TL, Galli M, de Groot PG (2009) Update of the guidelines for lupus anticoagulant detection. Subcommittee on Lupus Anticoagulant/Antiphospholipid Antibody of the Scientific and Standardisation Committee of the International Society on Thrombosis and Haemostasis. J Thromb Haemost 7(10):1737–1740
55. Pourrat O, Jollit C, Gombert JM, Boinot C, Pierre F (2006) Clinical relevance of the recent update of the classification criteria for definite antiphospholipid syndrome: an obstetric medicine clinic series of 107 patients. J Thromb Haemost 4(10):2276–2277
56. Reber G, Tincani A, Sanmarco M, de Moerloose P, Boffa MC (2004) Proposals for the measurement of anti-beta2-glycoprotein I antibodies. Standardization group of the European Forum on Antiphospholipid Antibodies. J Thromb Haemost 2(10):1860–1862
57. Rees JD, Lanca S, Marques PV, Gomez-Puerta JA, Moco R, Oliveri C, Khamashta MA, Hughes GR, D'Cruz DP (2006) Prevalence of the antiphospholipid syndrome in primary systemic vasculitis. Ann Rheum Dis 65(1):109–111
58. Ruffatti A, Olivieri S, Tonello M, Bortolati M, Bison E, Salvan E, Facchinetti M, Pengo V (2008) Influence of different IgG anticardiolipin antibody cut-off values on antiphospholipid syndrome classification. J Thromb Haemost 6(10):1693–1696
59. Ruffatti A, Tonello M, Del RT, Cavazzana A, Grava C, Noventa F, Tona F, Iliceto S, Pengo V (2006) Antibody profile and clinical course in primary antiphospholipid syndrome with pregnancy morbidity. Thromb Haemost 96(3):337–341
60. Ruffatti A, Tonello M, Visentin MS, Bontadi A, Hoxha A, De CS, Botta A, Salvi S, Nuzzo M, Rovere-Querini P, Canti V, Mosca M, Mitic G, Bertero MT, Pengo V, Boffa MC, Tincani A (2011) Risk factors for pregnancy failure in patients with anti-phospholipid syndrome treated with conventional therapies: a multicentre, case-control study. Rheumatology (Oxford) 50(9):1684–1689
61. Ruiz-Irastorza G, Cuadrado MJ, Ruiz-Arruza I, Brey R, Crowther M, Derksen R, Erkan D, Krilis S, Machin S, Pengo V, Pierangeli S, Tektonidou M, Khamashta M (2011) Evidence-based recommendations for the prevention and long-term management of thrombosis in antiphospholipid antibody-positive patients: report of a task force at the 13th International Congress on antiphospholipid antibodies. Lupus 20(2):206–218
62. Salmon JE, Girardi G (2008) Antiphospholipid antibodies and pregnancy loss: a disorder of inflammation. J Reprod Immunol 77(1):51–56
63. Solano C, Lamuno M, Vargas A, Amezcua-Guerra LM (2009) Comparison of the 1999 Sapporo and 2006 revised criteria for the classification of the antiphospholipid syndrome. Clin Exp Rheumatol 27(6):914–919
64. Swadzba J, Iwaniec T, Szczeklik A, Musial J (2007) Revised classification criteria for antiphospholipid syndrome and the thrombotic risk in patients with autoimmune diseases. J Thromb Haemost 5(9):1883–1889
65. Swadzba J, Musial J (2009) More on: the debate on antiphospholipid syndrome classification criteria. J Thromb Haemost 7(3):501–502
66. Tripodi A (2008) More on: criteria to define the antiphospholipid syndrome. J Thromb Haemost 6(6):1049–1050
67. Wahl D, Thiebaugeorges O, Regnault V, Dalloul A, Lecompte T (2008) Pursuing the debate on the serologic criteria that define the antiphospholipid syndrome. J Thromb Haemost 6(8):1433–1435
68. Weber M, Hayem G, Meyer O (2001) The Sapporo criteria for antiphospholipid syndrome: comment on the article by Lockshin et al. Arthritis Rheum 44(8):1965–1966
69. Wilson WA, Gharavi AE, Koike T, Lockshin MD, Branch DW, Piette JC, Brey R, Derksen R, Harris EN, Hughes GR, Triplett DA, Khamashta MA (1999) International consensus statement on preliminary classification criteria for definite antiphospholipid syndrome: report of an international workshop. Arthritis Rheum 42(7):1309–1311

Non-classification Criteria

6

Maria Gerosa and Francesca Rovelli

6.1 Introduction

Antiphospholipid syndrome (APS) is an acquired autoimmune disease mainly characterized by vascular thrombosis and/or pregnancy complications in association with autoantibodies belonging to the antiphospholipid antibody family (aPL).

The laboratory classification criteria for APS require the presence of lupus anticoagulant (LA, detected by a clotting assay) and of medium/high positivity for anticardiolipin (aCL) antibodies (IgM or IgG isotype) or anti-β2-glycoprotein I antibodies (IgM or IgG isotype), which must be confirmed twice, at least 12 weeks apart [1, 2]. Several other autoantibodies have been described in APS patients that are not included in the formal criteria as their diagnostic and prognostic value is still unclear.

The clinical criteria include a history of arterial or venous thrombosis, early or late pregnancy loss, or severe prematurity due to (pre-)eclampsia or placental failure (which are the major features of obstetric APS) [3]. Deep venous thrombosis of the lower limbs is one of the most common manifestations of APS, and it can be complicated by pulmonary thromboembolism. Arterial involvement is less common and often involves the central nervous system circulation [2].

The clinical spectrum of APS has markedly broadened from the first description of APS and a variety of other clinical manifestations has been reported in aPL-positive patients in addition to thrombosis and obstetric morbidity. However, the

M. Gerosa, MD (✉)
Division of Rheumatology, Department of Clinical Sciences and Community Health, Ospedale Gaetano Pini, University of Milan, via Pini 9, Milan 20122, Italy
e-mail: Maria.gerosa@unimi.it

F. Rovelli, MD
Division of Rheumatology, Ospedale Gaetano Pini, University of Milan, via Pini 9, Milan 20122, Italy
e-mail: frencir@hotmail.com

© Springer International Publishing Switzerland 2015

P.L. Meroni (ed.), *Antiphospholipid Antibody Syndrome: From Bench to Bedside*, Rare Diseases of the Immune System, DOI 10.1007/978-3-319-11044-8_6

formal classification criteria do not include these clinical findings because of their low prevalence or because they are not specific for APS, being common manifestations of other diseases [1].

6.2 Non-classification Laboratory Assays

Besides the three aPL assays currently included in the laboratory criteria for formal APS classification, several additional laboratory tests have been proposed for APS diagnosis [4, 5] (Table 6.1).

6.2.1 Anti-prothrombin Antibodies

Prothrombin (PT, also known as clotting factor II) is a vitamin K-dependent proenzyme that induces the conversion of fibrinogen to fibrin, via a prothrombinase complex. PT was first reported by Loeliger in 1959 as a possible cofactor for LA. Since then, many other authors have suggested that antibodies binding to PT could contribute to LA phenomenon and, at the present time, they are largely considered as one of the most important causes of the elongation of clotting time due to LA positivity, together with anti-β_2GPI antibodies [6, 7].

Table 6.1 Noncriteria laboratory assays

Test	Distinctive features
Anti-PS/PT antibodies	Strong correlation with LA
	Association with obstetric or thrombotic manifestations not definitely demonstrated
Anti-DI antibodies	Association with triple positivity
	Association with thrombosis (in few studies)
	Controversial data in OAPS
Anti-PE antibodies	No association with additional aPL laboratory tests
	Proposed as a possible serological marker of seronegative APS
Ab against negatively charged PLs[a]	aCL cross-react with aPS, aPA, and aPI
	Mainly recognize β2GPI complexed with anionic aPL
	Conflicting data regarding association with pregnancy morbidity
Annexin A5 resistance assay	Association with anti-DI
	Found in a significantly higher proportion of APS patients in comparison to controls
Anti-annexin 2	Described in patients with APS and severe thrombosis and/or pregnancy morbidity
IgA aCL and/or IgA anti-β2GPI	Reported in seronegative patients with a history of thrombosis and pregnancy morbidity

[a]Ab against negatively charged PLs: anti-phosphatidylserine (aPS), anti-phosphatidylinositol (aPI), and anti-phosphatidic acid (aPA)

Antibodies against prothrombin are usually detected by two different ELISAs (enzyme-linked immunosorbent assay) that employ human PT coated onto irradiated plates (aPT) or PT in complex with phosphatidylserine (aPS/PT) as antigen. These two assays seem to display different diagnostic and prognostic power, possibly attributable to their different ability to offer the antigen to antibody binding [6–8]. The real prevalence of aPT is still unknown, as it widely varies among studies, as a result of the variability of detection methods and the poor standardization among different laboratories. Also the clinical significance of aPT in both primary and secondary APS is still debated, as an apparent association with obstetric or thrombotic manifestations has not been definitely demonstrated [6]. On the other hand, aPS/PT antibodies strongly correlate with the presence of LA and are suggested to be highly specific for the diagnosis of APS [7, 8].

Most of the studies addressing the clinical significance of aPS/PT antibodies have demonstrated a significant association with thrombotic manifestations of APS, venous thrombosis above all, while the association with obstetric manifestations is still controversial. Actually, even if some authors reported that aPS/PT can be predictive of pregnancy morbidity in patients with systemic autoimmune diseases, most of the studies did not confirm this finding [9, 10].

Several studies have clearly demonstrated that multiple positive aPL tests are stronger predictor of thrombosis and pregnancy complications than single positivity. Accordingly, it has been suggested that the combination of routinely tested aPL (aCL, anti-β2GPI, and LA) with new (non-criteria) aPL assays would lead to a better risk stratification of patients. Among 23 possible combinations of six aPL assays (LA, aCL, anti-β2GPI, aPT, aPS/PT, and anti-phosphatidylethanolamine antibodies), the association of LA plus anti-β2GPI plus aPS/PT antibodies has recently been identified to display the best diagnostic accuracy for both vascular and obstetric APS [11].

A very recent and exhaustive review of the literature showed that both aPT and anti-PS/PT positivity increase the risk of thrombosis but that aPS/PT display the highest odds ratio (5.11 (95 % CI 4.2–6.3) vs 1.82 (95 % CI 1.44–2.75)). In line, the studies directly comparing aPT and aPS/PT and their odds ratio for thrombosis in 1196 patients demonstrate that aPS/PT antibodies are more strongly associated with both arterial and venous thrombosis than aPT antibodies [12].

Even if aPS/PT represent a very promising biomarker of APS, the lack of harmonization and standardization of the detection procedures and the low reproducibility of the results among laboratories are still unsolved problems. Promising data have been recently reported by Amengual et al. who have compared different assays for the detection of aPS/PT and found a good accuracy of both homemade and commercial ELISA kits and a high concordance of the results [13].

6.2.2 Antibodies to β2GPI Domains

β2GPI is a large anionic plasma glycoprotein, consisting of 326 amino acids, organized in five domains [14]. This protein is highly immunogenic, and it has been demonstrated that autoimmune patients can produce antibodies against several epitopes of the molecule, located in different domains. Antibodies directed to different β2GPI domains seem to display higher or lower clinical significance [15]. Anti-domain I (DI) antibodies were firstly described in 2002, but their importance has clearly emerged more recently [16]. Actually, even if there is growing evidence that domain I represents the immunodominant epitope of β2GPI, the clinical significance of anti-DI antibodies is still debated. De Laat et al. have shown that anti-β2GPI antibodies with DI specificity are associated with LA and that anti-DI positivity correlates with vascular thrombosis, with an OR for venous thrombosis ranging from 3.5 to 6.7 in different studies [17, 18]. In one of these studies, the group found a correlation between anti-DI antibodies and obstetric APS manifestations, even though to a lesser extent than with thrombosis [18]. However, the results of this study have to be carefully evaluated, as it showed no correlation between LA and miscarriages, conflicting with several previous publications and the known clinical LA predictive value for miscarriages [19, 20].

Moreover in a recent study by our group, a high prevalence of anti-DI antibodies was detected in both thrombotic and obstetric primary APS, albeit anti-DI IgG were not found to be predictive of these complications [21].

Antibodies directed to the other domains of β2GPI seem to have lesser predictive value for APS. For example, anti-domain IV (DIV) and domain V (DV) antibodies have been found in patients with chronic infections, such as leprosy, in children with atopic dermatitis and in aPL-positive asymptomatic carriers [22].

Thus, definite conclusions on the diagnostic and prognostic value of anti-DI antibodies cannot be drawn at present, as the data regarding the association with thrombosis are not univocal among different studies [17, 18, 21]. Moreover, a small but relevant proportion of anti-β2GPI-positive APS patients do not display anti-DI antibodies, suggesting that the assay for the whole molecule cannot be substituted up to now [21].

It has been proposed that the ratio between anti-β2GPI-DI and anti-β2GPI-D IV/V IgG antibody reactivities could add important information to discriminate between relevant anti-β2GPI positivity associated with an autoimmune disease (such as APS) and antibodies occurring in association with other pathologies, with less diagnostic and pathogenic value. If confirmed in larger studies, this finding would suggest that tests for antibodies against the different domains could help in the risk stratification of anti-β2GPI antibody-positive patients [23].

There are different methodologies that can be employed to detect these antibodies. Besides the two-step assay, three ELISAs and a CIA using different DI molecules or peptides have been reported [23, 24].

6.2.3 Other Antiphospholipid Antibodies

Phosphatidylethanolamine (PE) is a neutral phospholipid that constitutes the inner leaflets of biological membranes. PE has anticoagulant properties and the finding that PE can interfere with clotting time prolongation raised the hypothesis that aPE might be responsible for the LA phenomenon, even if a significant association between aPE and LA has not been demonstrated [25].

In in vitro experiments, PE has been found to be an essential cofactor for the protein C anticoagulant pathway. Moreover PE is an inhibitor of the factor Xa-prothrombin system [26].

Antibodies targeting PE have been reported in up to 43 % of APS patients [25]. In a population of women with a history of recurrent early pregnancy loss, aPE prevalence has been reported to range between 23 and 31.7 % [27]. In another study, the rate of aPE positivity in a population of patients with otherwise unexplained thrombotic events was 18 % when detected by ELISA and 30.5 % when tested using thin-layer immunostaining [25, 28]. Moreover, in a multicenter study on 270 thrombotic patients, 63 % of 40 aPE-positive subjects had no additional aPL laboratory tests [25]. On the basis of these data, some authors have proposed aPE as serological markers of seronegative APS. However, given the limited number of studies, the small sample size, and poor ELISA standardization, the clinical role of aPE is still not clear and aPE testing is still not recommended.

The diagnostic and prognostic role of several autoantibodies against negatively charged PLs (other than CL) have been also studied. Among them, most data regard phosphatidylserine (PS), phosphatidylinositol (PI), and phosphatidic acid (PA). In the past, aCL has been shown to cross-react with antibodies targeting both PS and PI. Further studies have demonstrated that aPS, aPI, and aPA antibodies mainly recognize a complex consisting of β2GPI, coupled to these negatively charged aPL [28]. Therefore, most of the cross-reactivity is due to autoantibodies actually reacting with β_2GPI [5, 29].

There are no recent studies demonstrating that aPS, aPI, and aPA antibody testing significantly improves the diagnosis of APS [5]. Nevertheless, aPS antibody detection has been suggested to be useful in the context of pregnancy-related morbidity [29]. Recent available literature reports conflicting results. In one study aPS was not associated with recurrent pregnancy loss, while in another aPS IgG but not IgM were related to obstetric morbidity [5]. Moreover, in a cohort of women with a history of recurrent miscarriage, aPS was the only autoantibody detectable in 3.6 % of subjects [30]. The significant role of aPS in obstetric APS is also supported by in vivo studies on animal models. Two murine monoclonal antibodies targeting PS have been demonstrated to decrease human chorionic gonadotropin (hCG) secretion and to inhibit trophoblast invasion [30, 31]. Notably, one of these two aPS reacted with PS only, while the other was able to recognize both CL and PS, but no information about a possible cross-reactivity with β2GPI was available [30, 31]. More recently, active immunization with β2GPI-dependent aPS was able to induce fetal resorption in a murine model of APS [5]. However, data on humans are inconsistent and aPS assays are still not included in classification criteria.

Recently, a novel aPL assay (APhL IgG/IgM ELISA), using a mixture of negatively charged phospholipids as antigen (including PS, phosphatidic acid, and β2GPI), has been tested in APS patients [32]. Positivity for this commercial ELISA kit has been reported to be more predictive for APS than aCL. Particularly, APhL test showed higher positive and negative predictive values for APS in comparison to two commercially available aCL assays. Moreover, in the same study, antibodies against APhL have been associated with arterial events in a cohort of SLE patients. The authors suggest that the routine use of this assay could implement specificity, without losing sensitivity for APS [32].

Annexins are a family of proteins that bind Ca^{++} and phospholipids and display several different functions, including inhibition of coagulation processes in the vasculature and on trophoblasts [33]. Annexin V (AnnA5) is present on the intervillous surface of the placenta, forming a shield that prevents the activation of the coagulation cascade [33, 34]. Several studies have reported a significant reduction of annexin V binding on the placental tissue from patients with obstetric APS in comparison with normal controls. In addition, aPL have been shown to displace annexin V from both trophoblast and endothelial cell monolayers in in vitro studies [33, 34].

Recently, the determination of resistance to the anticoagulant effects of AnnA5 (AnnA5 resistance) has been proposed as a marker of APS. AnnA5 resistance has been found in a significantly higher proportion of APS patients in comparison to controls. Moreover, a significant reduction of AnnA5 anticoagulant activity was detected in a cohort of SLE children in comparison to pediatric controls [35]. Notably, the same cohort of patients displayed a significant increased prevalence of anti-DI antibodies ($p=0.014$) compared to controls, and resistance to AnnA5 anticoagulant activity was found to inversely correlate with titers of anti-DI IgG antibodies [35]. Even if these promising data suggest that AnnV resistance could play a role in the identification of specific subsets of pathogenic aPL antibodies, further studies are needed to confirm this preliminary finding.

Annexin 2 (AnnA2) has been proposed as a target of aPL. Several studies have suggested that AnnA2 could represent a receptor mediating β2GPI binding to endothelial cells (ECs) [36]. Autoantibodies against AnnA2 have been described in patients with APS and severe thrombosis and/or pregnancy morbidity but also in some other autoimmune conditions (such as SLE and RA). Their clinical significance is unclear at the moment [36].

The clinical significance of aCL and anti-β2GPI antibodies of the IgA isotype in PAPS is still a controversial issue. IgA aCL and/or IgA anti-β2GPI antibodies have been reported in seronegative patients with a history of thrombosis and pregnancy morbidity. Particularly, IgA anti-β2GPI antibodies can potentially identify APS in patients who possess the clinical features of the disease but do not meet current laboratory criteria. In mouse models these antibodies were able to induce significantly larger thrombi and higher tissue factor levels compared to controls, demonstrating their pathogenic role. In a recent study of Mattia et al. on 84 PAPS patients, IgA aCL and IgA anti-β2GPI antibodies were found, respectively, in 19 and 50 % of patients. The mean titers of both IgA aCL and IgA anti-β2GPI antibodies were higher in the thrombotic patients, but only IgA anti-β2GPI were significantly associated with thrombosis. Isolated IgA anti-β2GPI antibody positivity was significantly prevalent in seven of the seronegative patients [37]. There are several reasons to explain why a number of studies failed to prove the usefulness of adding IgA aCL and IgA anti-β2GPI testing. In fact, these autoantibodies have a low prevalence and are mostly found in association with other aPL. Moreover, few accurate diagnostic tests are available for their detection [38]. Recently, Ruiz-García et al. found that mean levels of IgG, IgM, and IgA, both aCL and anti-β2GPI, antibodies were significantly higher in patients with clinical features of APS than in controls on a total of 156 patients fulfilling clinical criteria for APS. IgA anti-β2GPI was the most prevalent antibody in these patients [39].

6.3 Non-criteria Clinical Manifestations

In addition to thrombosis and pregnancy morbidity, a number of clinical manifestations have been described in aPL-positive patients. Non-thrombotic neurological features, thrombocytopenia, heart valve disease, microangiopathic nephropathy, livedo reticularis, and skin ulcers are some of the possible features that are not yet considered as classification criteria because of their low specificity (Table 6.2).

6.3.1 Skin

Skin involvement is common in APS patients, being skin ulcers and livedo reticularis the most frequent cutaneous manifestations [40]. Livedo reticularis (LR) is a blanching erythematous to violaceous netlike vascular pattern on the skin that can be secondary to numerous conditions, including APS. LR is present in up to 20–25 % of APS patients and has been originally described in association with arterial thrombosis. However, the relationship of LR with stroke or other types of arterial occlusion is still not clear as several studies did not confirm this original observation [41].

About 30–40 % of APS patients develop skin ulcers. Skin lesions are usually situated in the lateral face of the ankle or in pretibial area, display sharp margins, and are usually very painful. The pathogenesis of these dermatological manifestations is linked to fibrin deposition in the superficial dermal vessels lumen [41]. Skin ulcers are mainly associated with catastrophic APS and are usually concomitant with non-inflammatory purpura with microvascular occlusion [42].

Other skin manifestations anecdotally reported in the setting of APS include anetoderma, chronic venous ulcers, pseudovasculitis, superficial thrombophlebitis, superficial skin bullae, infarcts and distal gangrene, acrocyanosis, and relapsing polychondritis [43].

Anetoderma is an elastolytic disorder of unknown origin characterized by localized areas of flaccid skin, which can appear atrophic or protuberant. The occurrence of anetoderma in a skin region with no prior pathology (primary anetoderma) has been reported to be very suggestive for the presence of aPLs. In a study on 9 patients with primary anetoderma, aPLs were found in all 9 patients, with 4 patients also having APS [44].

Table 6.2 Non-criteria clinical manifestations

Clinical manifestations	Distinctive features
Skin	
Livedo reticularis	Original association with arterial thrombosis not confirmed in prospective studies
	Prevalence: 20–25 % in PAPS patients
Ulcers	Frequently observed in the catastrophic APS (CAPS)
	Prevalence around 33 % in PAPS patients
Heart valve disease	Possibly an additional risk for secondary thromboembolism
	Frequency: 12–33 % in PAPS patients
Kidney	
Renal artery stenosis	Resulting in severe renovascular hypertension, renal infarcts
	Prevalence: 26 % of aPL+patients with uncontrolled hypertension
APS nephropathy	Association with pregnancy complications, extrarenal vascular thrombosis and higher risk of chronic renal failure among SLE patients
	Prevalence in PAPS: 35 % (data from small series, with hypertension or signs suggestive of nephropathy)
Thrombocytopenia	Usually mild
	No protective effect on thrombotic risk
	Prevalence: 20–25 % in PAPS patients
Central nervous system	
Migraine/headache	Controversial association with aPL because of the high prevalence in the general population
	Prevalence in PAPS: 20 %
Epilepsy	In many but not all cases secondary to ischemic events
	Conflicting data on relationship between aPL and seizure in SLE
	Prevalence in PAPS: 6–7 %
MS-like disease	No definite data regarding prevalence because of the difficult differential diagnosis
Cognitive impairment	Mostly involving attention and verbal fluency
	Prevalence in PAPS: 38 %
Dementia	Resulting from chronic or recurrent ischemic events
	Prevalence: 2.5–56 %
Transverse myelopathy	Strong correlation with aPL in SLE patients
	Prevalence around 1 %

6.3.2 Heart

Heart valve involvement has been reported in APS patients, with a prevalence ranging from 10 to 40 % of aPL-positive patients [45]. The prevalence can be even higher, up to 80 %, if highly sensitive techniques such as transesophageal echocardiography are used. Valve involvement can be characterized by several different alterations, including vegetations, valve thickening, and valvular dysfunction mainly affecting mitral and aortic valve [45]. Most patients are asymptomatic, but cerebrovascular accidents are more prevalent among patients with significant valve lesions [46].

Longitudinal studies have suggested that a small but significant proportion (7–25 %) of patients suffering from both primary and SLE-associated APS can develop valve vegetations or thickening during the course of disease but also that these alterations can disappear overtime [5]. Disease duration and a diagnosis of SLE-APS were independent factors associated with valvular disease progression in a cohort of 82 patients suffering from primary APS, SLE-APS, aPL-positive SLE, and SLE negative for aPL, followed up for 10 years. In this study, anticoagulation was not able to prevent the worsening of valvular involvement [47].

Less frequent cardiac manifestations are ventricular hypertrophy and dysfunction and pulmonary hypertension [48].

6.3.3 Kidney

Renal involvement is not very common in APS. However, thrombosis of the renal artery or its main branches has been reported [49]. The most typical non-ischemic renal manifestation of APS is a small artery vasculopathy, involving both arterioles and glomerular capillaries, defined as aPL-associated nephropathy (aPLN). This histological entity has been described both in primary APS and SLE-APS. In the latter group it has been associated with pregnancy complications, extrarenal vascular thrombosis, and higher risk of renal failure [49]. aPLN can be clinically silent or manifest with systemic hypertension, proteinuria, and inconstant hematuria [5].

6.3.4 Thrombocytopenia

Thrombocytopenia is one of the most common laboratory abnormalities found in patients with APS [40, 48]. A variable degree of thrombocytopenia is observed in up to 40 % of patients with aPL [48]. As a low platelet count can manifest in a variety of autoimmune and non-autoimmune disease, this feature has not been included in the APS formal criteria [1]. Moderate thrombocytopenia is frequent in APS and generally does not modify the policy for treatment of thrombosis as several authors have clearly demonstrated that thrombocytopenia does not display a protective effect on the thrombotic risk of aPL [50]. Severe thrombocytopenia is relatively uncommon and it is seldom associated with bleeding events. A recent task force on non-criteria APS manifestations has concluded that thrombocytopenia should be incorporated in the clinical criteria of APS and that an international registry of aPL-positive patients with thrombocytopenia ("hematologic APS") could be very useful. Moreover, the task force has proposed a multicentric, international, prospective long-term follow-up study on aPL-positive patients with thrombocytopenia, to assess the risk of thrombosis in this type of patients [51].

6.3.5 Neurological Manifestations

A wide variety of neurological manifestations has been described in association with aPL, in addition to cerebral ischemia [52]. Headache and migraine are common in APS, but the real correlation with aPL is still debated as these manifestations are very frequent also in the general population. In the past, several studies have reported a high incidence of seizures in APS patients, particularly in SLE-APS, and aPL positivity has been considered a risk factor for epilepsy in SLE patients [53]. However, more recent studies on a very large cohort of SLE patients did not confirm these previous findings [54].

Additional manifestations that have been associated to aPL positivity are chorea, transverse myelopathy, and Guillain-Barré syndrome. Moreover a clinical syndrome resembling multiple sclerosis (MS) has also been described in APS. Such patients can display magnetic resonance imaging (MRI) lesions similar to those observed in MS that can make the differential diagnosis very difficult [52].

The presence of cognitive impairment in SLE patients has been associated with aPL in the past. However, this association was not confirmed in several recent studies on very large SLE cohorts [55]. In primary APS the data on the real incidence of cognitive dysfunction are very limited. Only two studies have evaluated cognitive functions in primary APS. Both studies demonstrate a high incidence of cognitive defects, mainly involving attention, verbal fluency, memory, and visual learning [56, 57]. Recently our group has demonstrated a high prevalence of cognitive defects in a very well-characterized population of strongly positive APS patients, mostly involving frontal functions [58].

On the contrary, the presence of dementia as a consequence of chronic or recurrent ischemic events affecting small or large cerebral vessels has been clearly demonstrated in APS patients, with a prevalence ranging from 10 to 56 % in different studies [52].

6.3.6 Other Manifestations

Several other manifestations, such as vertigo or hearing loss due to middle ear involvement, myocardial dysfunction, and diffuse alveolar hemorrhage, have been anecdotally reported in APS patients [48].

In addition to the classical manifestations included in the classification criteria for APS, several other obstetric complications have been associated with aPL, such as intrauterine growth restriction and placental abruption [48]. However, these clinical features have not been included in the classification criteria because they can be present in several different conditions.

aPLs have also been addressed as a possible cause of infertility. Actually, patients suffering from infertility or with recurrent implantation failure after in vitro fertilization (IVF) display a significantly higher prevalence of aPL in comparison to the general female fertile population (20–30 % versus 1–3 %). However, data of the literature are not univocal and a clear demonstration of aPL as a cause of infertility has not been provided [59].

In conclusion, there are several laboratory and clinical features of APS that have not been included in the classification criteria. Nevertheless these clinical and serological characteristics have to be carefully addressed as they could help to assess the risk of complication (i.e., thrombosis and pregnancy morbidity) and to choose the appropriate therapy for a single patient.

References

1. Miyakis S, Lockshin MD, Atsumi M et al (2006) International consensus statement on an update of the classification criteria for definite antiphospholipid syndrome (APS). J Thromb Hemost 4:295–306
2. Ruiz-Irastorza G, Crowter M, Branch W et al (2010) Antiphospholipid syndrome. Lancet 376:1498–1509
3. D'Ippolito S, Meroni PL, Koike T et al (2014) Obstetric antiphospholipid syndrome: a recent classification for an old defined disorder. Autoimmun Rev. 13:901–908
4. Bertolaccini ML, Amengual O, Andreoli L et al (2014) 14th International Congress on Antiphospholipid Antibodies Task Force. Report on antiphospholipid syndrome laboratory diagnostics and trends. Autoimmun Rev. 13:917–930
5. Meroni PL, Chighizola CB, Rovelli F, Gerosa M (2014) Antiphospholipid syndrome in 2014: more clinical manifestations, novel pathogenic players and emerging biomarkers. Arthritis Res Ther 16:209
6. Sciascia S, Khamashta MA, Bertolaccini ML (2014) New tests to detect antiphospholipid antibodies: antiprothrombin (aPT) and anti-phosphatidylserine/prothrombin (aPS/PT) antibodies. Curr Rheumatol Rep 16:415
7. Pregnolato F, Chighizola C (2014) Phospholipid autoantibodies (non anticardiolipin)-anti-prothrombin antibodies. In: Shoenfeld Y, Gershwin E, Meroni PL (eds) The autoantibodies, 3rd edn. Elsevier, New York, pp 741–749
8. Pregnolato F, Chighizola CB, Encabo S et al (2013) Anti-phosphatidylserine/prothrombin antibodies: an additional diagnostic marker for APS? Immunol Res 56:432–438
9. Zigon P, Čučnik S, Ambrožič A et al (2013) Detection of antiphosphatidylserine/prothrombin antibodies and their potential diagnostic value. Clin Dev Immunol 724592
10. Vlagea A, Gil A, Cuesta MV et al (2013) Antiphosphatidylserine/prothrombin antibodies (aPS/PT) as potential markers of antiphospholipid syndrome. Clin Appl Thromb Hemost 19:289–296
11. Sciascia S, Murru V, Sanna G et al (2012) Clinical accuracy for diagnosis of antiphospholipid syndrome in systemic lupus erythematosus: evaluation of 23 possible combinations of antiphospholipid antibody specificities. J Thromb Haemost 10:2512–2518
12. Sciascia S, Sanna G, Murru V et al (2014) Anti-prothrombin (aPT) and anti-phosphatidylserine/prothrombin (aPS/PT) antibodies and the risk of thrombosis in the antiphospholipid syndrome: a systematic review. Thromb Haemost 111:354–364
13. Amengual O, Horita T, Binder W et al (2014) Comparative analysis of different enzyme immunoassays for assessment of phosphatidylserine-dependent antiprothrombin antibodies. Rheumatol Int. 34:1225–1230
14. de Groot PG, Meijers JCM (2011) β2-Glycoprotein I: evolution, structure and function. J Thromb Haemost 9:1275–1284
15. Shoenfeld Y, Krause I, Kvapil F et al (2003) Prevalence and clinical correlations of antibodies against six b2-glycoprotein I-related peptides in the antiphospholipid syndrome. J Clin Immunol 23:377–383

16. Iverson GM, Reddel S, Victoria EJ et al (2002) Use of single point mutations in domain I of B2-glycoprotein I to determine fine antigenic specificity of antiphospholipid autoantibodies. J Immunol 169:7097–7103
17. De Laat B, Pengo V, Pabinger I et al (2009) The association between circulating antibodies against domain I of beta2-glycoprotein I and thrombosis: an international multicenter study. J Thromb Haemost 7:1767–1773
18. De Laat B, Derksen RH, Urbanus RT, de Groot PG (2005) IgG antibodies that recognize epitope Gly40-Arg43 in domain I of beta 2-glycoprotein I cause LAC, and their presence correlates strongly with thrombosis. Blood 105:1540–1545
19. Ruffatti A, Tonello M, Visentin MS et al (2011) Risk factors for pregnancy failure in patients with anti-phospholipid syndrome treated with conventional therapies: a multicentre case–control study. Rheumatology 50:1684–1689
20. Erkan D, Patel S, Nuzzo M et al (2008) Management of the controversial aspects of the antiphospholipid syndrome pregnancies: a guide for clinicians and researchers. Rheumatology 47:iii23–iii27
21. Andreoli L, Nalli C, Borghi MO et al (2013) Domain I is the main specificity of anti-beta2 GPI in systemic autoimmune diseases. Arthritis Rheum 65:S4
22. Andreoli L, Nalli C, Motta M et al (2011) AntiB2glycoprotein I IgG antibodies from 1-year old healthy children born to mothers with systemic autoimmune diseases preferentially target domain 4/5: might it be the reason for their 'innocent' profile? Ann Rheum Dis 70:280–283
23. Chighizola CB, Gerosa M, Meroni PL (2014) New tests to detect antiphospholipid antibodies: anti-domain I beta-2-glycoprotein-I antibodies. Curr Rheumatol Rep 16:402
24. Willis R, Mahler M, Pregnolato F et al (2013) Clinical evaluation of two anti-Beta2glycoprotein I Domain 1 autoantibody assays to aid in the diagnosis and risk assessment of the antiphospholipid syndrome. Arthritis Rheum 65:S3
25. Staub HL, Bertolaccini ML, Khamashta MA (2012) Anti-phosphatidylethanolamine antibody, thromboembolic events and the antiphospholipid syndrome. Autoimmun Rev 12:230–234
26. Zhixin L, Wells CW, North PE (2011) Phosphatidylethanolamine at the luminal endothelial surface–implications for hemostasis and thrombotic autoimmunity. Clin Appl Thromb Hemost 17:158–163
27. Sugi T, Matsubayashi H, Inomo A et al (2004) Antiphosphatidylethanolamine antibodies in recurrent early pregnancy loss and mid-to-late pregnancy loss. J Obstet Gynaecol Res 30:326–332
28. Conti F, Alessandri C, Sorice M et al (2012) Thin-layer chromatography immunostaining in detecting anti-phospholipid antibodies in seronegative anti-phospholipid syndrome. Clin Exp Immunol 167:429–437
29. Bertolaccini ML, Amengual O, Atsumi T et al (2011) 'Non-criteria' aPL tests: report of a task force and preconference workshop at the 13th International Congress on Antiphospholipid Antibodies, Galveston, TX, USA. Lupus 20:191–205
30. Nayfe R, Uthman I, Aoun J et al (2013) Seronegative antiphospholipid syndrome. Rheumatology 52:1358–1367
31. Yodfat O, Blank M, Krause I, Shoenfeld Y (1996) The pathogenic role of anti-phosphatidylserine antibodies: active immunization with the antibodies leads to the induction of antiphospholipid syndrome. Clin Immunol Immunopathol 78:14–20
32. Suh-Lailam BB, Cromar A, Davis KW, Tebo AE (2012) APhL antibody ELISA as an alternative to anticardiolipin test for the diagnosis of antiphospholipid syndrome. Int J Clin Exp Pathol 5:210–215
33. Meroni PL, Gerosa M, Raschi E et al (2008) Updating on the pathogenic mechanisms of the antiphospholipid antibodies-associated pregnancy loss. Clin Rev Allergy Immunol 34:332–337
34. Meroni PL, Borghi MO, Raschi E et al (2011) Pathogenesis of antiphospholipid syndrome: understanding the antibodies. Nat Rev Rheumatol 7:330–339

35. Wahezi DM, Ilowite NT, Wu XX et al (2013) Annexin A5 anticoagulant activity in children with systemic lupus erythematosus and the association with antibodies to domain I of β2-glycoprotein I. Lupus 22:702–711
36. Luo M, Hajjar KA (2013) Annexin A2 system in human biology: cell surface and beyond. Semin Thromb Hemost 39:338–346
37. Mattia E, Ruffatti A, Tonello M et al (2014) IgA anticardiolipin and IgA anti- β2 glycoprotein I antibody positivity determined by fluorescence enzyme immunoassay in primary antiphospholipid syndrome. Clin Chem Lab Med. 52:1329–1333
38. Meijide H, Sciascia S, Sanna G et al (2013) The clinical relevance of IgA anticardiolipin and IgA anti-β2 glycoprotein I antiphospholipid antibodies: a systematic review. Autoimmun Rev 12:421–425
39. Ruiz-García R, Serrano M, Martínez-Flores JÁ et al (2014) Isolated IgA anti-β2 glycoprotein I antibodies in patients with clinical criteria for antiphospholipid syndrome. J Immunol Res 2014:704395
40. Erkan D, Lockshin MD (2010) Non-criteria manifestations of antiphospholipid syndrome. Lupus 19:424–427
41. Frances C (2010) Dermatological manifestations of Hughes' antiphospholipid antibody syndrome. Lupus 19:1071–1077
42. Cervera R, Espinosa G (2012) Update on the catastrophic antiphospholipid syndrome and the CAPS registry. Semin Thromb Hemost 38:333–338
43. Thornsberry LA, LoSicco KI, English JC III (2013) The skin and hypercoagulable states. J Am Acad Dermatol 69:450–462
44. Hodak E, Feureman H, Molad Y et al (2003) Primary anetoderma: a cutaneous sign of antiphospholipid antibodies. Lupus 12:564–568
45. Zuily S, Huttin O, Mohamed S et al (2013) Valvular heart disease in antiphospholipid syndrome. Curr Rheumatol Rep 15:320–329
46. Cervera R (2005) Recent advances in antiphospholipid antibody-related valvulopathies. J Autoimmun 15:123–125
47. Kampolis C, Tektonidou M, Moyssakis I et al (2014) Evolution of cardiac dysfunction in patients with antiphospholipid antibodies and/or antiphospholipid syndrome: a 10-year follow-up study. Semin Arthritis Rheum 43(4):558–565
48. Cervera R, Piette JC, Font J et al (2002) Antiphospholipid syndrome: clinical and immunologic manifestations and patterns of disease expression in a cohort of 1,000 patients. Arthritis Rheum 46:1019–1027
49. Tektonidou MG (2009) Renal involvement in the antiphospholipid syndrome (APS)- nephropathy. Clin Rev Allergy Immunol 36:131–140
50. Atsumi T, Furukawa S, Amengual O et al (2005) Antiphospholipid antibody associated thrombocytopenia and the paradoxical risk of thrombosis. Lupus 14:499–504
51. Cervera R, Tektonidou MG, Espinosa G et al (2011) Task force on Catastrophic Antiphospholipid Syndrome (APS) and Non-criteria APS Manifestations (II): thrombocytopenia and skin manifestations. Lupus 20(2):174–181
52. Brey RL, Muscal E, Chapman J (2011) Antiphospholipid antibodies and the brain: a consensus report. Lupus 20:153–157
53. Sanna G, Bertolaccini ML, Cuadrado MJ et al (2003) Neuropsychiatric manifestations in systemic lupus erythematosus: prevalence and association with antiphospholipid antibodies. J Rheumatol 30:985–992
54. Hanly JG, Urowitz MB, Su L et al (2012) Seizure disorders in systemic lupus erythematosus results from an international, prospective, inception cohort study. Ann Rheum Dis 71:1502–1509
55. Hanly JG, Urowitz MB, Su L et al (2011) Autoantibodies as biomarkers for prediction of neuropsychiatric events in systemic lupus erythematosus. Ann Rheum Dis 70:1726–1732
56. Tektonidou MG, Varsou N, Kotoulas G et al (2006) Cognitive deficits in patients with antiphospholipid syndrome. Arch Intern Med 166:2278–2284

57. Kozora E, Erkan D, Zhang L et al (2014) Cognitive dysfunction in antiphospholipid antibody (aPL)-negative systemic lupus erythematosus (SLE) versus aPL-positive non-SLE patients. Clin Exp Rheumatol 32:34–40
58. Gerosa M, Poletti B, Pregnolato F et al (2009) Antiphospholipid syndrome and systemic lupus erythematosus: what's new about cognitive impairment. J Neurol 256:S190
59. Buckingham KL, Chamley LW (2009) A critical assessment of the role of antiphospholipid antibodies in infertility. J Reprod Immunol 80:132–145

7 Obstetric APS

Micaela Fredi and Angela Tincani

7.1 Antiphospholipid Syndrome and Pregnancy Loss

Antiphospholipid syndrome (APS) was first described in patients with obstetric morbidity, in particular midtrimester fetal losses [1], enlightening the impact of the obstetric manifestations in this condition.

When classification criteria of APS were defined in 1999 [2] and revised in 2006 [3], the obstetric manifestations were considered as one out of the two clinical aspects characterizing the syndrome. From a practical point of view, the right identification of the APS-related obstetric complications and the consequent application of an appropriate management had the greatest impact on the quality of life of these patients, returning to them, in the majority of cases, the possibility of having children.

The definition of obstetric APS (Table 7.1) includes different pathological manifestations: recurrent early pregnancy loss (REPL), fetal death, early severe preeclampsia with placental insufficiency and growth restriction, and even the HELLP syndrome (hemolysis, elevated liver enzymes, and low platelets), classified within the microangiopathic manifestations of APS [4]. In a multicenter prospective cohort of 1,000 patients with primary and secondary antiphospholipid syndrome followed for 10 years, the most frequent fetal complications were REPL, followed by fetal death and premature birth, whereas the most common maternal manifestations were preeclampsia, followed by eclampsia and abruptio placentae [5]. The wide spectrum of APS pregnancy complications implies that several pathogenic mechanisms might be involved, perhaps reflecting several possible interactions between antiphospholipid antibodies (aPL) and the uteroplacental unit (see Chap. 4). The observation that pregnancy losses tend to recur in a relevant percentage of the patients despite

M. Fredi • A. Tincani, MD (✉)
Rheumatology and Clinical Immunology, Spedali Civili, University of Brescia,
Piazzale Spedali Civili, 1, Brescia 25123, Italy
e-mail: elmic83@libero.it; angela.tincani@unibs.it

© Springer International Publishing Switzerland 2015
P.L. Meroni (ed.), *Antiphospholipid Antibody Syndrome: From Bench to Bedside*,
Rare Diseases of the Immune System, DOI 10.1007/978-3-319-11044-8_7

Table 7.1 Classification criteria for definite obstetric antiphospholipid syndrome proposed during the 11th International Congress on aPL held in Sydney in 2004

Criteria for obstetric APS
1. One or more unexplained deaths of a morphologically normal fetus at or beyond the 10th week of gestation, with normal fetal morphology documented by ultrasound or by direct examination of the fetus
2. One or more premature birth of a morphologically normal neonate before the 34th week of gestation because of eclampsia or severe preeclampsia or recognized features of placental insufficiency
3. Three or more unexplained consecutive spontaneous abortions before the 10th week of gestation, with maternal anatomic or hormonal abnormalities and paternal and maternal chromosomic causes excluded

From Miyakis et al. [3]

careful management and despite a treatment based on the actual guidelines suggests that part of aPL-mediated pregnancy damage remains still undefined and therefore not adequately prevented.

An additonal aspect that has to be considered is the clinical setting of patients with obstetric APS. The presence of aPL in a patient with a well-defined systemic autoimmune disease (mainly systemic lupus erythematosus) and obstetrical morbidity seems to be a different condition from that occurring in a patient with aPL and REPL or fetal death in the absence of other medical problems. It seems that these two conditions are hardly comparable and that the recurrence rate is probably higher in the first one [6]. Another well-established risk factor for recurrences is a previous history of thromboembolism that requires, beside a specific management during pregnancy, a careful prophylaxis not only to protect fetal well-being but also to avoid possible thrombotic events in the mother [7].

Antiphospholipid antibody profile has been also investigated as possible risk factor for pregnancy loss recurrence. A recent collaborative Italian study demonstrated that triple positivity of aPL antibodies (LA, aCL, and anti-β2GPI) is an independent risk factor for pregnancy poor outcome despite conventional treatment [6]. Conversely a multicenter American study enlightened the role of LA as primary predictor of adverse pregnancy outcome after 12 weeks of gestation in the pregnancies of aPL-positive mothers; in this study positivity for aCL and anti-β2GPI, if LA is not also present, did not predict adverse pregnancy outcome [6].

The aPL titer (aCL and anti-β2GPI) is also considered in the frame of aPL profile. According to international recommendation [8] IgG isotype at medium high titer is considered a higher risk factor for APS clinical manifestations compared to low titer and IgM isotype. In fact low titer is not recognized as formal classification criteria.

Nevertheless in obstetric APS also low titers were suggested to be of significance [9, 10] being associated with poor obstetric outcome. This particular aspect is still debated; a study from Israel showed a good pregnancy outcome in 77 % of patients with low aPL titers, compared to 35 % of good outcomes reported in patients with high aPL titers [9]. Instead a French study described poor pregnancy outcomes in untreated mothers with low aPL titers that were not significantly different from those observed in patients with medium-high titers [10]. Furthermore an English study showed that over 50 % of women with pure obstetric APS had low titer aCL and/or anti-β2GPI in the absence of LA. Approximately 27 % of these patients had clinical features of high-risk obstetric APS [11]. Indeed the impression is that in obstetric APS also low titer aPL may play a notable role. Accordingly, low titer aCL were already described to be of clinical significance for women with purely obstetric APS in a large prospective cohort of European patients [12] as well as in women with stillbirth in a recent collaborative report [13].

In addition to classical aPL antibodies, increasing evidence demonstrates that several other autoantibodies, such as antibodies against phosphatidylethanolamine (aPE), anti-annexin 5, antiprothrombin (aPT), and/or anti-phosphatidylserine/prothrombin complex (aPT/PS), can be found associated with pregnancy loss. Starting in the 1990s Yetman et al. reported non-criteria aPL, including aPE, in 10.1 % of women with REPL [14]. Further studies confirmed an increased incidence of aPE in patients with REPL, in fetal death, and in infertile women with recurrent implantation failures [15, 16]. However, aPE was not shown to be an independent risk factor for further miscarriage in patients with REPL [17], but the combinations of IgG aPE with other aPL detected by tests included in the Classification Criteria can be useful predictors of severe pregnancy-induced hypertension, with a 30.8 % sensitivity and a 99.2 % specificity [17].

The association of antiprothrombin antibodies and pregnancy morbidity is still not clear also because of the known difference between antibody binding to prothrombin alone (aPT) and antibodies binding to phosphatidylserine/prothrombin complex (aPS/PT). Several groups found that women with REPL, either idiopathic or within APS, display higher frequency of aPT compared to normal subjects [18]. Recently the prevalence of aPT was investigated in a cohort of patients negative for classical aPL with previous uteroplacental insufficiency complications, including severe preeclampsia, HELLP syndrome, placental abruption, and fetal death. A significantly 10-fold higher prevalence of aPT IgG was reported in cases compared to controls (OR, 95 % CI: 10.92, 4.52–26.38); the strongest statistical association was reached with fetal death [19]. The association between the aPS/PT antibodies and pregnancy morbidity is also still matter of discussion, with studies that have found low rate of aPS/PT positivity in patients with REPL without APS [20], while a recent paper reported high rate of antibodies against aPS/PT in patient with APS (with or without SLE) [21]. The authors reported that aPS/aPT antibodies were the strongest independent risk factor for obstetric complications in their cohort.

High rate of anti-annexin 5 antibodies was found in several retrospective studies [22]. However, in a large prospective cohort study, the detection of anti-annexin 5 at the beginning of pregnancy was not related to the occurrence of pregnancy loss [23]. In women with obstetric APS characterized by REPL, a higher prevalence of anti-annexin 5 antibodies has been observed compared to aPL-negative women with the same obstetrical complications or to general obstetric population [24]. Therefore, it is actually suggested that anti-annexin 5 antibodies do not represent an independent risk factor for REPL, while they could represent an additional risk factor possibly contributing to the disruption of the annexin 5 crystal shield [25].

To achieve a successful outcome in APS pregnancy, an optimal management strategy is required. This includes a proper treatment (as enlighten in the Chap. 16), but the experience has thought us that pharmacological treatment by itself is not sufficient. Success, defined as fetal survival, is the result of careful obstetric monitoring, proper delivery timing, and skilful neonatal care [26]. The careful surveillance conducted by a multidisciplinary team (obstetricians, rheumatologists, and neonatologists) and the progress in neonatal intensive care are as important as drugs to achieve a good obstetric outcome and to reduce the possible adverse consequences of premature delivery.

7.2 Nomenclature

A major problem in comparing the published data of obstetric APS has been and still is the lack of uniform definitions for pregnancy loss and pregnancy complications. Therefore, in the interest of the readers, we think important to share common definitions.

The nomenclature used for the definition of pregnancy loss can be quite outdated, and in this case it does not reflect the modern understanding of reproductive biology. Traditionally pregnancy loss occurring at less than 20 weeks of gestation have been grouped together as spontaneous abortions, while those occurring after 20 weeks gestation have been defined stillbirths. More recently nomenclature that accurately reflects our current knowledge of the developmental process and that is more aligned with pathophysiology or causes of pregnancy loss has been proposed [27]; these definitions are outlined in Table 7.2.

In the following pages we try to apply the new terminology; however, some of the reported data were published before its definition; therefore, we had to deal with various descriptions of pregnancy complications and adverse outcomes and some imprecision has to be taken into account.

7.3 Recurrent Early Pregnancy Loss

In a general obstetric population, 10–15 % of pregnancies end in spontaneous abortion, mainly occurring during the pre-embryonic (up to 5^{+6} weeks of gestation) or embryonic period (up to 9^{+6} weeks of gestation), while the rate of fetal death, after 10 weeks of gestation, is very low. In addition, the recurrence of early miscarriages in the general population is not unusual, being recorded in about 1 % of them. A recent critical review, including only four prospective studies performed on general population with REPL, reported aPL positivity in about 2 % of the women [28]. The selection of the included papers was limited to the studies including details allowing to verify the reliability of the findings and therefore might be near to the real picture.

Table 7.2 Proposed nomenclature

Proposed nomenclature	Definition	Previous nomenclature	Developmental stage
Early pregnancy loss (04^{+0}–09^{+6} weeks of gestation)	Either:	Early spontaneous abortion	Embryo
	Death of a conceptus measuring up to 29 mm in crown-rump length		
	Sonographic documentation of a dead conceptus consistent with a gestational age up to 9 weeks and 6 days gestation (crown-rump length up to 29 mm)		
	The embryo must be identified by ultrasound to rule out anembryonic pregnancy		
Fetal death (10^{+0}–19^{+6} weeks of gestation)	Either:	Spontaneous abortion	Fetus
	Passage of a conceptus measuring at least 30 mm in crown-rump length or		
(a) Early fetal death (10^{+0}–15^{+6} weeks gestation)	Sonographic documentation of a dead conceptus with crown-rump length consistent with a gestational age at least 10 weeks gestation		
(b) Late fetal death (16^{+0}–19^{+6} weeks of gestation)	Loss of the conceptus after documented fetal cardiac activity at or beyond 10 weeks gestational age The fetus is dead at the time of delivery with Apgar scores of zero at one and 5 min.		
Neonatal death	Death of a formed fetus alive at birth in the first 28 days of life	Neonatal death	Neonate
Stillbirth (at least 20 weeks of gestation)	Fetus at least 20 weeks of gestation that is dead at the time of delivery with Apgar scores of zero at one and 5 min.	Stillbirth	Fetus
Preeclampsia	Increased blood pressure associated with proteinuria in pregnancy Diagnostic blood pressures include either a systolic blood pressure ≥140 mmHg or a diastolic blood pressure ≥90 mmHg on at least two occasions (at least 4 h apart) Proteinuria is defined as the excretion of 300 mg of protein or greater in a 24-h specimen	Preeclampsia	
Early (<33 weeks)			
Late (≥34 weeks of gestation)			
Eclampsia	An acute and life-threatening complication of pregnancy characterized by the appearance of tonic–clonic seizures (convulsions)	Eclampsia	
HELLP syndrome	Hemolysis, elevated liver enzymes, and low platelet	HELLP syndrome	

Modified from Silver et al. [27]

The attribution of early recurrent miscarriages to aPL-mediated damage implies the exclusion of several other possible causes:

1. Chromosomal abnormalities, which often impair embryo formation, account for more than half of sporadic pre-embryonic or embryonic losses
2. Genetic abnormalities of the conceptus are less common in women with three or more consecutive miscarriages
3. Obstetric anomalies such as uterine anomalies, luteal phase insufficiency, and cervical infections
4. Endocrinological disorders such as thyroid hormone dysfunctions and undiagnosed celiac disease

The need for at least three REPL in the first 10 weeks of gestation to fulfill the classification criteria of APS is probably based on these observations and allows to exclude most of the losses due to genetic abnormalities that can confuse the clinical picture.

Nevertheless, REPL, often misdiagnosed because of their frequency in the general obstetric population, can be considered to be the most frequently occurring pregnancy losses associated with aPL. In fact according to a recent report of the 10-year follow-up of 1,000 APS patients [5], 188 pregnancies in 127 women were observed and despite prophylactic treatment, REPL occurred in 16.5 % of pregnancies, while fetal death in 5 %.

Many published studies reports a positive association between aPL and REPL, but they are highly heterogeneous concerning clinical events (number of previous pregnancy losses, gestational age of pregnancy losses, inclusion of early miscarriage, and late fetal death in the same analysis) and laboratory criteria (different cutoffs, inclusion of patients with low titers, and lack of confirmatory testing). A recent meta-analysis [29] tried to evaluate the previous papers that have analyzed this association in patients without systemic autoimmune disease. The authors underlined that the comparison between studies was difficult due to many methodological causes: poor standardization of assays testing for aPL, heterogeneity of studies regarding the definitions of cases (minimum number of consecutive losses required), and controls (not matched for parity, few studies with appropriate controls). No studies were found examining the association between lupus anticoagulant (LA) and anticardiolipin (aCL) IgM with pregnancy loss before 13 weeks of gestation, and the association between anti-β2 glycoprotein-I (aβ2GPI) and recurrent abortion before 13 weeks was not statistically significant. Instead they reported a positive association between low and moderate-high titers aCL IgG and REPL occurring at less than 13 weeks of gestation; however, only two studies, including 907 patients, could be evaluated in this analysis.

The recent report of the antiphospholipid antibodies taskforce [30] included only studies recording losses occurring within 10 weeks of gestation. Forty-six original studies investigating the frequency of positive aPL tests in patients with REPL were identified and included in the analysis. High percentage (nearly 80 %, 27 out of 34) of the case-control studies found a significant association of aPL and REPL. Results of LA and aCL antibodies were available in most of the studies, with only a small number of papers analyzing anti-β2GPI. Fourteen out of 27 studies reporting a positive association between aPL and REPL included a significant number of patients (>100). Conversely, a number of studies found no association between aPL and REPL. Notably, some of them published in the 1990s did not include the evaluation of patients by all the three tests. Panton et al. described a higher prevalence of aCL IgG among 177 women with REPL compared to 254 healthy blood donors [31], but the finding was not statistically significant. Two large studies [15, 32] published in the 2000s found no association between aPL and REPL. In the first LA and aCL IgG were studied in 273 patients [15], while the other considered aβ2GPI IgG and IgM in 172 patients [32]; data from both the works showed no significant difference in the frequency of aPL in patients compared to healthy controls. Finally a very recent reported no significant association between aCL or LA and REPL in 52 Pakistani women [33].

The heterogeneous results of the studies mentioned above can be partially explained by different inclusion criteria and definitions of positive laboratory tests. Many papers (26/46) investigating aPL in patients with REPL were published before the first international consensus on aPL [2] and most of them did not use the criteria currently accepted to classify patients with APS. More than three pregnancy loss was the criteria used only in two third of the studies (30/46), and the majority of the published studies did not mention if patients had consecutive pregnancy loss; only four papers [34–37] strictly followed the pregnancy morbidity criteria for REPL described in Sapporo/Sidney consensus ("Three or more unexplained consecutive spontaneous abortions before the 10th week of gestation"). The gestational age of the pregnancy loss used as inclusion criteria was also various among the publications with several studies including patients with both first and second trimester loss. Also the use of different cutoff in the diagnostic tests appears to have contributed to the discrepant findings, and the confirmation of aPL positivity was performed in only 8 out of 46 studies, increasing the risk of misclassification due to momentary aPL.

However the a majority of published studies identifie a positive association between aPL and REPL, they are highly heterogeneous concerning clinical events and laboratory criteria.

Evidence arising from clinical experience and the few relevant publications suggests that while the recurrent early pregnancy loss may be the most sensitive manifestations of obstetric APS, the specificity is uncertain because of the difficulty in excluding other known or suspected causes.

7.4 Fetal Death

Historically, repeated fetal deaths were the first pregnancy complication reported in patients with aPL with or without thrombosis [1, 38]. In the general population fetal death is a rare event, and only about 2 % of pregnancy losses seem to occur between 10 and 20 weeks of gestation [39]. It is estimated that up to 5 % of normal pregnancies end in loss during both fetal and neonatal periods [40].

However, in women with aPL positivity, late pregnancy failures are a frequent issue and represent one of the clinical classification criteria for APS; in the work of Cervera et al. [5], fetal death occurred in 16.9 % of the patients at time of the inclusion, and in nearly 5 % a recurrence despite treatment was reported during the 10 years of follow-up.

Among the formal classification criteria, fetal death is considered the most specific symptom defining obstetric APS [41]. In patients suffering recurrent pregnancy loss, the specificity of fetal death for the presence of aPL was shown to be up to 76 % compared with only 6 % for two or more pre-embryonic pregnancy losses [42]. Today, according to what is known about the biological development of the embryo, the fetal period is defined as starting at the 10th week of gestation and lasting until delivery.

Fetal damage may be reasonably due to the presence of aPL only after exclusion of other possible causes such as cervical insufficiency and infections. In this respect the role of heritable thrombophilia defects such as factor V or factor II Leiden mutation, antithrombin, and protein C or protein S deficiency is still debated. In fact heritable thrombophilia defects have been associated with fetal losses, but their role in the fetal damage is still unclear [43].

The association between fetal death and aPL has been evaluated in several studies, and a systematic review has been recently released [44]. According to this systematic review, fetal death, considered after 10 weeks of gestation, was shown to be associated with LA in 4 case-control studies and 3 cohort studies, aCL antibodies in 7 case control studies and 5 cohort studies, and anti-β2GPI in 2 cohort studies. However, the authors of this paper underlined several limitations of their work. First of all many studies included a small number of patients, so they were considerably underpowered to detect significant associations between aPL and fetal deaths. This observation is certainly pertinent from a methodological point of view, but does not consider that fetal death is rarer than early pregnancy loss and that APS is also un uncommon disease. Indeed, case control studies could include no more than 200–300 events of placenta-mediated complications (including but not limited to fetal deaths), and prospective studies on the pregnancy of general obstetric population could identify only few cases of fetal death. An additional limitation comes from the definition of fetal death itself that resulted to be widely different in the included studies. In fact, some cohorts called fetal death events occur after 8 weeks of gestations while others after 24. However, an association was found between aPL and both stillbirth (>20 weeks of gestation) and fetal death (>10 weeks of gestation), suggesting that antibody-mediated damage can similarly affect different pregnancy periods. Moreover wide methodological variability in aPL assays has been observed, as expected because of the well-known difficulties in the performance of aPL antibody tests. In the ELISA-based papers, the cutoff values applied to the different assays displayed significant variability, and frequently IgG- and IgM-positive values were merged, making impossible to evaluate isotypes separately. Lastly few papers included all the three criteria tests and the confirmation of positive results, as recommended by the international consensus [3]. After this systematic review a more recent large, multicenter, multiethnic prospective population-based study focused on the association between aPL and stillbirth [13], and this study showed that elevated levels of aCL and anti-β2GPI antibodies were associated with a 3- to 5-fold increased odds of stillbirth. Strengths of this study were the inclusion of a great number cases and the centralization of aCL and anti-β2GPI testing for homogeneous assessment of positive results. However, the lack of LA testing and the absence of any confirmation of aPL persistence are major limitations that do not allow the precise identification of the true-positive patients.

7.5 Preeclampsia and Placental Insufficiency

Pregnancy in women with positive aPL can also be complicated by uteroplacental insufficiency inducing intrauterine growth restriction (IUGR), premature delivery [45], and early preeclampsia; the early-onset, severe preeclampsia complicated by hemolysis, elevated liver enzymes, and low platelets (HELLP syndrome) was also reported in APS pregnant patients.

As already detailed elsewhere (Chap. 4), poor placentation has been demonstrated to impair the physiological change of spiral arteries into low-resistance vessels during the first half of pregnancy. The absence of this remodeling impairs uteroplacental blood flow and consequently does not allow a physiological fetal growth.

Preeclampsia (defined in Table 7.2) is a major obstetric problem leading to substantial maternal and perinatal morbidity and mortality worldwide. Maternal and perinatal outcomes in preeclampsia depend on one or more of the following situations: gestational age at time of onset, severity, presence or absence of preexisting medical disorders, and quality of management.

Preeclampsia generally affects 2–8 % of the pregnancies in general obstetric population [46], while in pregnant women with APS (with or without SLE), it is reported in 20–50 % of cases [47]. In particular there is a higher rate of early (<34 weeks of gestation) severe preeclampsia, whereas the late preeclampsia (near term), as seen in general population, is not associated with the presence of aPL [48, 49].

The association between severe preeclampsia at or before 34 weeks' gestation and aPL was first observed in 1989 [50], but the real linkage between aPL and preeclampsia is still debatable [47]. Several studies report high frequency of preeclampsia in patients with primary or secondary APS, and in the obstetric population with preeclampsia, aPL antibodies are often observed to confirm the linkage between these conditions [47]. This topic was recently revised by two meta-analysis: the main finding of the first [51] was the observation of an association between aPL and severe preeclampsia in pregnant patients without autoimmune disease, but again significant methodological limitations of the included studies were underlined. In the second meta-analysis [44] that focus on late fetal loss, preeclampsia, and IUGR, the authors conclude that only fetal loss are significantly associated with aPL.

IUGR is defined as a fetus with an abdominal circumference below the 5th percentile according the gestational age (assessed with ultrasound), and it is an established cause of perinatal mortality and severe morbidity in surviving infants. This complication is common in APS pregnancies, occurring in approximately 30 % of the women [45, 52, 53], while it is usually observed in only 3–10 % of the general obstetric population. In women without a prior diagnosis of APS, the presence of IUGR in the setting of preeclampsia may increase the likelihood of a positive test for aPL [47].

Regarding the association between aPL and IUGR, few studies have specifically addressed this issue. Positive tests for aPL occur in 25 % of women delivering IUGR fetuses [54], and aPL has been associated with IUGR in pregnancies complicated by preeclampsia [55]. In a prospective study conducted by Yasuda et al. [56], 12 % of women from a general obstetric population testing positive for aCL had infants who were small for gestational age, compared to 2 % of women testing negative. However, in two other prospective studies, investigators found no correlation between aPL and IUGR [57, 58].

Conclusion

Since the first description of obstetric APS, in the 1980s, great improvement has been achieved in the practical approach to pregnancy. However, after nearly 30 years from the identification of the syndrome and nearly 15 years from the publication of the clinical and laboratory criteria, uncertainties still abound regarding the association of each of the current clinical obstetric criteria for APS and aPL antibodies. New and more informative studies could be drawn taking into account the modern definitions of the events, the use of the three diagnostic tests, and the need to confirm the serological positivity. Nevertheless we have to admit that it will be always difficult to draw large trials in these relatively rare pregnancy complications or losses.

Despite these considerations, the key role of aPL in the occurrence of pregnancy morbidity is well established in the "real life." Today, the identification of an appropriate treatment and strict multidisciplinary management before and during pregnancy has allowed to achieve a good pregnancy outcome approximately by 80 % of the women. A precise classification of the events will allow the development of more targeted treatments possibly helping the 20 % of patients with obstetric APS that still have fetal losses regardless the current treatments.

References

1. Soulier JP, Boffa M (1980) Recurrent abortion, thrombosis and circulating antithromboplastin type anticoagulant. Nouv Presse Med 9:859–864
2. Wilson WA, Gharavi AE, Koike T et al (1999) International consensus statement on preliminary classification for definite antiphospholipid syndrome. Arthritis Rheum 42:1309–1311
3. Miyakis S, Lockshin MD, Atsumi T et al (2006) International consensus statement on an update of the classification criteria for definite antiphospholipid syndrome(APS). J Thromb Haemost 4:295–306
4. Asherson RA (2006) New subsets of the antiphospholipid syndrome in 2006: "PRE-APS" (probable APS) and microangiopathic antiphospholipid syndromes ("MAPS"). Autoimmun Rev 6:76–80

5. Cervera R, Serrano R, Pons Estel GJ et al (2014) Morbidity and mortality in the antiphospholipid syndrome during a 10-year period: a multicenter prospective study of 1000 patients. Ann Rheum Dis. doi: 10.1136/annrheumdis-2013-204838. [Epub ahead of print]
6. Ruffatti A, Tonello M, Visentin M et al (2011) Risk factors for pregnancy failure in patients with anti-phospholipid syndrome treated with conventional therapies: a multicentre, case–control study. Rheumatology 50:1684–1689
7. Lockshin MD et al (2012) Prediction of adverse pregnancy outcome by the presence of lupus anticoagulant, but not anticardiolipin antibody, in patients with antiphospholipid antibodies. Arthritis Rheum 64:2311–2318
8. Pierangeli SS, De Groot PG, Dlott J et al (2011) 'Criteria'aPL tests: report of a task force and preconference workshop at the 13th International Congress on Antiphospholipid Antibodies, Galveston, Texas, April 2010. Lupus 20(2):182–190
9. Mekinian A, Loire-Berson P, Nicaise-Roland P et al (2012) Outcomes and treatment of obstetrical antiphospholipid syndrome in women with low antiphospholipid antibody levels. J Reprod Immunol 94(2):222–226
10. Simchen MJ, Dulitzki M, Rofe G et al (2011) High positive antibody titers and adverse pregnancy outcome in women with antiphospholipid syndrome. Acta Obstet Gynecol Scand 90(12):1428–1433
11. Gardiner C, Hills J, Machin S et al (2013) Diagnosis of antiphospholipid syndrome in routine clinical practice. Lupus 22(1):18–25
12. Boffa MC, Boinot C, De Carolis S et al (2009) Laboratory criteria of the obstetrical antiphospholipid syndrome. Data from a multicentric prospective European women cohort. Thromb Haemost 102(1):25–28
13. Silver RM, Parker CB, Reddy UM et al (2013) Antiphospholipid antibodies in stillbirth. Obstet Gynecol 122(3):641–657
14. Yetman DL, Kutteh WH (1996) Antiphospholipid antibody panels and recurrent pregnancy loss: prevalence of anticardiolipin antibodies compared with other antiphospholipid antibodies. Fertil Steril 66:540–546
15. Matsubayashi H, Sugi T, Arai T et al (2001) Different antiphospholipid antibody specificities are found in association with early repeated pregnancy loss versus recurrent IVF-failure patients. Am J Reprod Immunol 46:323–329
16. Sanmarco M, Bardin N, Camoin L et al (2007) Antigenic profile, prevalence, and clinical significance of antiphospholipid antibodies in women referred for in vitro fertilization. Ann N Y Acad Sci 1108:457–465
17. Yamada H, Atsumi T, Kobashi G et al (2009) Antiphospholipid antibodies increase the risk of pregnancy-induced hypertension and adverse pregnancy outcomes. J Reprod Immunol 79: 188–195
18. Sater MS, Ramzi RF, Farah MA et al (2012) Anti-phosphatidylserine, anti-cardiolipin, anti-beta 2 glycoprotein I and anti-prothrombin antibodies in recurrent miscarriage at 8–12 gestational weeks. Eur J Obstet Gynecol Reprod Biol 163:170–174
19. Marozio L, Curti A, Botta G et al (2011) Antipropthrombin antibodies are associated with adverse pregnancy outcome. Am J Reprod Immunol 66:404–409
20. Tsutsumi A, Atsumi T, Yamada H et al (2001) Anti-phosphatidylserine/prothrombin antibodies are not frequently found in patients with unexplained recurrent miscarriages. Am J Reprod Immunol 46:242–244
21. Žigon P, Čučnik S, Ambrožič A et al (2013) Detection of antiphosphatidylserine/prothrombin antibodies and their potential diagnostic value. Clin Dev Immunol 2013
22. Sater MS, Finanb RR, Mustafa FE et al (2011) Anti-annexin V IgM and IgG antibodies and the risk of idiopathic recurrent spontaneous miscarriage. J Reprod Immunol 89:78–83
23. Bizzaro N, Antico A, Musso M et al (2005) A prospective study of 1038 pregnancies on the predictive value of anti-annexin V antibodies for foetal loss. Ann N Y Acad Sci 1050: 348–356
24. Alijotas-Reig J, Ferrer-Oliveras R, Rodrigo-Anoro MJ et al (2010) Anti-annexin A5 antibodies in women with spontaneous pregnancy loss. Med Clin (Barc) 134:433–438

25. Rand JH, Wu XX, Quinn AS et al (2010) The annexin A5-mediated pathogenic mechanism in the antiphospholipid syndrome: role in pregnancy losses and thrombosis. Lupus 19:460–469
26. Zatti S, Biasini Rebaioli C, Lojacono A et al (2006) Antiphospholipid syndrome and pregnancy. Womens Health 2:873–880
27. Silver RM, Branch DW, Goldenberg R et al (2011) Nomenclature for pregnancy outcomes: time for a change. Obstet Gynecol 118(6):1402–1408
28. Andreoli L, Chighizola CB, Banzato A et al (2013) Estimated frequency of antiphospholipid antibodies in patients with pregnancy morbidity, stroke, myocardial infarction, and deep vein thrombosis: a critical review of the literature. Arthritis Care Res 65(11):1869–1873
29. Opatrny L, David M, Kahn SR et al (2006) Association between antiphospholipid antibodies and recurrent fetal loss in women without autoimmune disease: a metaanalysis. J Rheumatol 33(11):2214–2221
30. de Jesus GR, Agmon-Levin N, Andrade C et al (2014) 14th International Congress on Antiphospholipid Antibodies Task Force report on obstetric antiphospholipid syndrome. Autoimmun Rev. 13(8):795–813
31. Panton JA, Kilpatrick DC (1997) Anti-cardiolipin antibodies in sexual partners of recurrent aborters. Hum Reprod 12(3):464–467
32. Zammiti W, Mtiraoui N, Hidar S et al (2006) Antibodies to beta2-glycoprotein I and annexin V in women with early and late idiopathic recurrent spontaneous abortions. Arch Gynecol Obstet 274(5):261–265
33. Hossain N, Shamsi T, Khan N et al (2013) Thrombophilia investigation in Pakistani women with recurrent pregnancy loss. J Obstet Gynaecol Res 39(1):121–125
34. Lee RM, Branch DW, Silver RM (2001) Immunoglobulin A anti-beta2-glycoprotein antibodies in women who experience unexplained recurrent spontaneous abortion and unexplained fetal death. Am J Obstet Gynecol 185(3):748–753
35. Alijotas-Reig J, Ferrer-Oliveras R, Rodrigo-Anoro MJ et al (2010) Anti-beta(2)-glycoprotein-I and anti-phosphatidylserine antibodies in women with spontaneous pregnancy loss. Fertil Steril 93(7):2330–2336
36. Mtiraoui N, Fekih M, Zammiti W et al (2007) Lupus anticoagulant and antibodies to beta 2-glycoprotein I, annexin V, and cardiolipin as a cause of recurrent spontaneous abortion. Fertil Steril 88(5):1458–1461
37. Lee RM, Emlen W, Scott JR et al (1999) Anti-beta2-glycoprotein I antibodies in women with recurrent spontaneous abortion, unexplained fetal death, and antiphospholipid syndrome. Am J Obstet Gynecol 181(3):642–648
38. Carreras LO, Vermylen J, Spitz B et al (1981) Lupus anticoagulant and inhibition of prostacyclin formation in patients with repeated abortion, intrauterine growth retardation and intrauterine death. Br J Obstet Gynaecol 88:890–894
39. Goldstein SR (1994) Embryonic death in early pregnancy: a new look at the first trimester. Obstet Gynecol 84:294–297
40. Frias AE, Luikenaar RA, Sullivan AE et al (2004) Poor obstetric outcome in subsequent pregnancies in women with prior fetal death. Obstet Gynecol 104:521–526
41. Tincani A, Bazzani C, Zingarelli S et al (2008). Lupus and the antiphospholipid syndrome in pregnancy and obstetrics: clinical characteristics, diagnosis, pathogenesis, and treatment. In: Seminars in thrombosis and hemostasis, vol. 34, no. 3. Stratton Intercontinental Medical Book Corporation, New York, pp 267–273, c1974-
42. Oshiro BT, Silver RM, Scott JR et al (1996) aPL and fetal death. Obstet Gynecol 87:489–493
43. Battinelli EM, Marshall A, Connors JM (2013) The role of thrombophilia in pregnancy. Thrombosis 2013
44. Abou-Nassar K, Carrier M, Ramsay T et al (2011) The association between antiphospholipid antibodies and placenta mediated complications: a systematic review and meta-analysis. Thromb Res 128(1):77–85
45. Lima F, Khamashta MA, Buchanan NM et al (1996) A study of sixty pregnancies in patients with the antiphospholipid syndrome. Clin Exp Rheumatol 14:131–136

46. Costedoat-Chalumeau N, Guettrot-Imbert G, Le Guern V et al (2012) Pregnancy and antiphospholipid syndrome. Revue de Medecine Interne 33:209–216
47. Clark EA, Silver RM, Branch DW (2007) Do antiphospholipid antibodies cause preeclampsia and HELLP syndrome? Curr Rheumatol Rep 9(3):219–225
48. Moodley J, Bhoola V, Duursma J et al (1995) The association of antiphospholipid antibodies with severe early-onset preeclampsia. S Afr Med J 85:105–107
49. Allen JY, Tapia-Santiago C, Kutteh WH (1996) Antiphospholipid antibodies in patients with preeclampsia. Am J Reprod Immunol 36:81–85
50. Branch DW, Andres R, Digre KB et al (1989) The association of antiphospholipid antibodies with severe pre-eclampsia. Obstet Gynecol 73:541–545
51. do Prado AD, Piovesan DM, Staub HL et al (2010) Association of anticardiolipin antibodies with preeclampsia: a systematic review and meta-analysis. Obstet Gynecol 116(6):1433–1443
52. Branch DW, Silver RM, Blackwell JL et al (1992) Outcome of treated pregnancies in women with antiphospholipid syndrome: an update of the Utah experience. Obstet Gynecol 80:614–620
53. Caruso A, de Carolis S, Ferrazzani S et al (1993) Pregnancy outcome in relation to uterine artery flow velocity waveforms and clinical characteristics in women with antiphospholipid syndrome. Obstet Gynecol 1993(82):970–977
54. Polzin WJ, Kopelman JN, Robinson RD et al (1991) The association of aPL with pregnancies complicated by fetal growth restriction. Obstet Gynecol 1991(78):1108–1111
55. Sletnes KE, Wisloff F, Moe N et al (1992) Antiphospholipid antibodies in pre-eclamptic women: relation to growth retardation and neonatal outcome. Acta Obstet Gynecol Scand 1992(71):112–117
56. Yasuda M, Takakuwa K, Tokunaga A et al (1995) Prospective studies of the association between anticardiolipin antibody and outcome of pregnancy. Obstet Gynecol 86:555–559
57. Pattison NS, Chamley LW, McKay EJ et al (1993) Antiphospholipid antibodies in pregnancy: prevalence and clinical associations. Br J Obstet Gynaecol 100:909–913
58. Lynch A, Marlar R, Murphy J et al (1994) Antiphospholipid antibodies in predicting adverse pregnancy outcome: a prospective study. Ann Intern Med 1994(120):470–475

APS and the Nervous System

8

Cecilia Beatrice Chighizola, Davide Sangalli, Barbara Corrà, Vincenzo Silani, and Laura Adobbati

8.1 Introduction

Antiphospholipid syndrome (APS) is a systemic autoimmune disease; the revised Sapporo criteria for the diagnosis of APS require either pregnancy morbidity or at least one episode of vascular thrombosis in any tissue or organ (demonstrated by appropriate imaging studies or histopathology) as well as the occurrence of circulating antiphospholipid antibodies (aPL) on two or more occasions at least 12 weeks apart. Three laboratory tests are considered in the same APS diagnostic criteria, namely, antibodies against β2-glycoprotein I (anti-β2GPI antibodies) and cardiolipin (aCL), together with a functional assay, lupus anticoagulant (LA) [1]. aPL-related vascular thrombosis might affect the venous and the arterial district of all anatomical sites, regardless of their size. In the Euro-Phospholipid Project Group study, which included 1,000 APS patients, stroke emerged as the most frequent vascular clinical manifestation at disease onset, being the most common presenting event after deep venous thrombosis [2]. In the follow-up study conducted over a 10-year period, stroke and transient ischemic attack were the most common aPL-related clinical events [3]. The importance of neurological manifestations in APS was first stressed in the early 1980s, when Graham Hughes reported the association of aPL with a

C.B. Chighizola (✉)
Department of Clinical Sciences and Community Health, University of Milan, Via Festa del Perdono 7, Milan 20122, Italy

Immunology Research Laboratory, IRCCS Istituto Auxologico Italiano, Via Zucchi 18, Cusano Milanino, Milan 20095, Italy
e-mail: cecilia.chighizola@unimi.it

D. Sangalli • B. Corrà • V. Silani • L. Adobbati
Department of Neurology – Stroke Unit, IRCCS Istituto Auxologico Italiano, University of Milan, P. Brescia 20, Milan 20149, Italy

© Springer International Publishing Switzerland 2015

P.L. Meroni (ed.), *Antiphospholipid Antibody Syndrome: From Bench to Bedside*, Rare Diseases of the Immune System, DOI 10.1007/978-3-319-11044-8_8

Table 8.1 Non-criteria neurological manifestations of APS and level of evidence of their association with aPL [1]

Clinical manifestation	Association	Level of evidence
Dementia	Association between LA and dementia	Level II
Cognitive dysfunction	Association between aPL and cognitive dysfunction	Level I
Migraine	No association between migraine and aPL	Level I
Multiple sclerosis	No association between aPL and clinical outcome	Level I
Myelopathy	Association between aPL and transverse myelitis in SLE	Level IV
Epilepsy	Association between aPL and epilepsy	Level II

Level I: Prospective study in a broad spectrum of the representative population or meta-analysis of randomized-controlled trials. *Level II:* Prospective study in a narrow spectrum of the representative population or well-designed cohort or case–control analytic study or retrospective study in a broad spectrum of the representative population. *Level III:* Retrospective study in a narrow spectrum of the representative population. *Level IV*: Study design where predictor is not applied in a blinded fashion or descriptive case series or expert opinion

spectrum of neuropsychiatric manifestations in the original description of the syndrome [4]. Indeed, besides cerebrovascular events, a wide range of "non-criteria" neurological manifestations has been associated with aPL. Dementia, migraine, multiple sclerosis, myelopathy, and epilepsy are regarded as clinical features undoubtedly frequent but not specific for APS diagnosis (Table 8.1, [1]). Many of these manifestations can be hardly explained by mere pro-thrombotic mechanisms, suggesting that aPL may exert a direct effect on brain cells, disrupting their function.

As a whole, the neurological involvement is responsible for a consistent burden of morbidity and mortality in APS, making rather relevant to promptly formulate the correct diagnosis. Therefore, clinicians should be aware of the constellation of neurological manifestations associated with aPL, in order to best manage these conditions.

8.2 aPL-Mediated Mechanisms of Neurological Damage

It is still not clear why aPL display such a particular tropism for the cerebral circulation, even though the mechanism of nervous system involvement in APS is considered to be primarily thrombotic. aPL exert a thrombogenic effect by interfering with both soluble components and cells involved in the coagulation cascade. These autoantibodies have been found to bind to some members of the serine protease family, which enlists proteins involved in hemostasis (procoagulant factors as thrombin, prothrombin, factors VIIa, IXa, and Xa and anticoagulants as protein C) as well as in fibrinolysis (plasmin and tissue plasminogen activator). aPL induce a proinflammatory and procoagulant endothelial phenotype upregulating cellular adhesion molecules, promoting the synthesis of endothelial nitric oxide synthase and proinflammatory cytokines as interleukin (IL)-6 and tumor necrosis factor (TNF)-α. In both endothelial cells and monocytes, aPL significantly increase the expression of tissue factor, the major initiator of the clotting cascade. Further, they promote aggregation and activation of platelets. It should be noted that aPL are necessary but not sufficient to trigger thrombosis in vivo: according to the two-hit hypothesis, the antibodies (first hit) induce a thrombophilic condition but clotting takes place in the presence of another thrombophilic condition (second hit). This theory might explain why aPL-positive subjects develop thrombotic events only occasionally despite aPL persistency [5].

It has been hypothesized that aPL tropism for cerebral circulation might be attributed to the peculiar morphological and functional features of brain microvascular endothelium compared to other anatomical districts. Indeed, brain microvascular endothelial cells display tight junctions, lack of fenestrations, and low active fluid-phase transport. In addition, these cells produce a very high amount of energy, necessary to activate transport of nutrients via receptor-dependent mechanisms, with a higher electrical resistance compared to that of endothelial monolayers from other districts. Notably, the brain microvasculature has been shown not to express the anticoagulant thrombomodulin while it exposes consistent amounts of β2GPI, the main antigenic target of aPL [6, 7].

Further mechanisms other than vascular thrombosis have been advocated to explain such tropism. It has been postulated that impairment in the blood–brain barrier (BBB) facilitates the passage of pathogenic autoantibodies into the brain with detrimental consequences. Such disruption of the BBB might be ascribed to proinflammatory cytokines as IL-6, which are produced by the damaged endothelium in response to aPL. Once gained the access to the central nervous system (CNS), aPL have been demonstrated to bind to various cells: in animal models anti-β2GPI antibodies have been found to adhere to the surface of not only endothelial cells but also neurons and astrocytes. aPL binding to CNS target cells leads to deregulation of their functions, thus causing peculiar clinical manifestations. At this regard, aPL have been demonstrated to depolarize synaptic brain extracts and to interfere with glutamatergic pathways in cerebellar granule cells, leading to neurotoxicity [8, 9]. Besides aPL, other autoantibodies might be involved in the pathogenesis of CNS involvement. Most recently, antibodies against an extracellular epitope located in the N-terminal domain of the NR1 subunit of the N-methyl-D-aspartate receptor NR2 (anti-NR2) have been described in 33 % of 15 unselected patients with primary APS [10]. Anti-NR2 antibodies can cause neuronal damage via an apoptotic pathway; in addition, it has been suggested that a decrease of NMDA receptors in inhibitory GABAergic neurons and glutamatergic synapses causes disinhibition of excitatory pathways and an increase in extracellular glutamate, resulting in a frontostriatal syndrome and disinhibition of brainstem central pattern generators, thus causing complex elaborate movements and dyskinesias [11].

8.3 Cerebrovascular Manifestations

The association between cerebrovascular disease and aPL was already reported in the early description of the syndrome and later confirmed in many prospective studies. In the Euro-Phospholipid Project Group study, 19.8 % of patients presented with stroke and 11.1 % with transient ischemic attack [2]. In the follow-up study, stroke was the most common APS clinical manifestations (5.3 % of the total cohort), followed by transient ischemic attacks (4.7 %) [3]. Individuals with stroke and aPL positivity are significantly younger compared to aPL-negative subjects: aPL are believed to mediate approximately one third of strokes occurring in individuals before 45 years, with a serious social impact [12]. In particular, the risk of cerebral infarction has been estimated to be 2.3 times higher in patients with positive aPL than in those testing negative [13]. Patients with stroke and aPL are also more likely to be female: in the Framingham study, high serum aCL titers were identified as an independent predictor of the risk of future stroke in females but not in males [14]. Conversely, Brey and coworkers found the risk of stroke to be 1.5 times higher in males carrying aCL than those without [15]. In a case–control study focusing on risk factors for stroke in women in the general population younger than 50 years of age, 17 % of the patients with stroke were positive for LA, as compared with 0.7 % of controls. The risk was further increased by taking oral contraceptive pills or smoking [16]. Even though aCL are a well-recognized risk factor for stroke, it is still debated whether aPL positivity at the time of the first event increases the risk of recurrence in unselected populations [17]. Indeed, aPL positivity in patients with ischemic stroke was not predictive of an increased risk of subsequent vascular occlusive events over a 2-year period [18]. However, it should be mentioned that studies not confirming the association between recurrent stroke and aPL used a very low cutoff to define aCL positivity (e.g., the APASS study considered aCL titers higher than 10 GPL [19]). Consistently, when stratifying patients upon aCL titers, it clearly emerges that those with higher titers (aCL >40 GPL) carry a higher risk of developing subsequent thrombo-occlusive events in the cerebral circulation [13, 19].

The clinical manifestations of stroke depend on the location and the caliber of the occluded vessel. The territory of the middle cerebral artery is more commonly affected. Transient episodes of cerebral ischemia can present with amaurosis fugax, transient paresthesia, muscle weakness, vertigo, and transient global ischemia [20].

The occlusion of cerebral vessels can occur on a thrombotic or embolic basis. Embolisms typically originate from aortic or mitral valve vegetations composed of platelets and fibrin, and particularly left-sided valvular vegetations provide a frequent finding in APS patients [21]. Therefore, a complete evaluation of young patients with aPL and cerebral embolism should include transthoracic and transesophageal echocardiography to rule out valvular abnormalities. On the other hand, arterial thrombotic events are relatively common in the general population and are suggestive of APS when they occur in individuals with no identifiable risk factors. Indeed, family history, age, smoking, hyperlipidemia, hypertension, diabetes mellitus, and other vascular risk factors should be evaluated in patients with cerebrovascular disease and aPL: the presence of these frequent conditions does not exclude APS diagnosis but certainly makes it difficult to fully attribute a stroke to the pathogenic potential of aPL. Surely, the association between aPL and stroke holds a particular clinical significance in young patients presenting additional features of APS and/or with a diagnosis of systemic lupus erythematosus (SLE) or other systemic autoimmune diseases.

Stroke provides the most severe complication of APS, and patients present a considerable stroke-related morbidity burden. Indeed, aPL-related stroke carries a poor prognosis: in the European APS cohort, stroke accounted for 13 % of deaths, at a mean age of 42 years [2].

The association of cerebrovascular disease with livedo reticularis is named Sneddon's syndrome. More than 40 % of the patients with Sneddon's syndrome have APS, suggesting an association between these two conditions [22]. Although clinical and magnetic resonance imaging findings are similar in the two diseases, the clinical course of Sneddon's syndrome is more severe, and patients present a more pronounced cognitive deterioration and a greater number of disabilities [23]. In addition, patients with Sneddon's syndrome more often display leukoaraiosis and small lacunar infarcts, whereas patients with APS usually develop main cerebral artery territory infarction [24].

8.4 Cognitive Impairment and Dementia

aPL-related cognitive dysfunction varies from global dysfunction in the context of multi-infarct dementia to subtle cognitive deficits in otherwise asymptomatic patients with aPL.

Chronic and recurrent ischemic events, affecting small vessels, predispose patients to early-onset multi-infarct dementia [25]. The prevalence of multi-infarct dementia in patients with APS has been reported to be around 2.5 % [2]. aPL-associated dementia cannot be easily differentiated from other forms of dementia such as Alzheimer's disease, senile dementia, and metabolic or toxic conditions involving the brain. The most common clinical manifestations enlist memory loss, language impairment, impaired concentration, impaired judgment, and shortened attention span. Memory loss is not severe in most patients and often improves once anticoagulant therapy is initiated [12]. In a 2005 review of the characteristics of 30 patients with APS-associated dementia, the mean age of patients was 49 years; 47 % of cases had primary APS, 30 % had SLE, and 23 % had lupus-like syndrome [26]. As a whole, aPL testing is surely recommended in young individuals with no apparent reason for dementia.

The application of formal neuropsychological assessment has allowed the recognition of subtle forms of cognitive dysfunction, indicating a probable preclinical phase of neurological involvement: these patients frequently complain of poor memory and difficulty in concentrating and in verbal fluency. The association between cognitive dysfunction and aPL has been confirmed in cross-sectional as well as prospective longitudinal studies [25].

The potential pathogenicity of aPL in inducing cognitive impairment has been clearly shown in vivo: passive immunization of mice with β2GPI leads to memory and learning deficits more evident 4–5 months after single immunization without signs of ischemic damage in tissue specimen. When mice received intraventricular injection of IgG aPL purified from patients' serum, antibodies were found to bind to specific areas of the brain, as hippocampus, cortex, and choroid plexus [27]. Depression and psychosis have been also associated with aPL, but some authors suggested they may emerge as a reaction to neuroleptic drugs. Moreover it is clearly difficult to determine whether psychiatric symptoms are due to a psychological reaction, to steroid therapy or to aPL itself.

8.5 Headache

Chronic headache, including migraine, is a common finding in patients with APS: in a large cohort of 1,000 aPL-positive patients, 20.2 % complained of migraine [2]. Headache in APS can vary from classic intermittent migraine to almost continuous incapacitating headache. It can persist for years before APS is diagnosed. It is often untreatable, since it does not respond to narcotics or analgesics [16]. Despite the high prevalence among aPL carriers, the association between migraine and aPL is still controversial. Few authors reported an association between migraine and LA or aCL, while other investigators observed no association. Similarly, in SLE cohort patients with aPL are more likely to develop headache than those aPL negative, even though no association between aPL positivity and particular type of headache could be detected. This heterogeneity across studies might be attributed to the high prevalence of chronic headache in the general population and in the different definitions of migraine used. Interestingly, there are some anecdotal reports of the beneficial effect of anticoagulation in APS patients with migraine [28].

8.6 Multiple Sclerosis-Like Disease

Multiple sclerosis is a demyelinating inflammatory disease of the CNS. Clinical syndromes resembling multiple sclerosis, mainly in its relapsing–remitting pattern, were first reported in APS patients back in 1994 [29]. The diagnostic process is complicated by the fact that white-matter lesions are common findings in APS as well as in multiple sclerosis, in both cases usually small and located in periventricular and subcortical areas. The clinical significance of these lesions, which are hyperintense on T2-weighted MRI sequences, in APS is still matter of debate. These lesions are thought to be due to small vessel thrombi: the white matter of the brain is much more vulnerable than the gray matter to hypoxemia and ischemia because of widely spaced linear arterioles, few anastomoses, and sparse collateralization [30]. In an analysis of the characteristics of patients with APS and multiple sclerosis-like disease, APS patients were reported to have lower severity scores for lesions of the white matter, pons, and cerebellum and higher severity scores for lesions of the caudate nucleus and putamen compared to subjects with a diagnosis of multiple sclerosis [31].

Another controversial aspect concerns the high prevalence of aPL among subjects diagnosed with multiple sclerosis. Indeed, the prevalence of aPL positivity in patients with multiple sclerosis, without clinical manifestations of autoimmune disease or APS, has been shown to range from 8 to 33 % [32–36]. The prevalence of anti-β2GPI IgG and IgM has been reported to be higher among patients compared to controls; it is not clear whether this association displays a clinical significance or it is a mere epiphenomenon [37, 38]. Patients with a diagnosis of multiple sclerosis and persistently elevated aCL levels were reported to display a slower rate of progression and some atypical clinical features such as headaches and absence of oligoclonal bands in the cerebrospinal fluid. It has been proposed that aPL might affect response to treatment [39]; some authors even proposed that aPL might be involved in the pathogenesis of the neurological symptoms of multiple sclerosis, even suggesting that management should include antiplatelet or anticoagulant agents [40].

8.7 Myelopathy

Myelopathy is a rare manifestation of APS, with a prevalence of less than 1 % [2]. The association with aPL seems to be rather strong for transverse myelitis, an acute inflammatory process affecting a focal area of the spinal cord. It is clinically characterized by the development of neuromotor, sensory, and autonomic dysfunction. Since the first report back in 1985, many subsequent studies have confirmed the association of aPL with transverse myelitis. The age at disease onset varies widely, ranging from childhood to 80 years [41]. The correlation between aPL positivity and the occurrence of transverse myelitis holds significance even when considering SLE individuals only [17]. It has been proposed that the pathogenesis might involve not only a thrombotic process leading to ischemia but also a direct interaction between aPL and spinal cord phospholipids [42, 43].

8.8 Epilepsy

In a large European cohort of 1,000 APS patients, the prevalence of convulsions was 7.0 % [2]. Similarly, in a more recent series of 538 patients with APS, epilepsy was reported in 8.6 % of subjects [44]. The prevalence of IgG aCL was even higher in patients with focal epilepsy than in those with generalized epilepsy (14 versus 8 %) [45]. It has been suggested that the increased prevalence of autoantibodies described in epileptic patients might be secondary to antiepileptic drugs. Consistently, patients with partial epilepsy and a disease duration longer than 30 years were three times more likely to have aCL than subjects with recent onset [46]. However, even newly diagnosed patients with epilepsy were found to present a higher positivity rate of aCL IgG compared to controls [40]. Another hypothesis envisages that disease itself, through the production of proinflammatory cytokines such as IL-6, might induce autoantibody production [42]. As seizure and epilepsy are a relative common manifestation of SLE, it is not surprising that epilepsy is more common in patients with secondary APS than in those with primary APS (13.7 % versus 6 %, respectively) [44]. Consistently, patients with SLE and aPL are more prone to develop convulsions than those who are aPL negative [47].

At multivariate logistic regression analysis, thromboembolic events involving the CNS emerged as the strongest predictor of epilepsy, with an odds ratio of 4.

Indeed, convulsions are a well-recognized symptom of cerebral ischemia, and it is possible that many cases of convulsions in aPL-positive patients are caused by ischemic events triggering the development of an epileptic focus [47]. However, since thrombotic events may explain the occurrence of epilepsy in APS only partially, other mechanisms of damage have been investigated. In lupus patients with convulsions, aPL have been shown to impair the function of a gamma-aminobutyric acid receptor-mediated chloride channel in the myelin sheath [48], suggesting aPL might decrease the seizure threshold through a direct and reversible mechanism. These findings are in line with the increasing evidence of the association of epilepsy with specific autoantibodies targeting neuronal structures, such as antibodies against glutamic acid decarboxylase and against glutamate receptor GluR3 in some types of autoimmune encephalitis [49].

8.9 Sensorineural Hearing Loss

Several anecdotal reports have highlighted the association of sensorineural hearing loss with aPL [25]. Series carried out in otologic centers showed that 27 % of patients with sudden deafness or progressive sensorineural hypoacusia had positive aCL [50]. The etiology of sensorineural hearing loss in aPL carriers might be on a vascular basis, as certified by the improvement observed in some patients on anticoagulation [25].

8.10 Ocular Syndromes

Ocular vaso-occlusive disease is frequently found in patients with APS, with amaurosis fugax being the most common manifestation [51]. Severe vaso-occlusive retinopathy leads to poor visual outcomes with visual loss in 80 % of cases with neovascularization occurring in 40 % of cases [52]. Optic neuropathy is less frequent in APS than in SLE and usually monolateral rather than bilateral. It has been proposed that the underlying mechanisms are different, implying a pro-thrombotic milieu involving the ciliary vasculature in APS and an inflammatory vasculitis in SLE [53].

8.11 Chorea

Chorea has been described in 1.3 % of APS patients, being thus regarded as a rare manifestation of APS [2]. Chorea is a well-known phenomenon in patients with SLE and is strongly correlated with aPL positivity. Chorea has been described in association with primary APS in a number of patients, many of whom were children [41]. In a review of the clinical presentation of 50 APS patients presenting with chorea, 15 % had SLE, 12 % had lupus-like syndrome, and 30 % had primary APS. In addition, 66 % of the patients had experienced only one episode of chorea.

The chorea was bilateral in 55 % of cases, and imaging studies revealed cerebral infarction in 35 % [2]. Besides a vascular mechanism, aPL might cause chorea by binding phospholipids in the basal ganglia, leading to movement disorders [42].

8.12 Guillain–Barre' Syndrome

Guillain–Barre' syndrome is an acute demyelinating disorder of the peripheral nervous system. In the original description of the syndrome, Hughes reported the association of demyelinating polyradiculoneuropathy and APS [54]. The motor nerves are affected, with little or no involvement of the sensory nerves. On the other hand, some Guillain–Barre' syndrome patients produce autoantibodies to various phospholipids and nuclear antigens. However, nowadays such association is not considered solid: those autoantibodies are probably produced as a result of damage to the myelin rather than being the cause of the demyelination [54].

8.13 Peripheral Neuropathy

Peripheral nervous system involvement is rare in APS [55]; distal, asymmetric, axonal polyneuropathy (mononeuritis multiplex) is extremely rare. Peripheral neuropathy might provide a common asymptomatic abnormality in primary APS patients: in a study on 26 primary APS patients, 35 % presented abnormalities at nerve conduction studies, 15.5 % had pure sensory or sensorimotor distal axonal neuropathy, 4 % had sensorimotor demyelinating and axonal neuropathy involving upper and lower extremities, and 15.5 % showed isolated carpal tunnel syndrome [56]. The pathogenesis of peripheral neuropathy involves both immune and vascular mechanisms. The inflammation and lesion of nerves might be caused by autoantibodies or immune complex deposits or might be directly caused by vasculitis or thrombosis of the vasa nervorum [57].

8.14 Treatment

The management of stroke in APS patients is still rather controversial; therapeutic options include moderate- or high-intensity anticoagulant regimens as well as antiplatelet agents.

To date, two randomized controlled studies addressed the management of noncardioembolic stroke. In the earlier one, the 2004 APASS study, aspirin given at a dose of 325 mg daily was shown to be as effective as low-intensity anticoagulants in the secondary prevention of stroke among aPL-positive patients [13]. The APASS study is flawed by some limitations: aPL positivity was not confirmed 12 weeks apart, and patients were recruited even when aCL positivity was detected at low titers; the median INR in the patients receiving warfarin was 1.9, a value whose efficacy is unproven also for the treatment of thromboembolism. These biases preclude results extrapolation to patients with definite APS. However, it is generally accepted to consider prescribing low-dose aspirin (LDASA) to stroke patients without SLE and a low-risk aPL profile. In 2009, Okuma first shed light on the combination of LDASA with moderate-intensity anticoagulation as a therapeutic option in stroke patients with definite APS [58]. In this randomized controlled trial, a lower incidence of recurrent stroke was observed among patients treated with LDASA plus warfarin compared to those receiving LDASA alone, with a cumulative stroke-free survival of 74 % versus 25 %. However, this study is flawed by important limitations: firstly, the sample size was rather small, no details of the aPL profiles were provided, and limited information on the number and type of recurrent strokes in each group were available. Nevertheless, considering the high incidence of recurrent stroke in the monotherapy arm, this study suggests that LDASA alone might not be sufficient for secondary stroke prevention in patients with definite APS.

The optimum intensity of oral anticoagulation has been also a matter of debate, since a retrospective analysis suggested a beneficial effect of high-intensity anticoagulation. Therefore, two randomized trials by Crowther and Finazzi recruited APS patients with a history of thrombotic events in order to confirm these findings, even though arterial thrombosis were underrepresented compared to subjects experiencing venous thrombosis (24 % in the study by Crowther and 32 % in the trial promoted by Finazzi). These two studies didn't support a superiority of high intensity (INR 3–4) as compared to moderate-intensity anticoagulation (INR 2–3) [59, 60]. Consequently, a 2006 systematic review including only these randomized controlled trials recommended moderate anticoagulation [61]. Nevertheless a systematic review by Ruiz-Irastorza, who considered also observational studies, supported the utility of the high-intensity regimen [62]. This review concluded that oral anticoagulation to a standard target INR range of 2.0 to 3.0 was not sufficient in preventing recurrences among patients presenting with arterial events, with most of the new thrombotic events occurring at an INR below 3.0. Given this conflicting picture, an international task force could not reach a consensus about the optimal management of arterial thrombosis. Eight out of the 13 members of the task force suggested treatment with warfarin with an INR over 3.0 for patients with definite APS; the combination of moderate anticoagulation and aspirin was also listed as an option, while ASA was reserved to stroke patients with a low-risk profile and reversible thrombotic risk factors [63]. The guidelines issued in 2014 by the American Heart Association/American Stroke Association recommended antiplatelet therapy in patients with ischemic stroke or transient ischemic attack with aPL who don't fulfill the criteria for APS, but anticoagulant therapy might be considered for patients meeting the criteria for APS, depending on the perception of risk for recurrent thrombotic events and bleeding [64].

While ischemic manifestations of APS always imply the initiation of either antiplatelet drugs or long-term anticoagulants, no standard treatment is available for nonvascular neurological manifestations of APS. First-line treatment of aPL-related neurological manifestations follows the recommendation for the same manifestations outside APS field. In case of failure, the usage of steroids and other immunosuppressive agents might be justified by the probable flogistic/autoimmune mechanisms underlying these symptoms. Intravenous immunoglobulins, plasmapheresis, and rituximab have been occasionally reported to be effective in cases unresponsive to conventional drugs [28].

Conclusions

Besides cerebral ischemic events, several heterogeneous neurological manifestations have been identified as part of the spectrum of APS. An increasing body of evidence from experimental APS models as well as from patients currently suggests an immune-mediated pathogenesis underlying non-thrombotic manifestations of APS such as movement disorders and neuropsychiatric symptoms.

In consideration of the available literature, aPL might be worth testing in patients with autoimmune diseases and neuropsychiatric manifestations, in young individuals experiencing ischemic cerebral events without an underlying known disease, and in those with transverse myelitis or atypical seizures. Young subjects with atypical multiple sclerosis clinical features and those with multiple hyperintense lesions on brain MRI T2-weighted sequences, without other known causes, should also be tested for aPL. These complex and multifaceted neurological presentations represent a challenge for clinicians, who need to promptly recognize and effectively treat them in early stages, in order to avoid diagnostic and therapeutic delay. In fact some of these manifestations often improve drastically with the administration of anticoagulants at appropriate doses.

References

1. Miyakis S, Lockshin MD, Atsumi M et al (2006) International consensus statement on an update of the classification criteria for definite antiphospholipid syndrome (APS). J Thromb Haemost 4:295–306
2. Cervera R, Piette JC, Font J et al (2002) Antiphospholipid syndrome: clinical and immunologic manifestations and patterns of disease expression in a cohort of 1,000 patients. Arthritis Rheum 46:1019–1027
3. Cervera R, Serrano R, Pons-Estel GJ et al (2014) Morbidity and mortality in the antiphospholipid syndrome during a 10-year period: a multicentre prospective study of 1000 patients. Ann Rheum Dis. doi:10.1136/annrheumdis-2013-204838
4. Hughes GRV (1983) Thrombosis, abortion, cerebral disease and the lupus anticoagulant. Br Med J 287:1088–1089
5. Meroni PL, Chighizola C (2012) Pathophysiology of the antiphospholipid syndrome (APS). Rev Med Interne 33(S2):A2–A4
6. Meroni PL, Tincani A, Sepp N et al (2003) Endothelium and the brain in CNS lupus. Lupus 12:919–928
7. Ishii H, Salem HH, Bell CE et al (1986) Thrombomodulin, an endothelial anticoagulant protein, is absent from the human brain. Blood 67:362–365
8. Carecchio M, Cantello R, Comi C (2014) Revisiting the molecular mechanism of neurological manifestations in antiphospholipid syndrome: beyond vascular damage. J Immunol Res 2014:239398
9. Riccio A, Andreassi C, Eboli ML (1998) Antiphospholipid antibodies bind to rat cerebellar granule cells: the role of N-methyl-D-aspartate receptors. Neurosci Lett 257:116–118

10. Pregnolato F, Gerosa M, Chighizola C et al (2010) Anti-NR2 antibodies and primary antiphospholipid syndrome: a preliminary study. Ann Rheum Dis 69:665
11. Lancaster E, Martinez-Hernandez E, Dalmau J (2011) Encephalitis and antibodies to synaptic and neuronal cell surface proteins. Neurology 77:179–189
12. Hughes GR (2003) Migraine, memory loss, and "multiple sclerosis". Neurological features of the antiphospholipid (Hughes') syndrome. Postgrad Med J 79:81–83
13. Group APASS (1997) Anticardiolipin antibodies and the risk of recurrent thrombo-occlusive events and death. Neurology 48:91–94
14. Janardhan V, Wolf PA, Kase CS et al (2004) Anticardiolipin antibodies and risk of ischaemic stroke and transient ischemic attack: the Framingham cohort and offspring study. Stroke 35:736–744
15. Brey RL, Stallworth CL, McGlasson DL et al (2002) Antiphospholipid antibodies and stroke in young women. Stroke 3:2396–2400
16. Urbanus RT, Siegerink B, Roest M et al (2009) Antiphospholipid antibodies and risk of myocardial infarction and ischaemic stroke in young women in the RATIO study: a case-control study. Lancet Neurol 8:998–1005
17. Sanna G, D'Cruz D, Cuadrado MJ (2006) Cerebral manifestations in the antiphospholipid (Hughes) syndrome. Rheum Dis Clin North Am 32:465–490
18. Levine SR, Brey RL, Tilley BC et al (2004) Antiphospholipid antibodies and subsequent thrombo-occlusive events in patients with ischemic stroke. JAMA 291:576–584
19. Levine SR, Salowich-Palm L, Sawaya KL et al (1997) IgG anticardiolipin antibody titer >40 GPL and the risk of subsequent thrombo-occlusive events and death. A prospective cohort study. Stroke 28:1660–1665
20. Asherson RA, Khamashta MA, Gil A et al (1989) Cerebrovascular disease and antiphospholipid antibodies in systemic lupus erythematosus, lupus-like disease, and the primary antiphospholipid syndrome. Am J Med 86:391–399
21. Tincani A, Rebaioli CB, Taglietti M et al (2006) Heart involvement in systemic lupus erythematosus, anti-phospholipid syndrome and neonatal lupus. Rheumatology (Oxford) 45:iv8–iv13
22. Frances C, Papo T, Wechsler B et al (1999) Sneddon syndrome with or without antiphospholipid antibodies: a comparative study in 46 patients. Medicine 78:209–219
23. Sun KH, Liu WT, Tsai CY et al (1992) Inhibition of astrocyte proliferation and binding to brain tissue of anticardiolipin antibodies purified from lupus serum. Ann Rheum Dis 51:707–712
24. Fetoni V, Grisoli M, Salmaggi A (2000) Clinical and neuroradiological aspects of Sneddon's syndrome and primary antiphospholipid antibody syndrome: a follow-up study. Neurol Sci 21:157–164
25. Sanna G, Bertolaccini ML, Cuadrado MJ (2003) Central nervous system involvement in the antiphospholipid (Hughes) syndrome. Rheumatology (Oxford) 42:200–213
26. Gomez-Puerta JA, Cervera R, Calvo LM et al (2005) Dementia associated with the antiphospholipid syndrome: clinical and radiological characteristics of 30 patients. Rheumatology (Oxford) 44:95–99
27. Shoenfeld Y, Nahum A, Korczyn AD et al (2003) Neuronal-binding antibodies from patients with antiphospholipid syndrome induce cognitive deficits following intrathecal passive transfer. Lupus 12:436–442
28. Rodrigues CEM, Carvalho JF, Shoenfeld Y (2010) Neurological manifestations of antiphospholipid syndrome. Eur J Clin Invest 40:350–359
29. Scott TF, Hess D, Brillman J (1994) Antiphospholipid antibody syndrome mimicking multiple sclerosis clinically and by magnetic resonance imaging. Arch Intern Med 154:917–920
30. Tektonidou MG, Varsou N, Kotoulas G et al (2006) Cognitive deficits in patients with antiphospholipid syndrome: association with clinical, laboratory, and brain magnetic resonance imaging findings. Arch Intern Med 13:2278–8224
31. Cuadrado MJ, Khamashta MA, Ballesteros A et al (2000) Can neurologic manifestations of Hughes (antiphospholipid) syndrome be distinguished from multiple sclerosis? Analysis of 27 patients and review of the literature. Medicine (Baltimore) 79:57–68

32. Miserocchi E, Baltatzis S, Foster S (2001) Ocular features associated with antibodies: a descriptive study. Am J Ophthalmol 131:451–456
33. Tourbah A, Clapin A, Gout O et al (1998) Systemic autoimmune features and multiple sclerosis: a 5-year follow-up study. Arch Neurol 55:517–521
34. Sastre-Garriga J, Reverter JC, Font J et al (2001) Anticardiolipin antibodies are not a useful screening tool in a nonselected large group of patients with multiple sclerosis. Ann Neurol 49:408–411
35. Heinzlef O, Weill B, Johanet C et al (2002) Anticardiolipin antibodies in patients with multiple sclerosis do not represent a subgroup of patients according to clinical, familial, and biological characteristics. J Neurol Neurosurg Psychiatry 72:647–649
36. Koudriavtseva T, D'Agosto G, Mandoj C et al (2014) High frequency of antiphospholipid antibodies in relapse of multiple sclerosis: a possible indicator of inflammatory-thrombotic processes. Neurol Sci doi:10.1007/s10072–014–1823–4
37. Szmyrka-Kaczmarek M, Pokryszko-Dragan A, Pawlik B et al (2012) Antinuclear and antiphospholipid antibodies in patients with multiple sclerosis. Lupus 21:412–420
38. Renaud M, Aupy J, Uring-Lambert B et al (2014) Isolated anti-β2-glycoprotein I antibodies in neurology: a frontier syndrome between multiple sclerosis and antiphospholipid syndrome? Eur J Neurol 21:901–906
39. Zivadinov R, Ramanathan M, Ambrus J et al (2012) Anti-phospholipid antibodies are associated with response to interferon-beta1a treatment in MS: results from a 3-year longitudinal study. Neurol Res 34:761–769
40. Karussis D, Leker RR, Ashkenazi A et al (1998) A subgroup of multiple sclerosis patients with anticardiolipin antibodies and unusual clinical manifestations: do they represent a new nosological entity? Ann Neurol 44:629–634
41. Katzav A, Chapman J, Shoenfeld Y (2003) CNS dysfunction in the antiphospholipid syndrome. Lupus 12:903–907
42. Mok CC, Lau CS, Chan EY et al (1998) Acute transverse myelitis in systemic lupus erythematosus: clinical presentation, treatment, and outcome. J Rheumatol 25:467–473
43. Lavelle C, Pizarro S, Drenkard C et al (1990) Transverse myelitis: a manifestation of systemic lupus erythematosus strongly associated with antiphospholipid antibodies. J Rheumatol 17:34–37
44. Shoenfeld Y, Lev S, Blatt I et al (2004) Features associated with epilepsy in the antiphospholipid syndrome. J Rheumatol 31:1344–1348
45. Peltola J, Kulmala P, Isojarvi J et al (2000) Autoantibodies to glutamic acid decarboxylase in patients with therapy-resistant epilepsy. Neurology 55:46–50
46. Ranua J, Luoma K, Peltola J et al (2004) Anticardiolipin and antinuclear antibodies in a epilepsy population based cross-sectional study. Epilepsy Res 58:13–18
47. Cimaz R, Meroni PL, Shoenfeld Y (2006) Epilepsy as part of systemic lupus erythematosus and systemic antiphospholipid syndrome (Hughes syndrome). Lupus 15:191–197
48. Liou HH, Wang CR, Chou HC et al (1994) Anticardiolipin antisera from lupus patients with seizures reduce a GABA receptor-mediated chloride current in snail neurons. Life Sci 54:1119–1125
49. Xie XK, Tang LO (1990) Observation of anti-brain antibody in serum of 110 epileptics. Chin Med J (Engl) 103:71–75
50. Toubi E, Ben-David J, Kessel A et al (1997) Autoimmune aberration in sudden sensorineural hearing loss: association with anti-cardiolipin antibodies. Lupus 6:540–542
51. Wiechens B, Schroder JO, Potzsch B et al (1997) Primary antiphospholipid antibody syndrome and retinal occlusive vasculopathy. Am J Ophthalmol 123:848–850
52. Au A, O'Day J (2004) Review of severe vaso-occlusive retinopathy in systemic lupus erythematosus and the antiphospholipid syndrome: associations, visual outcomes, complications and treatment. Clin Experiment Ophthalmol 32:87–100
53. Reino S, Munoz-Rodriguez FJ, Cervera R et al (1997) Optic neuropathy in the 'primary' antiphospholipid syndrome: report of a case and review of the literature. Clin Rheumatol 16:629–631

54. Harris EN, Englert H, Derue G (1983) Antiphospholipid antibodies in acute Guillain-Barre syndrome. Lancet 2:1361–1362
55. Erten N, Saka B, Karan MA et al (2004) Catastrophic secondary antiphospholipid syndrome with peripheral nervous system involvement: a case report. Acta Med Okayama 58:107–110
56. Santos MSF, Carvalho JF, Brotto M et al (2010) Peripheral neuropathy in patients with primary antiphospholipid (Hughes') syndrome. Lupus 19:583–590
57. McCombe PA, McLeod JG, Pollard JD et al (1987) Peripheral sensorimotor and autonomic neuropathy associated with systemic lupus erythematosus. Clinical, pathological and immunological features. Brain 110:533–534
58. Okuma H, Kitagawa Y, Yasuda T et al (2010) Comparison between single antiplatelet therapy and combination of anti-platelet and anticoagulation therapy for secondary prevention in ischemic stroke patients with antiphospholipid syndrome. Int J Med Sci 7:15–18
59. Crowther MA, Ginsberg JS, Julian J et al (2003) A comparison of two intensities of warfarin for the prevention of recurrent thrombosis in patients with the antiphospholipid antibody syndrome. N Engl J Med 349:1133–1138
60. Finazzi G, Marchioli R, Brancaccio V et al (2005) A randomized clinical trial of high-intensity warfarin vs. conventional antithrombotic therapy for the prevention of recurrent thrombosis in patients with the antiphospholipid syndrome (WAPS). J Thromb Haemost 3:848–853
61. Lim W, Crowther MA, Eikelboom JW (2006) Management of antiphospholipid antibody syndrome. JAMA 295:1050–1057
62. Ruiz-Irastorza G, Hunt BJ, Khamashta MA (2007) A systematic review of secondary thromboprophylaxis in patients with antiphospholipid antibodies. Arthritis Rheum 57:1487–1495
63. Ruiz-Irastorza G, Cuadrado MJ, Ruiz-Arruza I et al (2011) Evidence-based recommendations for the prevention and long-term management of thrombosis in antiphospholipid antibody-positive patients: report of a task force at the 13th international congress on antiphospholipid antibodies. Lupus 20:206–218
64. Kernan WN, Ovbiagele B, Black HR et al (2014) Guidelines for the prevention of stroke in patients with stroke and transient ischemic attack: a guideline for healthcare professionals from the American Heart Association/American Stroke Association. Stroke 45:2160–2236

Antiphospholipid Syndrome (APS) and the Renal Involvement

9

Nicoletta Mezzina and Renato Alberto Sinico

9.1 Introduction

Even if hypertension (the most frequent clinical sign of APS renal involvement) has been described as a part of the spectrum of APS manifestations since the first publication on this syndrome [1], APS kidney involvement was probably underestimated and not well characterized until recently.

A possible explanation is that several manifestations of renal involvement (hypertension, haematuria, and proteinuria) were often neglected and that renal biopsy was rarely performed due to the frequent occurrence of thrombocytopenia and the use of anticoagulants among APS patients.

For these reasons the true prevalence of renal involvement in APS is difficult to establish. In the few retrospective studies on large cohorts of APS patients, a prevalence of approximately 9–10 % is reported [2, 3], but it could be speculated that it might be higher.

Renal involvement in APS is characterized by noninflammatory occlusion/thrombosis of renal vessels (arterial and venous) ranging in size from large vessels to intrarenal microvasculature. Indeed, a large spectrum of vascular manifestations have been described in association with antiphospholipid antibodies, such as renal artery stenosis/thrombosis, renal infarction, renal vein thrombosis, and a

N. Mezzina
Clinical Immunology and Renal Unit, Azienda Ospedaliera Ospedale San Carlo Borromeo/Università Statale di Milano, Via Pio II, 3/Via Festa del Perdono, Milan 20100, Italy
e-mail: nicoletta.mezzina@unimi.it

R.A. Sinico (✉)
Clinical Immunology Unit and Renal Unit, Azienda Ospedaliera Ospedale San Carlo Borromeo, Via Pio II, 3, Milan 20100, Italy
e-mail: renatoalberto.sinico@fastwebnet.it

© Springer International Publishing Switzerland 2015

P.L. Meroni (ed.), *Antiphospholipid Antibody Syndrome: From Bench to Bedside*, Rare Diseases of the Immune System, DOI 10.1007/978-3-319-11044-8_9

small-vessel vaso-occlusive nephropathy recently defined as "APS nephropathy" [4, 5]. In addition to vaso-occlusive abnormalities, other kinds of renal lesions such as glomerulonephritis have been reported in primary APS (PAPS) [2, 6]. This heterogeneity of renal involvement could be explained by the presence of different underlying pathogenetic mechanisms.

From a clinical point of view, the most frequent signs and laboratory characteristics of APS renal involvement include hypertension, hematuria, acute renal failure, and progressive chronic renal insufficiency with mild to nephrotic range proteinuria. APS can also cause end-stage renal disease (rare) and allograft vascular thrombosis [7].

This chapter reviews the range of renal abnormalities associated with APS, their diagnosis and treatment options.

9.2 Renal Artery Lesions

Renal artery involvement is well known and has been described in either SLE-related APS and primary APS (PAPS).

In 1990, Ostuni et al. [8] reported for the first time the occurrence of renal artery thrombosis and hypertension in a 13-year-old girl with high titers of aCL (anticardiolipin Ab). More recently, in 2003 Sangle et al. [9] showed how aPL-positive hypertensive patients, compared to young hypertensive controls and healthy individuals, had more frequently renal artery lesions detected by magnetic resonance renal angiography (26 vs. 8 %, $p<0.001$).

The defining characteristic of artery involvement associated with aPL is renal artery stenotic lesions which had two different patterns with some unique features: smooth well delineated and often noncritical stenosis distal to the ostium of the renal artery and, a less frequent pattern, similar to atherosclerotic lesion, characterized by stenosis proximal to the ostium, occasionally involving the aorta [9].

These occlusive lesions can be uni- or bilateral and their pathogenesis can be related with in situ thrombosis of the renal artery or emboli from heart valve lesions [9]. Moreover, it has been suggested that aPL leads to accelerated atherosclerosis as well as to increased endothelin levels with consequent vasoconstriction. Additional observations have suggested cross-reactivity between aPL and antibodies to Apo A-I, HDL, and oxidized LDL, which could indicate a possible link between thrombotic and atherosclerotic complications [10].

9.2.1 Clinical Manifestations and Diagnosis

The most common clinical manifestation of renal artery thrombosis is the onset of severe hypertension or a worsening of a preexisting systemic hypertension, sometimes associated with pain in the renal area, hematuria, or renal failure [5, 9]. This lesion can also lead to renal infarction, resulting from partial or total occlusion of renal artery or infrarenal aorta, or to ischemic acute renal failure, or to the slowly progressive ischemic chronic renal insufficiency.

Imaging techniques, for example, renal Doppler ultrasound as a first-line procedure followed, if necessary, by computed tomography (CT), renal angiography, renal scintigraphy, and gadolinium enhancement magnetic resonance angiography, should be used for the diagnosis and the evaluation of the extension of these lesions [11].

9.2.2 Treatment

For all aPL-positive patient, as general recommendations, it is important to control risk factors for atherosclerosis, such as obesity, smoking, hypertension, diabetes, and hyperlipidemia. The oral contraceptive pill and hormone replacement therapy should be avoided, given their association with thromboembolic events [7].

Regarding drugs therapy, a successful management with antihypertensive drugs, antiplatelet drugs, or anticoagulants has been reported. After the initial heparin treatment, the current recommendation for secondary thromboprophylaxis in APS patients is lifelong warfarin, because of the risk of recurrent events. But the intensity of anticoagulation is controversial because in randomized controlled trials (RCT), aimed at finding the appropriate INR levels for secondary thrombosis prevention, only a small proportion of the involved patients had arterial events. Although target INR levels of 2.0–3.0 should be enough for APS patients with vein thrombosis, for patients with renal artery thrombosis, an addition of antiplatelet agents to warfarin (target INR 2.0–3.0) or adoption of higher INR target ranges of 3.0–4.0 may be required [12].

Thrombolysis or transluminal balloon angioplasty with or without stenting has also been described [13] and may be considered. For severe lesions not amenable to angioplasty and stenting, surgical intervention is suggested [14].

9.3 Renal Vein Thrombosis

Thrombosis of the inferior vein cava and the main and/or minor renal veins has been described in patients with primary APS as well as SLE-related APS.

In 1993, Asherson et al. [15] reported for the first time the association of aPL and renal vein thrombosis in patients with SLE and positive lupus anticoagulant (LA).

Indeed this manifestation has been especially associated with LA positivity and occurs more frequently in APS patients with SLE than in those without SLE [11]. These associations suggest that aPL could play a role in renal vein thrombosis pathogenesis; however, other procoagulant conditions, such as trauma, extrinsic compression, pregnancy, oral contraceptive, and especially nephrotic syndrome, have to be ruled out in any cases of renal thrombosis in APS patients.

9.3.1 Clinical Manifestations and Diagnosis

The clinical manifestation depends on the extent of the renal thrombosis, but it is usually represented by nephrotic range proteinuria. Renal failure may also occur, especially in cases of bilateral thrombosis.

Consequently, if any patient with persistently positive aPL suddenly develops heavy proteinuria or presents an exacerbation of a previously stable proteinuria, careful doppler studies of the renal vasculature should be considered in order to rule out renal vein thrombosis [16].

9.3.2 Treatment

As assumed for arterial lesions, the control of risk factors for atherosclerosis is indicated in patients with venous renal thrombosis, and a lifelong thromboprophylaxis with warfarin (target INR 2.0–3.0) is mandatory for the high risk of recurrence. An adoption of higher INR target (3.0–4.0) or addition of antiplatelet agents may be required in recurrent cases [12].

9.4 Intrarenal Vascular Lesions "APS Nephropathy"

As it was previously stated, even if thrombosis may take place at any vascular site of the renal vasculature, the intrarenal lesions of APS were poorly recognized until recently.

The term "APS nephropathy" was coined in the near 1999 by Nochy et al. who first described in a systematic way the clinical and histopathologic lesions on renal biopsy of 16 cases of primary APS (PAPS). The patients had small-vessel acute thrombosis (thrombotic microangiopathy, TMA) associated with chronic vascular lesions such as fibrous intimal hyperplasia (FIH) or occlusion of intrarenal arteries and arterioles, organizing thrombi with or without recanalization, or focal cortical atrophy (FCA) [5] (Table 9.1).

APS nephropathy was also observed in SLE-related APS patients, independently of lupus nephritis, and in catastrophic APS (especially thrombotic microangiopathy) [17].

Thrombotic microangiopathy (TMA) in APS patients is the best-known feature of APS nephropathy as it was observed previously also by other authors [18, 19], and it is histopathologically characterized by the absence of inflammatory cells and of vascular immune deposits and by the presence of fibrin thrombi in glomeruli and in the entire intrarenal vascular circulation. Immunofluorescence studies reveal that fibrin is the main constituent of thrombi in the absence of immunoglobulins. These lesions resemble the histological picture of the other thrombotic microangiopathies such as thrombocytopenic purpura and hemolytic uremic

Table 9.1 Histologic characteristics of APS nephropathy

Acute lesions	Chronic lesions
Thrombotic microangiopathy (TMA)	Arterial fibrous intimal hyperplasia (FIH) or arterial occlusion by organized thrombi with or without recanalization
	Focal cortical atrophy (FCA)
	Tubular thyroidization

syndrome. TMA represents the most important vascular lesion threatening the renal prognosis in SLE-related APS [20], and it is the predominant renal lesion seen in catastrophic APS [17].

Fibrous intimal hyperplasia (FIH) is characterized by an intense myofibroblastic intimal cellular proliferation which reduces the arteriolar lumen. The intima tends to be much more cellular than that seen in typical arteriosclerosis of aging, assuming an onion-skin arrangement in biopsy cross sections. Sometimes the lumina could be obstructed by fibrous tissue and permeated with endothelialized channels indicative of recanalizing thromboses (organizing thrombi).

Focal cortical atrophy (FCA) involves the superficial cortex under the renal capsule, forming foci or triangles that led to retraction of the tissue, with a sharp border with the rest of the normal cortex, and it is accompanied by a depression of the contour of the remaining renal capsule.

In these atrophic areas all elements of the renal parenchyma are altered as a part of the ensemble of lesions comprising FCA: the glomeruli appear either small and sclerotic or large but virtually lacking the glomerular tuft, the tubules are atrophic and packed with eosinophilic casts, resembling thyroid tissue (tubular thyroidization), and the arterioles are occluded by fibrin microthrombi or by fibrous tissue.

The presence of identical lesions of FIH and tubular thyroidization in surgical nephrectomies performed for renal artery stenosis (in order to reduce hypertension secondary to unilateral stenosis) led to speculate that tissue ischemia and the activation of the renin-angiotensin system are possible causes of those lesions in APS [5].

9.4.1 Clinical Manifestations and Diagnosis

Clinical presentation of APS nephropathy can vary widely ranging from arterial hypertension, which is the prominent and sometimes the only clinical sign suggestive of nephropathy, to sudden acute renal failure or to mild and progressive chronic renal insufficiency with different levels of proteinuria. Lupus anticoagulant (LA) positivity seems to be more frequently present among APS patients with an intrarenal involvement (2).

In all APS patients with clinical and laboratory findings that suggest renal involvement (new onset of hypertension, proteinuria, hematuria, or renal insufficiency), renal biopsy should be performed [21].

On the other hand, every time it is found in a biopsy section, a combination of any two of three elements which represents a constellation more or less characteristic of APS (TMA, FIH, or FCA), the pathologist should be alerted to the possibility of PAPS diagnosis which has to be clinically confirmed [5].

Moreover, in patients with biopsy-proven APS nephropathy lesions and persistently positive aPL, the diagnosis of APS should be considered even without thrombotic events or pregnancy morbidity [21].

9.4.2 Treatment

Since no evidence-based recommendations are available, the optimum management of patients with only intrarenal vascular lesions (APS nephropathy), alone or in combination with SLE nephropathy, is unknown.

Several empirical therapeutic approaches have been used, ranging from the pharmacological management of hypertension, associated with aspirin and/or oral anticoagulants, with steroids, and in some cases with additional immunosuppressive treatment.

Pons-Estel et al. [7] on the basis of their personal experience recommend starting anticoagulation with an INR target of 2.0–3.0 (as for any other patient with thrombotic APS) and adding antiplatelet agents or increasing target INR levels to 3.0–4.0 if no improvement is achieved.

In other recent studies, a stabilization of renal function and proteinuria by use of rituximab is reported. These studies proposed that rituximab might have a function in the treatment of persistently aPL-positive patients with non-criteria manifestations of APS, by reducing the production of autoantibodies [22, 23].

9.5 Glomerular Disease

Besides the vaso-occlusive abnormalities of the intrarenal arteries and glomerular capillaries, other types of histological lesions have been also described in primary APS patients with renal involvement. These lesions include membranous glomerulonephritis (the most frequent), IgA nephropathy, pauci-immune crescentic glomerulonephritis, mesangial C3 nephropathies, vasculitis, and minimal change disease/focal segmental glomerulosclerosis [6, 2, 24].

Glomerulonephritis in PAPS can't be ascribed to thrombosis; instead other mechanisms such as immune complex deposition seem to be implicated. PAPS is considered a systemic autoimmune disease, and it has been described a number of different circulating autoantibodies and a different degree of complement reduction especially among patients who had PAPS with nephropathy.

The autoantibodies positivity, such as antinucleosome (anti-NSC) ab, and complement reduction found in renal PAPS support the idea of heterogeneity of renal involvement and suggest the presence of a continuum between SLE and PAPS.

As expected, anti-NCS antibodies are more frequently detected in PAPS with lupus-like disease, and patients with MN or proliferative glomerulonephritis, especially when C1q deposits and hypocomplementemia are present, should be considered at high risk for developing SLE. So a careful monitoring is mandatory in these patients [2].

9.5.1 Clinical Manifestations and Diagnosis

The clinical presentation is not different from APS nephropathy, with only a more frequent presence of nephrotic range proteinuria. As it was stated before, renal biopsy should be performed every time a renal APS involvement is suspected.

Moreover, a complete nephrologic workup should be performed especially in these kinds of patients, in which a differential diagnosis is very important to classify and treat them correctly.

9.5.2 Treatment

Since no evidence-based recommendations are available, several different therapeutic approaches have been used in these cases. The treatments usually consist in steroids, also IV pulses, associated with different immunosuppressive drugs, on the basis of the scheduled treatments for the same but not APS-related glomerulonephritis.

9.6 ESRD and Renal Transplantation

ESRD is a rare complication of primary APS. This was clearly revealed in different prospective and retrospective studies in which only few PAPS patients developed ESRD [2, 25]. Instead, several studies have revealed that there is a higher incidence of aPL positivity among patients with ESRD and on dialysis, than that found in the general population [26, 27]. This association of ESRD and aPL is irrespective of age, sex, type of dialysis membrane, drug treatment, and chronic B and C hepatitis. Possible causes include bioincompatibility problems as dialysis membranes, trauma to blood passing through the hemodialysis circuit, and induction by microbial agents or their products, for example, endotoxins present in the dialysate. However, it is still uncertain if these antibodies are truly pathogenic in ESRD patients or are just an epiphenomenon.

Moreover, evidence suggests that aPL-positive patients undergoing renal transplantation are at increased risk of renal and systemic vascular thrombosis and graft failure. For this reason, recently the somministration of perioperative immunosuppressives, given in addition to anticoagulation, has been proposed for aPL-positive patients undergoing renal transplantation [28].

In Table 9.2 the main reports from the literature concerning renal involvement in primary antiphospholipid syndrome are summarized.

APS and the renal involvement: key points
1. Probably underestimated
2. Hypertension, microscopic hematuria and proteinuria: most common clinical signs
3. New onset or worsening of hypertension and/or pain in the renal area suggest renal artery thrombosis/stenosis
4. New onset or worsening of proteinuria and/or pain in the renal area may be due to renal vein thrombosis
5. Positive LA is more closely associated with APS renal involvement
6. APS nephropathy: acute lesions (TMA)+chronic lesions (FCA, FIH)
7. Kidney biopsy crucial for diagnosis and management
8. APS as allograft rejection cause (higher RR in positive aCL patients)

Table 9.2 Main reports on renal involvement in primary antiphospholipid syndrome (PAPS)

Author, year	Type of study	$n°$ of patients	Result
D'Agati et al. (1990) [18]	Biopsy-documented report	3 patients:	In all pts:
		1 with PAPS	Active lesions → TMA involving arterioles and glomerular capillaries
		1 with SLE-APS	Renal thrombosis not associated with active endocapillary proliferative lupus nephritis
		1 with lupus-like syndrome	
Amigo et al. (1992) [19]	Case series	20 patients with PAPS:	In all pts:
		5 with renal involvement → renal biopsy performed	Active lesions → TMA involving both arterioles and glomerular capillaries
Levy et al. (1996) [24]	Case report	1 patient with PAPS and MN at renal biopsy	Peripheral blood lymphocytes from the patient transferred to a SCID mice, which developed renal lesion consistent with the human MN → role of aPL as possible inducers of renal damage
Nochy et al. (1999) [5]	Biopsy case series	16 patients with PAPS and renal manifestations undergone renal biopsy	"APS nephropathy"
			Active lesions → TMA in 5 cases (31 %)
			Chronic lesions → FCA in 10 cases (62 %) and FIH in 12 cases (75 %)
Fakhouri et al. (2003) [6]	Biopsy case series	29 biopsies performed in patients with PAPS	"APS nephropathy" (TMA + FCA + FIH) in 20 cases
			Glomerular diseases in 9 cases:
			MN in 3 cases
			MCD/FSGS in 3 cases
			Mesangial C3 nephropathy in 2 cases
			Pauci-immune crescentic GN in 1 case
Tektonidou et al. (2008) [17]	Biopsy case series	37 patients with biopsy-proven renal involvement:	"APS nephropathy"
		6 with CAPS	Acute lesions (TMA)
		8 with CAPS	CAPS: all patients (100 %)
		23 with SLE-APS	PAPS: in 3 of 8 (37.5 %) patients
			SLE-APS: 8 of 23 (35 %) patients
			Chronic lesions (FIH and FCA)
			Similar frequencies (66 % and 50, respectively) in all 3 groups

Table 9.2 (continued)

Author, year	Type of study	*n*° of patients	Result
Sinico et al. (2010) [2]	Retrospective study on PAPS patients	160 patients with PAPS:	"APS nephropathy" in 4 patients:
		14 (8.7 %) patients with renal manifestations → in 10 pts was performed a renal biopsy	Acute lesions (TMA) in 2 cases
			Chronic lesions (FCA + FIH) in 2 cases
			Glomerular diseases in 10 patients:
			MN in 4 cases
			Proliferative GN in 2 cases

SLE systemic lupus erythematosus, *TMA* thrombotic microangiopathy, *MN* membranous nephropathy, *aPL* antiphospholipid antibodies, *FCA* focal cortical atrophy, *FIH* fibrous intimal hyperplasia, *MCD/FSGS* minimal change disease/focal segmental glomerular sclerosis, *GN* glomerulonephritis, *CAPS* catastrophic antiphospholipid syndrome

References

1. Hughes GR (1983) Thrombosis, abortion, cerebral disease, and the lupus anticoagulant. Br Med J (Clin Res Ed) 87:1088–1089
2. Sinico RA, Cavazzana I, Nuzzo M et al (2010) Renal involvement in primary antiphospholipid syndrome: retrospective analysis of 160 patients. Clin J Am Soc Nephrol 5:1211–1217
3. Vlachoyiannopoulos PG, Kanellopoulos P, Tektonidou M et al (2001) Renal involvement in antiphospholipid syndrome. Nephrol Dial Transplant 16(Suppl 6):60–62
4. Piette JC, Kleinknecht D, Bach JF (1996) Renal manifestations in the antiphospholipid syndrome. In: Asherson RA, Cervera R, Piette JC, Shonfield Y (eds) The antiphospholipid syndrome. CRC Press, Boca Raton, pp 169–181
5. Nochy D, Daugas E, Droz D et al (1999) The intrarenal vascular lesions associated with primary antiphospholipid syndrome. J Am Soc Nephrol 10:507–518
6. Fakhouri F, Noel LH, Zuber J et al (2003) The expanding spectrum of renal diseases associated with antiphospholipid syndrome. Am J Kidney Dis 41:1205–1211
7. Pons-Estel GJ, Cervera R (2014) Renal involvement in antiphospholipid syndrome. Curr Rheumatol Rep 16:397
8. Ostuni PA, Lazzarin P, Pengo V et al (1990) Renal artery thrombosis and hypertension in a 13 year old girl with antiphospholipid syndrome. Ann Rheum Dis 49:184–187
9. Sangle SR, D' Cruz DP, Jan W et al (2003) Renal artery stenosis in the antiphospholipid syndrome (Hughes) syndrome and hypertension. Ann Rheum Dis 62:999–1002
10. Delgado AJ, Kumar S, Isenberg DA (2003) Cross-reactivity between anticardiolipin, anti-high-density lipoprotein and anti-apolipoprotein A-I IgG antibodies in patients with systemic lupus erythematosus and primary antiphospholipid syndrome. Rheumatology 42:893–899
11. Tektonidou MG (2009) Renal involvement in the antiphospholipid syndrome (APS)-APS nephropathy. Clin Rev Allergy Immunol 36:131–140
12. Lim W, Crowther MA, Eikelboom JW (2006) Management of antiphospholipid antibody syndrome: a systematic review. JAMA 295:1050–1057
13. Sangle SR, D' Cruz DP, Abbs IC et al (2005) Renal artery stenosis in hypertensive patients with antiphospholipid syndrome (Hughes syndrome): outcome following anticoagulation. Rheumatology 44:372–377
14. Rysana R, Zabka J, Peregin JH et al (1998) Acute renal failure due to bilateral renal artery thrombosis associated with primary antiphospholipid syndrome. Nephrol Dial Transplant 13: 2645–2647

15. Asherson MA, Khamashta MA, Hughes GRV (1993) Hypertension and the antiphospholipid antibodies. Clin Exp Rheumatol 11:465–467
16. D'Cruz DP (2005) Renal manifestations of the antiphospholipid syndrome. Lupus 14:45–48
17. Tektonidou MG, Sotsiou F, Moutsopoulos HM (2008) Antiphospholipid syndrome (APS) nephropathy in catastrophic, primary and systemic lupus erythematosus-related APS. J Rheumatol 35:1983–1988
18. D'Agati V, Kunis C, Williams G et al (1990) Anticardiolipin antibody and renal disease: a report of three cases. J Am Soc Nephrol 1:777–784
19. Amigo MC, Garcia-Torres R, Robles M et al (1992) Renal involvement in primary antiphospholipid syndrome. J Rheumatol 19:1181–1185
20. Banfi G, Bertani T, Boeri V et al (1991) Renal vascular lesions as a marker of poor prognosis in patients with lupus nephritis. Am J Kidney Dis 18:240–248
21. Cervera R, Tektonidou MG, Espinosa G et al (2011) Task force on Catastrophic Antiphospholipid Syndrome (APS) and non-criteria APS Manifestations (I): catastrophic APS, APS nephropathy and heart valve lesions. Lupus 20:165–173
22. Tsagalis G, Psimenou E, Nakopoulou L et al (2010) Effective treatment of antiphospholipid syndrome with plasmapheresis and rituximab. Hippokratia 14:215–216
23. Erkan D, Vega J, Ramon G et al (2013) A pilot open-label phase II trial of rituximab for non-criteria manifestations of antiphospholipid syndrome. Arthritis Rheum 65:464–471
24. Levy Y, Ziporen L, Gilburd B et al (1996) Membranous nephropathy in primary antiphospholipid syndrome: description of a case and induction of renal injury in SCID mice. Hum Antibodies Hybridomas 7:91–96
25. Erkan D, Yazici Y, Sobel R et al (2000) Primary antiphospholipid syndrome: functional outcome after 10 years. J Rheumatol 27:2817–2821
26. Gronhagen-Riska C, Teppo AM, Helantera A et al (1990) Raised concentrations of antibodies to cardiolipin in patients receiving dialysis. BMJ 300:1696–1697
27. Garcia-Martin F, De Arriba G, Carrascosa T et al (1991) Anticardiolipin antibodies and lupus anticoagulant in end-stage renal disease. Nephrol Dial Transplant 6:543–547
28. Domingues V, Dadhania D, Hartona C et al (2013) Hospital for special surgery—Cornell protocol for antiphospholipid antibody positive patients undergoing renal transplantation. In: 14th International Congress on Antiphospholipid Antibodies, Rio de Janeiro, 2013

Non-Thrombotic Hematologic Manifestations in APS

10

Wilma Barcellini and Carolina Artusi

10.1 Introduction

Non-thrombotic hematologic manifestations have been largely reported in antiphospholipid syndrome (APS), although not included in the criteria for classification of this syndrome. The most common hematologic manifestation is thrombocytopenia, followed by hemolytic anemia and less frequently leukopenia [1, 2]. The underlying pathophysiology of these cytopenias is usually thought to be mediated by autoimmune mechanisms, even if more recently other factors are under investigation. Consistent with the autoimmune genesis are the demonstration of antibodies directed against platelets, erythrocytes, or leukocytes and the finding of compensatory hyperplasia of the respective bone marrow precursors. However, the diagnosis of "true" autoimmune cytopenia may be cumbersome due to the heterogeneity and the low sensitivity of the different methods available for the detection of autoantibodies, particularly for platelets and leukocytes. In addition, it may be important to distinguish between mild cytopenias in the context of APS and primary immune thrombocytopenia (ITP), autoimmune hemolytic anemia (AIHA), and chronic idiopathic neutropenia (CIN) which may be definite diseases associated with APS

In this chapter, we will describe these hematologic abnormalities, both considering the context of APS and the hematologic point of view.

W. Barcellini, MD (✉)
Anemia Physiopathology Unit, Onco-hematology Unit, Fondazione IRCCS Ca' Granda Ospedale Maggiore Policlinico, Via F. Sforza 35, Milan 20122, Italy
e-mail: wbarcel@policlinico.mi.it

C. Artusi
Division of Rheumatology – Istituto Ortopedico Gaetano Pini, Department of Clinical Sciences and Community Health, University of Milan, Milan 20122, Italy
e-mail: carolina.artusi@unimi.it

© Springer International Publishing Switzerland 2015
P.L. Meroni (ed.), *Antiphospholipid Antibody Syndrome: From Bench to Bedside*, Rare Diseases of the Immune System, DOI 10.1007/978-3-319-11044-8_10

10.2 Thrombocytopenia

Thrombocytopenia, defined by a platelet count lower than $100 \times 10^9/L$ [1], is reported in about 20–40 % of APS patients [3–5]. It is usually a chronic, mild form and is rarely associated with hemorrhagic complication [6]; in fact, most cases show platelets $>50 \times 10^9/L$ and only about 5–10 % platelets $<50 \times 10^9/L$ [7]. In the latter cases, bleeding manifestations may occur, although severe and life-threatening hemorrhages are reported for platelets $<5–10 \times 10^9/L$. In the last years, there is accumulating evidence about the risk of hemorrhage and platelet count in ITP, where treatment is recommended for platelets $<25–30 \times 10^9/L$. The different guidelines recommend that not only the "number" of platelets should be considered in the decision to treat but also age and lifestyle, comorbidities predisposing to bleeding, patient need for non-ITP medications that may create a bleeding risk, and surgery potentially causing major bleeding [8–10]. For example, a "safe" platelet count, in the absence of other risk factors for bleeding, was reported as $\geq 30 \times 10^9/L$ for simple dental extractions or low-risk procedures (bronchoscopy and endoscopy); $\geq 50 \times 10^9/L$ for complex dental extraction, biopsy of soft tissues, or minor surgery; $\geq 80 \times 10^9/L$ for major surgery; and $\geq 100 \times 10^9/L$ for neurosurgery, including epidural or spinal puncture [8]. Finally, it is worth underlining that patients with chronic thrombocytopenia are ~4- to 5-fold at risk for hemorrhage compared with the general population, but also ~4- to 5-fold at risk for infections, so that bleeding and infection contribute equally to mortality [11]. Moreover, there is emerging evidence that the thrombotic risk is increased in ITP, even at platelet count where the concern of the general practitioner is bleeding [12, 13]. This increased risk has also been attributed to the presence of antiphospholipid (aPL) antibodies, together with conventional prothrombotic risk factors (diabetes, hypertension, old age). Kim et al. [14] reported that 12.7 % of patients with ITP experienced a thromboembolic event (both arterial and venous), with a cumulative incidence rate ratio of 3.15 (95 % CI 1.21–8.17) in aPL antibodies-positive versus aPL antibodies-negative cases, after adjusting for age, hypertension, diabetes, dyslipidemia, smoking, and pregnancy/puerperium; moreover, hypertension and the presence of lupus anticoagulant (LA) emerged as independent risk factor for thrombosis.

10.2.1 Pathogenesis

The pathogenesis of thrombocytopenia in APS is not fully understood. There is a proposed role for aPL antibodies which can directly bind to platelet membrane anionic phospholipids, usually hidden in the inner membrane leaflet but exposed after activation [15]. Currently, there is a general agreement that aPL antibodies react with beta2 glycoprotein, which is a cationic protein that binds to negatively charged phospholipids exposed by activated platelets; consistently, it was demonstrated that aPL do not react with resting platelets [16].

Other studies have focused on antibodies directed against platelet glycoproteins (GP) IIb–IIIa and/or GPIb–IX, usually detected in 20–50 % of primary ITP by various techniques (ELISA, modified antigen-capture ELISA, flow cytometry, and immunoblot) [17–19]. These antibodies have been detected in 40 % of cases positive for aPL antibodies [17, 18] and in a fraction of small series of patients with aPL antibodies and thrombocytopenia [20]. On the other hand, aPL antibodies have been detected in primary ITP: aCL antibodies in 25–30 % [21], LA or aCL antibodies in 46 %, and both LA and aCL antibodies in 16 % [22]. More recently, a prospective study showed that 38 % of ITP patients were aPL antibodies positive at diagnosis and that half of them developed clinical features of APS after a median of 38 months [23]. These findings suggest that there is an overlapping pathogenic role for anti-GP and aPL antibodies in ITP and APS, although the former seem to have a major role. Of note, in ITP, it is well established that antibody-coupled platelets are removed by macrophages via FCγ receptors in the reticular endothelial system and spleen [24]. However, there is emerging evidence that antibodies react against bone marrow megakaryocytes, leading to apoptosis and therefore inadequate compensatory hematopoiesis. This mechanism of immune cytopenia has been hypothesized also for other autoimmune diseases, such as SLE [25].

10.2.2 Diagnosis

The diagnosis of thrombocytopenia in the context of the APS is usually simple, as it is based on the presence of platelets $<100 \times 10^9$/L. The diagnostic scenario is more complicated in patients with isolated aPL antibodies positivity and thrombocytopenia. In these cases, the diagnosis of ITP should be considered, according to the diagnostic workup proposed in the recently published guidelines [8–10, 26]. In fact, ITP is a diagnosis made after the exclusion of infectious (particularly Helicobacter pylori), liver, bone marrow, drug-associated, and inherited thrombocytopenias, since no "gold standard" test can reliably establish the diagnosis; even the test for antibodies directed against platelet GPIIb–IIIa and/or GPIb–IX is considered of potential utility only [26].

10.2.3 Therapy

Treatment of thrombocytopenia in the context of APS depends on clinical manifestations, serologic profile, comorbidities, and other thrombotic risk factors. While therapy for patients with an established ITP diagnosis is quite well defined, the treatment in case of aPL antibodies positivity in patients asymptomatic or with non-classification criteria is still a matter of debate. In the recent years, various guidelines have been published for the treatment of ITP, which usually starts at platelet values $25–30 \times 10^9$/L, provided that no other bleeding factors are present [8–10, 26]. This is of particular importance in APS patients, since aspirin and anticoagulants are frequent concurrent medications. In fact, a long-term oral anticoagulant therapy is suggested for APS patients with history of thrombosis [27, 28], and obstetric APS patients should be treated with low-dose aspirin associated to prophylactic dosage of low molecular weight heparin, increased at full therapeutic dose in case of previous thromboembolic events [27]. In these cases, treatment of thrombocytopenia should be considered at platelet count above the "classic" threshold, although it is not proven by a definite clinical study ad hoc: in the clinical practice, a platelet value of 50–60 × 10^9/L is considered "safe" enough to administer concurrent anticoagulant or antiaggregant therapy, and 90–100 × 10^9/L is required for double antiaggregant; finally, anticoagulation and antiaggregation with platelets <20 × 10^9/L require carefully discussion of pros and cons in the particular clinical context [29].

First-line treatment of ITP usually includes steroids alone or in combination with intravenous immunoglobulins (IVIG). Steroids may be administered orally (prednisone 1 mg/kg/day for 21 days then tapered off over a period of 3–4 months) or, in particularly severe cases, as intravenous bolus (methylprednisolone 5–10 mg/kg/day for 3–5 days, followed by oral prednisone). Recently, high-dose dexamethasone (40 mg/day for 4 days, for 4–6 cycles every 14 days) was proven effective as standard prednisone (about 80–85 % responses), with possible lower side effects [30, 31]. However, looking forward for ongoing randomized controlled studies aimed to demonstrate the better first-line steroid regimen, the current guidelines recommend longer rather than shorter courses of corticosteroids, because the former are associated with a better sustained response.

Regarding IVIG, their use is recommended in association to steroids for severe cases, in steroid-refractory patients, and as first line before steroids when the latter are clearly contraindicated. The most common regimens are 0.4 g/kg/day for 5 days or 1 g/kg for 1–2 days, the former being the more used and the latter recommended by the guidelines. It is worth reminding that platelet transfusion should never be denied in the presence of major hemorrhagic diathesis. Of note, the clinical practice is different in APS-associated ITP, where immunosuppressors such as azathioprine are given as steroid-sparing agents even as first-line treatment and IGIV are used as second-line treatment. Moreover, hydroxychloroquine is increasingly used in APS-associated ITP for its anti-inflammatory and antithrombotic properties and ability to reduce the expression of GpIIb/IIIa on activated platelets [32, 33]. On the contrary, in primary ITP, there is no clear recommendation about the sequence of second-line treatments, i.e., splenectomy, rituximab, immunosuppressors, and thrombopoietin (TPO) agonists. The guidelines for primary ITP recommend that the choice among various options should be individualized, and patient participation in decision-making should be paramount [8, 26]. Splenectomy provides the highest cure rate (60–70 % of primary ITP patients at 5 years) but is invasive, irreversible, and associated with postoperative complications and its outcome is currently unpredictable [8, 10, 26]. In APS-associated ITP, the outcome after splenectomy is even more controversial, both poor and good responses being seldom reported [27, 34]. Moreover, the increased rate of thrombotic events reported after splenectomy may further discourage this treatment option in APS [28].

Rituximab (375 mg m^2/weekly × 4 weeks) was reported effective in about 50–60 % of primary ITP cases, with 20 % sustained responses at 5 years; it is generally well tolerated, and its short-term toxicity is acceptable [8, 26]. TPO agonists induce platelet count >50 × 10^9/L in 90 % of adults with primary ITP, are well

Table 10.1 Most common treatment options for primary ITP

	Treatment	Response rate	Sustained response
First-line therapy	*Corticosteroids*	~70–85 %	20–30 %
	Prednisone 1 mg/kg/day p.o.		
	Methylprednisolone i.v. 5–10 mg/kg/day for 3–5 days		
	High-dose dexamethasone 40 mg/day for 4 days for 4–6 cycles every 14 days		
	IVIG	>80 % transient responses	Poor evidence
Further lines of therapy	*Immunosuppressive drugs* (azathioprine, cyclophosphamide, cyclosporine)	~40–60 %	Not available
	Rituximab standard dose (375 mg/m²/week × 4 weeks)	~50–60 %	20 % at 5 years
	Splenectomy	~80 %	60–70 % at 5 years
	Thrombopoietin agonists	~90 %	Not available

tolerated and show relatively little short-term toxicity, but need continuous administration [8, 26] and no data are available in APS-associated ITP.

The guidelines for primary ITP conclude that at one end of the spectrum, splenectomy may be the preferred option for younger patients, who have the best response and lowest complication rates; at the other end of the spectrum, splenectomy is not recommended in patients over 65–70 years of age because of higher complications and lower response rates, and in very frail cases, with significant surgical comorbidities, and history or risk of thrombosis. The latter should be kept in mind because abnormal elevation of platelet count and thrombotic events are increasingly reported in patients treated with TPO agonists [10].

The most common treatment options for primary ITP are shown in Table 10.1.

10.3 Autoimmune Hemolytic Anemia

Autoimmune hemolytic anemia (AIHA) was reported to occur in about 10 % of APS patients belonging to a large cohort of 1,000 patients [1]. Moreover, several studies report high frequencies of positive direct antiglobulin test (DAT) or Coombs test in patients with SLE-associated APS. A significant association between AIHA and the presence of aCL IgG was reported in 41 patients affected by SLE [35] and later confirmed in a larger retrospective study including 305 SLE patients [36]. Furthermore, aCL antibodies were found in eluates from erythrocytes of patients with AIHA and positivity for aCL antibodies [37], and anti-red cell binding activity present in eluates can be inhibited by absorption on phospholipid micelles [38]. More recently, the associations between AIHA and various manifestations of APS were evaluated in 308 patients with APS, confirming a prevalence of AIHA of 10.4 % [39]. The authors found that odds ratio for AIHA was increased in the presence of aCL antibodies and livedo reticularis and that AIHA was associated with cardiac valvular vegetations and thickening, arterial thrombosis, and CNS signs of epilepsy or chorea; in addition, AIHA may identify a subgroup of patients with a significant risk for subsequent development of SLE. Moreover, AIHA at the onset of SLE was independently associated with renal involvement, thrombocytopenia, and possibly thrombotic episodes during follow-up [35].

On the other hand, patients with AIHA, both idiopathic and associated with SLE, displayed higher titers of aCL antibodies [40]. The role of aPL antibodies with regard to the reported thromboembolic risk of AIHA has been investigated [41–43]. In particular, Pullarkat et al. [41] reported venous thromboembolic events in 27 % of AIHA patients and detected aPL antibodies in 63 % of them, of whom 30 % had a lupus anticoagulant and 57 % aCL antibodies. There was a statistically significant association between presence of LA and occurrence of venous thromboembolic events. The target red cell antigen of aCL antibodies on red cells is still undefined: since cardiolipin is not present in the inner leaflet of erythrocytes, some authors have hypothesized a cross reactivity against negatively charged phospholipids (such as phosphatidylcholine) [43].

Clinically, AIHA may develop gradually, with concomitant physiologic compensation, or may have a fulminant presentation with rapid onset of profound, life-threatening anemia. Clinical features are determined by the rate and type of hemolysis, which mainly depend on the autoantibody's characteristics (Ig class, thermal amplitude, affinity, efficiency in activating complement) and on the efficacy of the erythroblastic response. In particular, cases with reticulocytopenia are often more severe and require high transfusion support; in these cases, an anti-erythroblast reactivity has been hypothesized to occur, with consequent intramedullary death or apoptosis of red cell precursors [44].

10.3.1 Diagnosis

The diagnosis of AIHA is based on the presence of hemolytic anemia and serologic evidence of anti-erythrocyte autoantibodies, detected by the DAT, and identified in the serum and/or eluate obtained from the patient's red blood cells (RBCs) [44]. DAT tube, the traditional agglutination technique, is usually performed with broad-spectrum Coombs reagents. Clinically, it is important to perform the test with monospecific antisera, to distinguish "warm" (WAIHA), "cold" (cold hemoagglutinin disease, CHD), and "mixed" forms. The former are due to IgG which generally react at 37 °C, are usually directed against epitopes of the Rh system, and mainly determine extravascular hemolysis. Cold forms are due to IgM, which are able to fix complement more efficiently than other isotypes, have an optimal temperature of reaction at 4 °C, are directed against the I/i system, and prevalently cause intravascular hemolysis. The presence of cold IgM autoantibodies can easily be revealed by the spontaneous agglutination of RBCs at 20 °C. It should be reminded that there are rare cases of warm AIHA caused by IgM "warm" autoantibodies that have more severe hemolysis and more fatalities than patients with other types of AIHA. This may be related to the amount of RBC destruction by intravascular hemolysis, calculated in 200 mL of RBCs in one hour, versus extravascular hemolysis which is 10-fold lesser [44].

It is important to remind that DAT with polyspecific or anti-IgG and anti-C antisera may yield false-negative results due to the presence of IgA, low-affinity autoantibodies, or numbers of RBC-bound IgG molecules below the threshold of the test (400 molecules per RBC). For the former two conditions, the use of monospecific antisera against IgA and low ionic strength solutions (LISS) or cold washings can overcome the DAT negativity; small amounts of RBC-bound IgG can be detected employing more sensitive but less specific techniques, such as microcolumn and solid-phase antiglobulin tests that are suitable for automation, or other more sophisticated techniques, such as the complement fixation antibody consumption test, the enzyme-linked and radiolabeled tests, and the flow cytometry, that are not routine in the majority of laboratories. The latter deserves a particular mention because of its high sensitivity, being able to detect up to 30–40 molecules of anti-RBC autoantibodies. Finally, the mitogen-stimulated (MS) DAT has been proposed as a functional and quantitative method for the detection of anti-RBC antibodies in mitogen-stimulated whole-blood cultures, which may facilitate the diagnosis of some DAT-negative AIHA cases [45].

Despite the numerous tests available for the detection of antibodies against RBCs, and the development of additional more sensitive techniques, about 10 % of AIHA remains DAT negative, and the diagnosis is made after exclusion of other causes of hemolysis and on the basis of the clinical response to therapy [44].

It is worth reminding that DAT positivity may be due not only to autoantibodies, but also to alloantibodies, possibly present in transfused subjects and in multiparous females, and responsible severe hemolytic reactions in case of RBC transfusion. Moreover, false-positive DAT have been reported in patients with hypergammaglobulinaemia or following high-dose immunoglobulin therapy [46]. Finally, 0.007–0.1 % of the healthy population and 0.3–8 % of hospitalized patients have a positive DAT without AIHA.

10.3.2 Treatment

The treatment of AIHA is still not evidence based as there are no randomized studies and only a few prospective phase 2 trials. Conventional therapy of WAIHA includes administration of corticosteroids as first-line therapy, which is expected to provide a response in 70–80 % of patients. Second-line therapy for APS-associated AIHA is mainly represented by immunosuppressive agents, such as azathioprine, cyclophosphamide, and cyclosporine, which generally provide a 40–60 % response rate. There is growing interest in the use of mycophenolate mofetil in patients with warm AIHA, particularly children; although limited to small series of patients, good responses are reported in almost all cases both idiopathic and secondary to SLE [47, 48]. More recently, rituximab (375 mg m^2/weekly ×4 weeks) has been shown to be effective in about 60–80 % of cases, either in monotherapy or in combination with corticosteroids and immunosuppressors, and regardless of prior therapy. The time to response varies considerably, with some patients responding very quickly and others taking weeks or even months to achieve their maximum response. Finally, rituximab re-treatment may be effective, and some patients responded to re-treatment more than once [49]. In attempt to minimize side effects and reduce costs, first-line treatment with low-dose rituximab (100 mg fixed dose×4 weeks) plus a short course of steroids was reported equally effective as standard doses, with an overall response in 89 % (complete response 67 %) and 68 % relapse-free survival at 3 years [50, 51].

IVIG are frequently used in AIHA, alone or in combination with prednisone, probably because of their proven effectiveness in primary ITP and the relatively low incidence of adverse effects. However, only small case series have been reported [44, 52], and the only large retrospective study of 73 patients [53] showed a response in 40 % of cases, only 15 % achieving hemoglobin levels of 10 g/dL or greater.

It is noteworthy that steroids are poorly useful in cold forms, whereas rituximab is able to induce a complete response in 10–15 % and a partial in 50 % of patients; this compares favorably with the next best treatment regimens which give about 15–20 % of partial responses [54–56]. Recently, fludarabine-rituximab combination therapy was reported very effective, resulting in 75 % response rate, complete remissions in about 20 %, and more than 66 months estimated response duration [57].

The effectiveness of other options, such as plasmapheresis and danazol, is controversial and mostly anecdotal [54, 55]. High-dose cyclophosphamide was effective in 4/5 patients, all of whom were previously treated with corticosteroids [58]. Other "last option" treatments include alemtuzumab, bortezomib, and eculizumab which have been shown to be of some efficacy in few cases [54, 59–61]. Moreover, the administration of erythropoietin was successfully used in patients with therapy-refractory AIHA, particularly in the presence of reticulocytopenia [62]. Finally, both autologous and allogenic bone marrow transplantation were reported in immune cytopenias, including severe AIHA and Evans syndrome [63].

Splenectomy, although not performed in APS-associated cytopenias, is considered the most effective second-line treatment for primary warm AIHA, with early responses in around 70 % of cases and persistent remissions without need of medical intervention for years [54].

The most common treatment options for idiopathic AIHA are shown in Table 10.2.

10.4 Leukopenia

It is known that antibodies anti-beta2-GPI may bind neutrophils [64]; however, the association between leukopenia and aPL antibodies is reported only in few studies. Cervera et al. analyzed the clinical and immunologic manifestations of APS in a cohort of 100 patients and reported that patients with APS secondary to SLE more frequently exhibited neutropenia than primary APS patients (38 % versus 2 %) [65]. This finding was confirmed by Vienna et al. [66] in a subsequent study on 56 patients

Table 10.2 Most common treatment options for idiopathic AIHA

	Treatment	Response rate	Sustained response
First line therapy	*Corticosteroids* (prednisone 1 mg/kg/day p.o.)	~70–80 % in WAIHA	30 % once the drug is discontinued, 40–50 % require maintenance doses, 20–30 % need additional second-line therapies
		~20 % in CHD	
Further lines of therapy	*Immunosuppressive drugs* (azathioprine, cyclophosphamide, cyclosporine)	~40–60 %	Not available
	Rituximab standard dose (375 mg/m^2/week × 4 weeks)	~60–80 % in WAIHA	>3 years in some cases
	Rituximab low dose (100 mg/week × 4 weeks)	~15 % CR, 50 % PR in CHD	~70 % at 2 and 3 years (similar for WAIHA and CHD)
		100 % WAIHA, 60 % CHD	
	Splenectomy	~70 % in WAIHA ineffective in CHD	20–60 % at 4–7 years

WAIHA warm autoimmune hemolytic anemia, *CHD* cold hemoagglutinin disease, *CR* complete response (Hb ≥ 12 g/dL and normalization of all hemolytic markers), *PR* partial response (Hb ≥ 10 g/dL or at least 2 g/dL increase in hemoglobin, and no transfusion requirement)

with APS plus SLE and 58 with APS. At variance, in both studies, lymphopenia does not correlate with aPL antibodies. These data suggest that in these patients, neutropenia is due to other factors involved in the pathogenesis of SLE, rather than to the direct role of aPL antibodies.

Recently, we prospectively studied 56 adult patients with idiopathic neutropenia (manuscript submitted) to investigate the incidence of infections and the risk of evolution in hematologic malignancies. Results showed that neutropenia was mild in 35 patients (median 1.36×10^3/μL), moderate in 14 (median 0.49×10^3/μL), and severe in 7 (median 0.3×10^3/μL); monocytosis was observed in 10 patients, lymphocytosis in 5, and MGUS in 6; antineutrophil antibodies were positive in 19 cases, and splenomegaly was found in 11. During the 4-years follow-up, mean neutrophils were stably under the normal range, with a great intersubject variability but without significant intra-subject variations. Mean neutrophils were lower in patients with antineutrophil antibodies, in males, and in cases with MGUS. A grade 2 infection occurred in 13 patients without relationship with neutrophil values. Eleven patients evolved into chronic NK expansion ($N=4$), hairy cell leukemia ($N=4$), and myelodysplasia (1 chronic myelomonocytic leukemia, 1 refractory cytopenia with unilineage dysplasia, and 1 with multilineage dysplasia). The median time to the evolution was 30 months. These data suggest that idiopathic neutropenia in adults is a benign disease without occurrence of severe infections, despite the concern of the general practitioner. However, a hematologic follow-up is advisable considering the possible evolution into clonal hematologic diseases.

Conclusions

Non-thrombotic hematologic manifestations have been largely reported in APS and are caused by antibodies directed against blood cells. Among them, thrombocytopenia is the most frequent, followed by autoimmune hemolytic anemia and few cases of leukopenia/neutropenia. Most information on these cytopenias come from primary ITP guidelines and studies on idiopathic forms of AIHA and neutropenia that should be put into the context of APS. Several diagnostic aspects are important, such as the distinction between warm and cold AIHA forms, which has therapeutic implications. For mild forms, which are the most frequent ones, treatment is simple and effective and mostly based on drugs that are already used in APS or SLE, such as steroids, IVIG, immunosuppressors, and rituximab. However, for severe and refractory cases of these largely heterogeneous diseases, a particular experienced attention by clinicians is required, and a tight and constructive collaboration with hematologists is advisable.

Take Home Messages

- Thrombocytopenia (platelets $<100 \times 10^9$/L) is the most frequent hematologic manifestation of APS (20–40 % of cases) and is generally mild and without hemorrhagic manifestations, in contrast with primary immune thrombocytopenia (ITP).
- No specific treatment for ITP is generally required for platelets >25–30×10^9/L.
- Steroid-refractory ITP in the context of APS is mostly treated with immunosuppressors and poorly responsive to splenectomy, at variance with primary ITP.
- Autoimmune hemolytic anemia (AIHA) occurs in about 10 % of APS patients and it is particularly heterogeneous from a clinical point of view.
- Warm (direct antiglobulin test + for IgG) and cold forms (IgM, C) of AIHA have different responses to available treatments.
- Both primary ITP and AIHA display a thrombotic diathesis, which should be carefully considered in the context of APS.

References

1. Cervera R, Piette JC, Font J, Khamashta MA, Shoenfeld Y, Camps MT, Jacobsen S, Lakos G, Tincani A, Kontopoulou-Griva I, Galeazzi M, Meroni PL, Derksen RH, de Groot PG, Gromnica-Ihle E, Baleva M, Mosca M, Bombardieri S, Houssiau F, Gris JC, Quéré I, Hachulla E, Vasconcelos C, Roch B, Fernández-Nebro A, Boffa MC, Hughes GR, Ingelmo M, Euro-Phospholipid Project Group (2002) Antiphospholipid syndrome: clinical and immunologic manifestations and patterns of disease expression in a cohort of 1,000 patients. Arthritis Rheum 46(4):1019–1027
2. Hughes GR (1993) The antiphospholipid syndrome: ten years on. Lancet 342(8867):341–344
3. Cuadrado MJ, Mujic F, Muñoz E, Khamashta MA, Hughes GR (1997) Thrombocytopenia in the antiphospholipid syndrome. Ann Rheum Dis 56(3):194–196
4. Galli M, Finazzi G, Barbui T (1996) Thrombocytopenia in the antiphospholipid syndrome. Br J Haematol 93(1):1–5

5. Italian Registry of Antiphospholipid Antibodies [IR-APA]. Thrombosis and thrombocytopenia in antiphospholipid syndrome [idiopathic and secondary to SLE]: first report from the Italian Registry (1993). Haematologica 78(5):313–8
6. Uthman I, Godeau B, Taher A, Khamashta M (2008) The hematologic manifestations of the antiphospholipid syndrome. Blood Rev 22(4):187–194
7. Lechner K, Pabinger-Fasching I (1985) Lupus anticoagulants and thrombosis. A study of 25 cases and review of the literature. Haemostasis 15(4):254–262
8. Cuker A, Cines DB (2010) Immune thrombocytopenia. Hematology Am Soc Hematol Educ Program 2010:377–384
9. Neunert C, Lim W, Crowther M, Cohen A, Solberg L Jr, Crowther MA, American Society of Hematology (2011) The American Society of Hematology 2011 evidence-based practice guideline for immune thrombocytopenia. Blood 117(16):4190–4207
10. Ghanima W, Godeau B, Cines DB, Bussel JB (2012) How I treat immune thrombocytopenia: the choice between splenectomy or a medical therapy as a second-line treatment. Blood 120(5):960–969
11. Portielje JE, Westendorp RG, Kluin-Nelemans HC, Brand A (2001) Morbidity and mortality in adults with idiopathic thrombocytopenic purpura. Blood 97(9):2549–2554
12. Enger C, Bennett D, Forssen U, Fogarty PF, McAfee AT (2010) Comorbidities in patients with persistent or chronic immune thrombocytopenia. Int J Hematol 92(2):289–295
13. Nørgaard M, Jensen AØ, Engebjerg MC, Farkas DK, Thomsen RW, Cha S, Zhao S, Sørensen HT (2011) Long-term clinical outcomes of patients with primary chronic immune thrombocytopenia: a Danish population-based cohort study. Blood 117(13):3514–3520
14. Kim KJ, Baek IW, Yoon CH, Kim WU, Cho CS (2013) Thrombotic risk in patients with immune thrombocytopenia and its association with antiphospholipid antibodies. Br J Haematol 161(5):706–714
15. Bevers EM, Smeets EF, Comfurius P, Zwaal RF (1994) Physiology of membrane lipid asymmetry. Lupus 3(4):235–240
16. Pierangeli SS, Chen PP, Raschi E, Scurati S, Grossi C, Borghi MO, Palomo I, Harris EN, Meroni PL (2008) Antiphospholipid antibodies and the antiphospholipid syndrome: pathogenic mechanisms. Semin Thromb Hemost 34(3):236–250
17. Galli M, Daldossi M, Barbui T (1994) Anti-glycoprotein Ib/IX and IIb/IIIa antibodies in patients with antiphospholipid antibodies. Thromb Haemost 71(5):571–575
18. Fabris F, Steffan A, Cordiano I, Borzini P, Luzzatto G, Randi ML, Girolami A (1994) Specific antiplatelet autoantibodies in patients with antiphospholipid antibodies and thrombocytopenia. Eur J Haematol 53(4):232–236
19. Macchi L, Rispal P, Clofent-Sanchez G, Pellegrin JL, Nurden P, Leng B, Nurden AT (1997) Anti-platelet antibodies in patients with systemic lupus erythematosus and the primary antiphospholipid antibody syndrome: their relationship with the observed thrombocytopenia. Br J Haematol 98(2):336–341
20. Godeau B, Piette JC, Fromont P, Intrator L, Schaeffer A, Bierling P (1997) Specific antiplatelet glycoprotein autoantibodies are associated with the thrombocytopenia of primary antiphospholipid syndrome. Br J Haematol 98(4):873–879
21. Harris EN, Gharavi AE, Hegde U, Derue G, Morgan SH, Englert H, Chan JK, Asherson RA, Hughes GR (1985) Anticardiolipin antibodies in autoimmune thrombocytopenic purpura. Br J Haematol 59(2):231–234
22. Stasi R, Stipa E, Masi M, Oliva F, Sciarra A, Perrotti A, Olivieri M, Zaccari G, Gandolfo GM, Galli M (1994) Prevalence and clinical significance of elevated antiphospholipid antibodies in patients with idiopathic thrombocytopenic purpura. Blood 84(12):4203–4208
23. Diz-Küçükkaya R, Hacihanefioğlu A, Yenerel M, Turgut M, Keskin H, Nalçaci M, Inanç M (2001) Antiphospholipid antibodies and antiphospholipid syndrome in patients presenting with immune thrombocytopenic purpura: a prospective cohort study. Blood 98(6):1760–1764
24. Cines DB, Liebman H, Stasi R (2009) Pathobiology of secondary immune thrombocytopenia. Semin Hematol 46(1 Suppl 2):S2–S14

25. Park SH, Kim JY, Kim SK, Choe JY, Kim SG, Ryoo HM (2010) Regulatory T-cells in systemic lupus erythematosus-associated thrombocytopenia: a comparison with idiopathic thrombocytopenic purpura. Lupus 19(7):888–889
26. Provan D, Stasi R, Newland AC, Blanchette VS, Bolton-Maggs P, Bussel JB, Chong BH, Cines DB, Gernsheimer TB, Godeau B, Grainger J, Greer I, Hunt BJ, Imbach PA, Lyons G, McMillan R, Rodeghiero F, Sanz MA, Tarantino M, Watson S, Young J, Kuter DJ (2010) International consensus report on the investigation and management of primary immune thrombocytopenia. Blood 115(2):168–186
27. Galindo M, Khamashta MA, Hughes GR (1999) Splenectomy for refractory thrombocytopenia in the antiphospholipid syndrome. Rheumatology (Oxford) 38(9):848–853
28. Boyle S, White RH, Brunson A, Wun T (2013) Splenectomy and the incidence of venous thromboembolism and sepsis in patients with immune thrombocytopenia. Blood 121(23): 4782–4790
29. Matzdorff A, Beer JH (2013) Immune thrombocytopenia patients requiring anticoagulatio--aneuvering between Scylla and Charybdis. Semin Hematol 50(Suppl 1):S83–S88
30. Cheng Y, Wong RS, Soo YO et al (2003) Initial treatment of immune thrombocytopenic purpura with high-dose dexamethasone. N Engl J Med 349(9):831–836
31. Mazzucconi MG, Fazi P, Bernasconi S et al (2007) Therapy with high-dose dexamethasone [HDDXM] in previously untreated patients affected by idiopathic thrombocytopenic purpura: a GIMEMA experience. Blood 109(4):1401–1407
32. Ruiz-Irastorza G, Crowther M, Branch W et al (2010) Antiphospholipid syndrome. Lancet 376:1498–1509
33. Giannakopoulos B, Krilis SA (2013) The pathogenesis of the antiphospholipid syndrome. N Engl J Med 368:1033–1044
34. Hall S, McCormick JL Jr, Greipp PR, Michet CJ Jr, McKenna CH (1985) Splenectomy does not cure the thrombocytopenia of systemic lupus erythematosus. Ann Intern Med 102(3): 325–328
35. Kokori SI, Ioannidis JP, Voulgarelis M, Tzioufas AG, Moutsopoulos HM (2000) Autoimmune hemolytic anemia in patients with systemic lupus erythematosus. Am J Med 108(3):198–204
36. Sultan SM, Begum S, Isenberg DA (2003) Prevalence, patterns of disease and outcome in patients with systemic lupus erythematosus who develop severe haematological problems. Rheumatology (Oxford) 42(2):230–234
37. Hazeltine M, Rauch J, Danoff D et al (1998) Antiphospholipid antibodies in systemic lupus erythematosus: evidence of an association with positive Coombs and hypocomplementemia. J Rheumatol 15:80–86
38. Del Papa N, Meroni PL, Barcellini W, Borghi MO, Fain C, Khamashta M, Tincani A, Balestrieri G, Hughes GR (1992) Antiphospholipid antibodies cross-reacting with erythrocyte membranes. A case report. Clin Exp Rheumatol 10(4):395–399
39. Rottem M, Krause I, Fraser A, Stojanovich L, Rovensky J, Shoenfeld Y (2006) Autoimmune hemolytic anaemia in the antiphospholipid syndrome. Lupus 15(7):473–477
40. Lang B, Straub RH, Weber S, Röther E, Fleck M, Peter HH (1997) Elevated anticardiolipin antibodies in autoimmune haemolytic anaemia irrespective of underlying systemic lupus erythematosus. Lupus 6(8):652–655
41. Pullarkat V, Ngo M, Iqbal S, Espina B, Liebman HA (2002) Detection of lupus anticoagulant identifies patients with autoimmune haemolytic anaemia at increased risk for venous thromboembolism. Br J Haematol 118(4):1166–1169
42. Hendrick AM (2003) Auto immune haemolytic anaemia—a high-risk disorder for thromboembolism? Hematology 8(1):53–56
43. Cabral AR, Cabiedes J, Alarcón-Segovia D (1990) Haemolytic anaemia related to an IgM autoantibody to phosphatidylcholine that binds in vitro to stored and to bromelain-treated human erythrocytes. J Autoimmun 3(6):773–787
44. Petz LD, Garratty G (2004) Immune hemolytic anemias, 2nd edn. Churchill Livingstone, Philadelphia

45. Barcellini W, Clerici G, Montesano R, Taioli E, Morelati F, Rebulla P, Zanella A (2000) In vitro quantification of anti-red blood cell antibody production in idiopathic autoimmune haemolytic anaemia: effect of mitogen and cytokine stimulation. Br J Haematol 111:452–460
46. Valent P, Lechner K (2008) Diagnosis and treatment of autoimmune haemolytic anaemias in adults: a clinical review. Wien Klin Wochenschr 120(5–6):136–151
47. Alba P, Karim MY, Hunt BJ (2003) Mycophenolate mofetil as a treatment for autoimmune haemolytic anaemia in patients with systemic lupus erythematosus and antiphospholipid syndrome. Lupus 12:633–635
48. Kotb R, Pinganaud C, Trichet C, Lambotte O, Dreyfus M, Delfraissy JF et al (2005) Efficacy of mycophenolate mofetil in adult refractory auto-immune cytopenias: a single center preliminary study. Eur J Haematol 75:60–64
49. Barcellini W, Zanella A (2011) Rituximab therapy for autoimmune haematological diseases. Eur J Intern Med 22:220–229
50. Barcellini W, Zaja F, Zaninoni A, Imperiali FG, Di Battista ML, Bona E et al (2012) Low-dose rituximab in adult patients with idiopathic autoimmune hemolytic anemia: clinical efficacy and biological studies. Blood 119:3691–3697
51. Barcellini W, Zaja F, Zaninoni A, Imperiali FG, Di Bona E, Fattizzo B et al (2013) Sustained response to low-dose rituximab in idiopathic autoimmune hemolytic anemia. Eur J Haematol 91:546–551
52. Barros MM, Blajchman MA, Bordin JO (2010) Warm autoimmune hemolytic anemia: recent progress in understanding the immunobiology and the treatment. Trans Med Rev 24: 195–210
53. Flores G, Cunningham-Rundles C, Newland AC, Bussel JB (1993) Efficacy of intravenous immunoglobulin in the treatment of autoimmune hemolytic anemia: results in 73 patients. Am J Hematol 44:237–242
54. Lechner K, Jager U (2010) How I treat autoimmune hemolytic anemias in adults. Blood 16:1831–1838
55. Crowther M, Chan YL, Garbett IK, Lim W, Vickers MA, Crowther MA (2011) Evidence-based focused review of the treatment of idiopathic warm immune hemolytic anemia in adults. Blood 118:4036–4040
56. Berentsen S, Tjønnfjord GE (2012) Diagnosis and treatment of cold agglutinin mediated autoimmune hemolytic anemia. Blood Rev 26:107–115
57. Berentsen S, Randen U, Vagan AM, Hjorth-Hansen H, Vik A, Dalgaard J et al (2010) High response rate and durable remissions following fludarabine and rituximab combination therapy for chronic cold agglutinin disease. Blood 116:3180–3184
58. Moyo VM, Smith D, Brodsky I, Crilley P, Jones RJ, Brodsky RA (2002) High-dose cyclophosphamide for refractory autoimmune hemolytic anemia. Blood 100:704–706
59. Carson KR, Beckwith LG, Mehta J (2010) Successful treatment of IgM-mediated autoimmune haemolytic anemia with bortezomib. Blood 115:915
60. Roth A, Huttmann A, Rother RP, Duhrsen U, Philipp T (2009) Long-term efficacy of the complement inhibitor eculizumab in cold agglutinin disease. Blood 113:3485–3486
61. Wouters D, Stephan F, Strengers P, de Haas M, Brower C, Hagenbeek A et al (2013) C1-esterase inhibitor concentrate rescues erythrocytes from complement-mediated destruction in autoimmune hemolytic anemia. Blood 121:1242–1244
62. Arbach O, Funck R, Seibt F, Salama A (2012) Erythropoietin may improve anemia in patients with autoimmune hemolytic anemia associated with reticulocytopenia. Transfus Med Hemother 39:221–223
63. Snowden JA, Saccardi R, Allez M, Ardizzone S, Arnold R, Cervera R, Denton C, Hawkey C, Labopin M, Mancardi G, Martin R, Moore JJ, Passweg J, Peters C, Rabusin M, Rovira M, van Laar JM, Farge D, EBMT Autoimmune Disease Working Party [ADWP]; Paediatric Diseases Working Party [PDWP] (2012) Haematopoietic SCT in severe autoimmune diseases: updated guidelines of the European Group for Blood and Marrow Transplantation. Bone Marrow Transplant 47(6):770–790

64. Arvieux J, Jacob MC, Roussel B, Bensa JC, Colomb MG (1995) Neutrophil activation by anti-beta 2 glycoprotein I monoclonal antibodies via Fc gamma receptor II. J Leukoc Biol 57(3):387–394
65. Cervera R, Font J, López-Soto A, Casals F, Pallarés L, Bové A, Ingelmo M, Urbano-Márquez A (1990) Isotype distribution of anticardiolipin antibodies in systemic lupus erythematosus: prospective analysis of a series of 100 patients. Ann Rheum Dis 49(2):109–113
66. Vianna JL, Khamashta MA, Ordi-Ros J, Font J, Cervera R, Lopez-Soto A, Tolosa C, Franz J, Selva A, Ingelmo M et al (1994) Comparison of the primary and secondary antiphospholipid syndrome: a European Multicenter Study of 114 patients. Am J Med 96(1):3–9

Heart and APS

11

Gentian Denas and Vittorio Pengo

Hell is empty, all the devils are here.

W. Shakespeare

11.1 Introduction

The antiphospholipid syndrome is an autoimmune disease characterized by the presence of antiphospholipid antibodies (aPL) and a hypercoagulable state associated with vascular thrombosis and pregnancy loss [1]. Thrombosis mainly occurs in the venous district, but arterial thrombosis is also common. Due to this vascular nature, a number of organs are affected in APS, and among these, the heart (Table 11.1).

Cardiovascular complications in APS may be directly related to the presence of autoantibodies or secondary to thrombotic vessel occlusion. These pathological mechanisms produce valvular damage due to the deposition of immune complexes; left ventricular diastolic and systolic dysfunction due to microvessel injury, atherosclerosis of the great vessels and coronary artery disease, myocardial infarction, and endocavitary thrombi; and right heart failure due to pulmonary hypertension. Both valvular abnormalities and coronary artery disease account for more than two-thirds of the cardiac manifestations in APS. Other cardiac manifestations, such as pericarditis and myocarditis, have mild subclinical features and may go undiagnosed in APS patients. Accelerated atherosclerosis is another feature of APS-mediated vascular damage. The pathological process may be mediated by the direct or indirect mechanisms related with the presence of antiphospholipid antibodies [2]. This review will focus on the cardiac presentations in APS patients: the pathological mechanisms, clinical presentation and diagnostic tools, and therapeutic considerations.

G. Denas • V. Pengo (✉)
Department of Cardiologic Thoracic and Vascular Sciences, Padua University Hospital, Via Giustiniani, 2, Padua 235121, Italy
e-mail: gentian.denas@unipd.it; vittorio.pengo@unipd.it

© Springer International Publishing Switzerland 2015

P.L. Meroni (ed.), *Antiphospholipid Antibody Syndrome: From Bench to Bedside*, Rare Diseases of the Immune System, DOI 10.1007/978-3-319-11044-8_11

Table 11.1 Cardiovascular manifestations in primary and secondary APS

	Features
Arterial	Atherosclerosis of aorta, carotid, iliofemoral, coronary arteries
	Thrombosis of the aorta or axillary, carotid, hepatic, iliofemoral, mesenteric, pancreatic, popliteal, splenic, or subclavian artery
Valve involvement	Valve abnormalities including leaflet thickening, vegetations, nonbacterial thrombotic endocarditis, Libman-Sacks endocarditis
Myocardial involvement	Ventricular hypertrophy, diastolic and systolic dysfunction, myocarditis, heart failure
Coronary artery disease	Embolization or atherosclerosis, angina, myocardial infarction, microvascular damage
Intracavitary thrombi	Peripheral embolization, myocardial microthrombi
Pulmonary hypertension	Pulmonary emboli, pulmonary arterial in situ thrombosis

11.2 Pathogenesis

APS is a prothrombotic disease caused by antiphospholipid antibodies (aPLs). The term antiphospholipid is a misnomer, because the antibodies itself are directed against plasma proteins, specifically the DmI of the β2GPI molecule [3]. The mechanisms by which this interaction causes the cardiac involvement are multiple and not fully understood. They are related not only to thrombosis [4] but also to the deposition of immune complexes in various sites and the cross-reactivity between antibodies and other self-antigens [5].

11.2.1 Valvular Involvement

Valvular involvement in APS is the most frequent finding. The pathological role has been attributed to the circulating aPL antibodies that may bind the valvular endothelium leading to superficial thrombosis or subendocardial inflammatory infiltration. One possible hypothesis for the genesis of aPL antibodies is the molecular mimicry; in fact, APS may be unleashed by streptococcal infections, and cross-reactivity between the streptococcal M-protein and aPLs has been reported [6] raising the possibility for an infectious origin of APS. In a study seeking to find the β2GPI-related target epitopes recognized by the self-antibodies on the valves, one of the β2GPI-related synthetic peptides was a specific target for anti-β2GPI antibodies deposited on the valves of APS patients [7]. This synthetic peptide was able to displace the anti-β2GPI anti-idiotypic antibodies by a competition assay [7].

The histological analysis on valve specimens in patients with APS revealed that the noninflammatory lesions were characterized by superficial or intravalve fibrin deposits, vascular proliferation, laminar or verrucous superficial thrombosis, intravalve capillary thrombosis, and calcification [6, 8, 9]. Microscopy revealed positive staining for aCL (mainly IgG), for immunoglobulins, and for complement (C1q, C3c, and C4) all appearing along the surface of the leaflets and cusps as a continuous ribbonlike layer with complement deposits being more granular [10]. On the other hand, control valves from aPL-negative patients and control tissue specimens from an APS patient do not demonstrate such deposits [10]. The deposition of aPL antibodies in the subendothelial layer of the valve initiates an inflammatory process [11] with upregulation of markers of endothelial cell activation while the inflammatory exudate was scant. α3β1 integrin, laminin, fibronectin, and a thick layer of collagen IV are present in the deformed valves, while controls did not express the integrin and had only a thin subendothelial band of collagen IV [12].

The two-hit model [13], the most accredited pathophysiologic mechanism relating the presence of aPLs to the clinical features in APS, can be used to explain the valvular damage in APS. Microinjuries in hemodynamically vulnerable sites expose negative phospholipids on the surface of valvular structures or on endothelial cells of intravalvular capillaries [14]. β2GPI changes conformation exposing the DmI to the immune system and is recognized by its antibodies; the resulting complexes cause cell activation and tiny spots of coagulation. Microinjuries, fibrosis, and calcification result in valve thickening and rigidity leading to valvular dysfunction.

A few words should be spent on Libman-Sacks endocarditis. This entity is associated with SLE and, although used interchangeably with APS, is strictly speaking distinct pathological entity. Unlike the bland lesions of APS, Libman-Sacks endocarditis is a true valvulitis replete with inflammatory cell infiltration [15].

11.2.2 Accelerated Atherosclerosis

Accelerated atherosclerosis has been found in APS patients more frequently than in the general population [16]. Data come from retrospective studies and case series. No prospective studies confirm an increased risk in APS. Some have postulated a protective role of aPLs against atherosclerosis [17]; however, most of the literature supports the pathological role of aPLs in the development of premature atherosclerosis. Direct and indirect mechanisms are held responsible about this pathological process. aPLs exert a direct proinflammatory and procoagulant activity on endothelial cells; on the other hand, indirect inflammatory/immune mechanisms are mediated by autoantibody cross-reaction [18, 19]. β2GPI is a major antigenic target for antiphospholipid antibodies.

Other than the abovementioned mechanisms, oxidative stress has a key role in atherogenesis [20]. Oxidized low-density lipoprotein (oxLDL) is the principal lipoprotein found in atherosclerotic lesions, and it colocalizes with β2GPI and immunoreactive CD4 lymphocytes. The oxLDL/β2GPI complexes are internalized by macrophages via IgG anti-β2GPI antibody-mediated phagocytosis [21] to form foam cells [22] leading to the formation of fatty streaks and atheromatous plaques. β2GPI specifically binds to oxLDL, but not to native LDL [23]. oxLDL/β2GPI complexes acting as an autoantigen [24] are closely associated with autoimmune-mediated atherogenesis. IgG anti-oxLDL/β 2GPI-complex autoantibodies and their immune complexes were detected only in SLE/APS patients and in its animal model and were strongly associated with arterial thrombosis [21]. Moreover, IgG autoantibodies against oxLDL/β2GPI were significantly elevated in about 40 % of patients with APS as compared to SLE patients without APS [24, 25]. The immune response triggered by immunization with these autoantigens leads to the progression of atherosclerosis [26]. In contrast, immunization with IgM anti-oxLDL antibodies derived from hyperlipidemic mice reduced the incidence of atherosclerosis [21]. These findings confirm the complexity of the atherogenic mechanisms in APS and a different significance of the classes and subclasses of anti-oxLDL antibodies (IgG and IgM). Other chemo-mediators, such as pattern-recognition receptors (Toll-like receptors and scavenger receptors), cytokines (such as IL-1, IL-6, and TNF-alpha), chemokines, and pentraxins (such as CRP and PTX3), have been correlated with atherogenesis [27].

The whole inflammatory response that derives from the above described pathological mechanisms leads to the enhanced production of mediators that stimulate leukocyte adhesion and recruitment to the vessel wall and proliferation of monocyte/macrophages and of vascular endothelial and smooth muscle cells. The production of matrix-degrading proteases and tissue factor by macrophages eventually leads to plaque rupture and thrombus formation [28].

11.2.3 Ventricular Involvement

The pathogenesis of ventricular dysfunction in APS in the absence of valvular or coronary artery disease is unclear. The histological findings range from microvascular thrombosis to endomyocardial fibrosis [29–31]. Several reports have related the presence of aPLs with otherwise unexplained (by conventional risk factors) ventricular dysfunction especially in young individuals [29, 31–33]. Histological evidence of inflammation, intramyocardial arteriolar immune deposits, and widespread thrombosis, with surrounding areas of microinfarction, has been reported [34–36]. Diastolic dysfunction of the right and left ventricle is a more prominent feature in patients with APS or PAPS compared to systolic dysfunction [37, 38]. Myocardial ischemia mediated by antiphospholipid antibody may slow isometric relaxation and impair left ventricular filling, in the same manner as reported in patients with coronary heart disease. Regional wall motion abnormalities in the left ventricle have been correlated to the presence of high titers of antiphospholipid antibodies [39] and might be related to myocardial necrosis due to microvascular damage or myocardial infarction from coronary artery disease. Moreover, microvascular thrombosis may contribute to myocardial hypertrophy [40]. Finally, endomyocardial fibrosis is a rare cause of myocardial dysfunction in patients with APS [30].

11.2.4 Intracardiac Thrombi

While intracardiac thrombi on the surface of prosthetic or morphologically abnormal native heart valves are often seen in patients with APS, intracardiac thrombi on either structurally normal valve leaflets or unrelated to cardiac valves and involving mural endomyocardium appear to be uncommon.

Although antibodies are thought to contribute to intracardiac thrombus formation, the exact mechanism is still unclear. One of the proposed mechanisms is the disturbance of the physiologic fibrinolysis by aPLs, which, in presence of predisposing factors, brings about thrombus formation on the endocardial surface [41]. Other authors have speculated that disturbances in intracardiac blood flow pattern might contribute to thrombosis [42]. Echocardiographic studies have reported the presence of spontaneous echo contrast in APS patients [43]. Spontaneous echo contrast is caused by reversible red cell agglutination produced by intracardiac stasis rather than by activation of the clotting cascade [44]. How aPLs may contribute to it, is another unexplained issue.

11.2.5 Pulmonary Hypertension

The pathophysiology of the pulmonary hypertension in APS is strongly related to embolism from the veins of the lower limbs, to in situ thrombosis, or rarely to emboli derived from the right heart chambers. Chronic thromboembolic pulmonary hypertension (CTEPH) then builds up over time. Pulmonary embolism alone is not the only actor in the pathophysiology of CTEPH, as the vast majority of the thrombi resolve within a few weeks of the acute event [45]. Although venous thromboembolism (VTE) is the initial event in the vast majority of cases, in situ thrombosis in the pulmonary vasculature may also have an important role, especially during the course of the disease. In situ thrombi are histologically indistinguishable from thromboemboli and thus their role is difficult to be established. On the other hand, a causative role for aPL in the development of CTEPH other than the increased risk for VTE has to be established. One of the proposed mechanisms is an interaction between aPL and endothelial cells on the pulmonary vasculature, leading to vascular remodelling. The whole process may be enhanced by the implication of endothelin-1, a peptide that induces vasoconstriction and stimulates the proliferation of vascular muscle cells, high levels of which have been found in plasma of patients with APS and arterial thrombosis [46].

11.3 Clinical Presentation and Diagnosis

11.3.1 Valvular Involvement

Almost a third of the patients with primary APS present valve abnormalities [47–49]. However, variability in the studied population, APS testing, and different echocardiography techniques (transesophageal echocardiography which is more sensitive than transthoracic echocardiography) account for a big variability in the prevalence of valvulopathy. APS-related valvulopathy is defined as the echocardiographic detection of valvular regurgitation or stenosis in patients with aPLs in the presence of valvular apparatus involvement including valve thickness of more than 3 mm involving the leaflet's proximal or middle portion and/or irregular nodules on the atrial face of the edge of the mitral valve and/or the vascular face of the aortic valve [1].

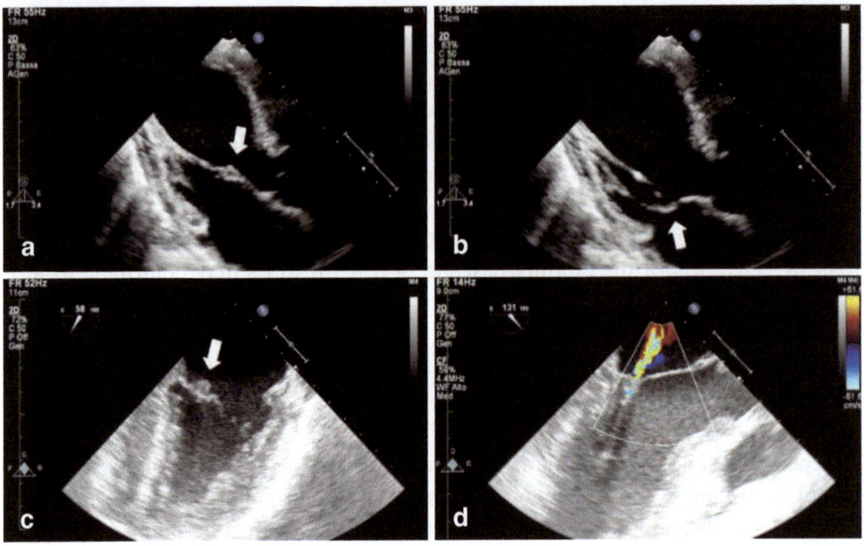

Fig. 11.1 (**a**, **b**) TTE showing thickening of the anterior mitral valve leaflet on its midportion (*arrow*) in a primary APS patient; chordal apparatus is not involved. (**c**) TEE showing typical vegetation on the atrial surface (*arrow*) of the mitral valve. (**d**) The same patient (as in **c**) had mild mitral insufficiency due to the valvular affection (Source: Echocardiography Laboratory, Cardiology Clinic, Padua University Hospital)

In a review [50] of the largest echocardiographic studies including 168 primary APS patients, the prevalence of valvular involvement as assessed with transthoracic echocardiogram was 32–38 % as compared to 0–5 % in the controls. Left-sided valves were most frequently affected, with mitral valve being involved more frequently than the aortic valve [43, 51, 15]. A rationale behind this distinction might be that the left-sided valves are more vulnerable to microinjuries due to stress, jet effect, and turbulence. This suggests that although the initial valve pathology may be simple nodular thrombi especially on the coapting site, the underlying inflammatory process leads to fibrosis [52]. In general, tricuspid valve seems to be seldom affected [47]. Subvalvular thickening and chordal apparatus involvement is also rare [53]. Heart valve lesions include irregular valve thickening that may evolve to vegetations and rarely lead to clinically significant valvular dysfunction (Fig. 11.1). Peculiarities of the nodular abnormalities resulting from thrombi at the coapting site of the leaflets are the focal localization and symmetry [52]. The extent of fibrosis may determine the degree of valve thickening as well as valve retraction or mobility. Mitral valve thickness can increase to up to 2.5 times that of controls [54].

Vegetations are seen less often but might be present in up to 40 % of the patients with aPLs as detected by transesophageal echocardiography [47] and are usually solitary but may be multiple. They present an irregular shape and are predominantly thrombotic but can be inflammatory or mixed, may be mobile or not, and change in appearance, resolve, or reappear over time [52, 55, 56]. Vegetations appear generally on the atrial surface of the mitral valve, while aortic valve vegetations have been described on both the ventricular and the vascular surface of the valve [57].

Valvular involvement is generally subclinical and leads to hemodynamically significant valvular dysfunction only in 3–5 % of patients [58, 51]. The valvular dysfunction results from an improper closure mechanism caused by fibrosis/thickening, valve deformity, and nodular vegetations, resulting in regurgitation. Valvular stenosis is seldom encountered in primary APS patients [43, 59].

Valvular abnormalities may be a risk factor for stroke, particularly with primary APS [60]. In fact, the presence of both stroke and valvulopathy was found in 77.4 % of all patients in one study [59], while thromboembolism in coronary arteries occurs less frequently (20–25 %) [47].

Considering echocardiographic studies, it is still unclear whether patients with primary APS have a higher prevalence of valvular abnormalities with respect to patient with SLE with or without associated aPL. Several studies using Doppler echocardiography have shown a higher prevalence of valve defects in patients with primary APS and SLE with aPL than in patients without these antibodies [51, 49, 43]. In fact, in large echocardiography study of 200 patients with SLE [61], aPL antibody positivity (IgG subtype) was most frequently associated with mitral valve nodules and the presence of moderate to severe mitral regurgitation. No correlation between aPL antibodies and aortic valve involvement was found [61]. The incidence of valve abnormalities in primary APS was as high as 82 % in one study [43]. In the same study, the authors confirmed that mitral valve thickening is most commonly found (63 %), followed by aortic and tricuspid valve thickening (32 and 8 %, respectively) [43]. Valve involvement in secondary APS has similar characteristics [15]. Localized thickening is generally confined to the base or midportion of the affected leaflet [62]. Vegetations, occurring in 10–40 % of the patients [47], are irregular in shape, broad based, and immobile [62, 39]. Lesions are also typically located on the atrial surface of the mitral valve and the vascular side of the aortic valve, with a predilection for the leaflet base [62].

11.3.2 Differential Diagnosis

Due to the nature and characteristics of the valvular lesions in APS, it might become clinically and therapeutically important to distinguish them from infective endocarditis (Table 11.2) and rheumatic disease (Table 11.3).

Noteworthy, aPLs may be present in some infectious diseases and even infective endocarditis [63]. On the other hand, culture-negative patients presenting with fever, and aPLs, can pose significant diagnostic challenges. Echocardiography becomes an important tool for the differential diagnosis as valvular lesions have discriminating echocardiographic features.

Vegetations of infective endocarditis tend to be solitary, asymmetric, of uniform echogenicity, and highly mobile [64]. In contrast to the vegetations of APS, they typically affect the low-pressure sides of the valves; they are typically found on the atrial surface of the mitral valve and on the ventricular side of the aortic valve. Furthermore, the adjoining leaflet or cusp is usually damaged in infective endocarditis. Anatomically, unlike the sterile vegetations of APS, infective endocarditis is characterized by a

Table 11.2 Differential diagnosis with infective endocarditis (see text for a detailed description)

Echocardiographic feature	IE	APS
Vegetation mobility	Mobile (pedunculated)	Mobile or immobile (broad based)
Tissue destruction	Present	Absent
Vegetation location	Usually near leaflet-free margins	Base to mid (especially SAPS) or free margin (especially PAPS)
Lesion number	Vegetations usually solitary	Single or multiple (e.g., kissing vegetations)
Echogenicity	Usually homogeneous	Usually heterogeneous
Symmetry	Asymmetric	Usually symmetric
Leaflet thickening	Absent	Often present
Mitral valve surface	Atrial	Atrial; occasionally ventricular
Aortic valve surface	Ventricular	Ventricular or vascular

Table 11.3 Differential diagnosis with rheumatic heart disease (see text for a detailed description)

Echocardiographic feature	Rheumatic valve disease	APS
Valves involved	Typically the mitral	Both may be involved, usually the mitral
Vegetations	Absent	Present
Increased leaflet thickness	Free margins toward base	Base to midportion
Chordal lesions	Frequent	Rare
Calcifications	Present	Absent
Leaflet fusion	Present	Absent
Valve stenosis	Frequent	No

combination of vegetations, destructive lesions, and abscess formation, resulting in severe early complications of the disease like chordal rupture and valvular destruction leading to acute heart failure [64].

Valvular involvement may be encountered in both rheumatic heart disease and APS, but their echocardiographic characteristics are different [65]. Moreover, other characteristics of valvular involvement in rheumatic heart disease, and that are unlikely in APS, are thickening of the subvalvular apparatus chordal structures, leaflet restrictions, commissure fusion, and leaflet and annular calcification; all these features are commonly found together especially in the advanced stages of the disease. In addition, unlike the valvular dysfunction in APS, rheumatic valvular disease usually progresses to stenosis rather than regurgitation. Another peculiar distinction is that unlike APS, leaflet thickening in rheumatic valvular disease generally progresses from the free margin towards the leaflet base. The chordae and subvalvular apparatus are typically thickened, fused, and foreshortened in rheumatic heart disease, while in APS, nodules may be seen attached to otherwise normal chordal structures [15].

Papillary fibroelastomas, a rarely encountered cardiac tumor, can also enter differential diagnosis with APS vegetations. These are typically solitary highly mobile vegetations, with a characteristic shimmering or vibratory appearance, and are typically located on virtually all endocardial surfaces [66].

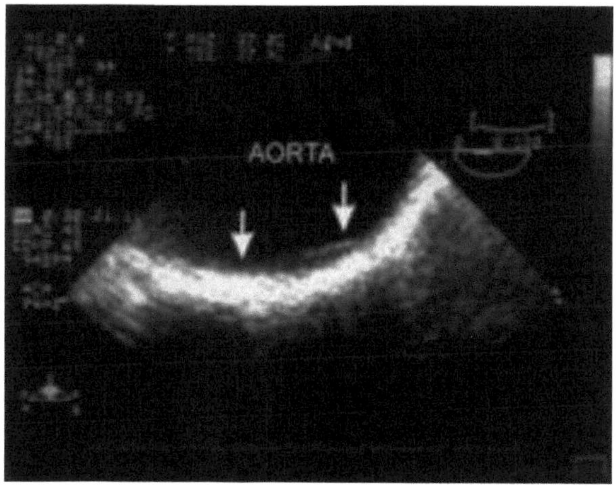

Fig. 11.2 Atherosclerotic lesion (*arrows*) on the abdominal aorta of a young patient with primary APS

11.3.3 Accelerated Atherosclerosis

Although premature or accelerated atherosclerosis has been associated with the presence of aPLs and APS [16], atherosclerosis in patients with primary APS has not been widely assessed. Existing studies are scarce and have dealt with a relatively small number of patients. Most studies have included both patients with primary and secondary APS. A higher number of carotid plaques have been linked to SLE-associated APS in comparison to primary APS [28]. In addition, secondary APS patients also had a higher prevalence of traditional risk factors for CVD [67].

Despite being frequently of subclinical entity, accelerated atherosclerosis is an important concern in primary APS because it may become clinically relevant rapidly in the young individuals [68, 2] and contributes to important cardiovascular morbidity (Fig. 11.2). In fact, premature atherosclerosis is a possibility in primary APS patients starting in their fourth decade of life [69], and most importantly intimal-medial thickness has been linked to a 3-fold higher risk for stroke in patients with primary APS patients as compared to patients without intimal-medial thickness [68].

Traditional (Framingham) risk factors for cardiovascular disease, such as hyperlipidemia, diabetes mellitus, smoking, obesity, arterial hypertension, and sedentary lifestyle, do not account for the increased risk for accelerated atherosclerosis in APS patients as their prevalence in APS patients is no different from that of the general population [19]. The increased risk might be explained by considering additional risk factors such as inflammation and autoimmunity (as described in the Sect. 11.2 of this chapter). Carotid arteries are most commonly affected, but peripheral artery disease evolving to claudication is not uncommon (Fig. 11.2).

Few specific studies aimed at the detection of atherosclerosis in APS have been performed and current information comes from cohorts assessing other cardiovascular manifestations of APS. Imaging techniques are sensitive enough to detect subclinical atherosclerosis by assessing early endothelial dysfunction, abnormalities of circulation, or atherosclerotic plaques [2]. Carotid intimal-medial thickness (IMT) is considered an early sensitive marker of generalized atherosclerosis [70]. In one

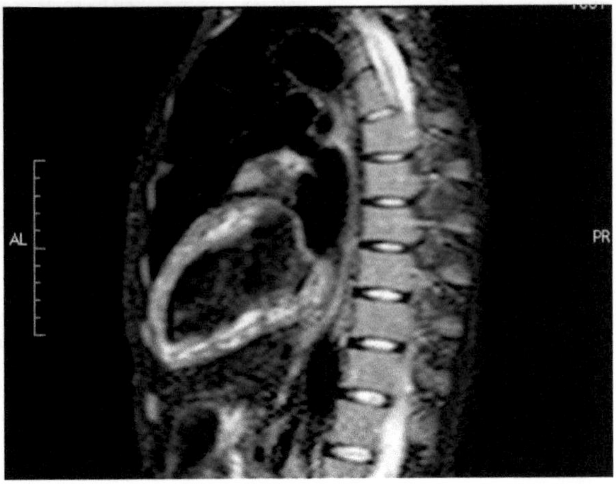

Fig. 11.3 STIR sequence images on a cardiac magnetic resonance in a patient with primary APS and diffuse myocardial ischemia, as documented by the diffuse subendocardial LGE, due to microvascular involvement

study, primary APS patients had significantly higher carotid intimal-medial thickness and reduced internal lumen diameter as compared to controls [68]. The authors [68] suggest that atherosclerosis in patients with primary APS develops primarily by generalized IMT rather than by atherosclerotic plaques. In the presence of continuous stressing factors, one of them being the persistence of aPLs, these lesions progress to manifest atherosclerosis [71].

Imaging studies have confirmed an increased incidence of early endothelial dysfunction and increased common carotid intimal-medial thickness in patients with APS [2]. An increased incidence of premature atherosclerosis was found in premenopausal women with APS undergoing vascular ultrasound; an increased prevalence of carotid and femoral plaques not related to any other predictors of atherosclerosis tested including age, lipid levels, or cumulative corticosteroid use was found [2]. Overall, patients with primary APS have a high prevalence of increased carotid artery intimal-medial thickness and lumen diameter decrease, with or without clinically relevant atherosclerosis. It may be easily detected with Doppler carotid ultrasound. Its detection may have important prognostic and therapeutic values, as this condition is related with an increased risk for stroke.

11.3.4 Coronary Artery Disease and Myocardial Infarction

Patients with APS have an increased risk of developing coronary artery disease. The mechanism of epicardial coronary artery involvement in APS is related to the risk of accelerated atherosclerosis; however, myocardial infarction can occur in patients with normal coronary arteries, due to thromboembolism or microvascular thrombosis (Fig. 11.3). Unlike the classic coronary syndrome, myocardial infarction in APS manifests in the young patients. Almost all the patients have structurally normal coronary arteries, while coronary artery abnormalities are seldom encountered and might be merely incidental findings.

In one of the largest cohorts of APS patients [72], myocardial infarction was a presenting manifestation in 2.8 % of the patients and appeared during the follow-up in 5.5 % of the cohort. However, the risk of myocardial infarction associated with aPLs in the general population remains unclear. There is still controversy as whether aCLs and aβ2GPI antibodies are associated with an increased risk of myocardial infarction and coronary artery disease in different settings of APS [73, 74].

Some authors have suggested a positive correlation between aβ2GPI and myocardial infarction in the setting of secondary APS. In a study on patients with cardiovascular disease, less than 2.6 % of patients were positive for aCLs, as compared to 36 % testing positive for anti-β2GPI [75]. The relative infrequency of aCLs in patients with CAD and APS without underlying autoimmune disease was confirmed in another prospective study [76]. The presence of aCL antibodies is also associated with typical chest pain and significant coronary artery stenosis on angiography and is predictive of myocardial infarction [49]. Despite the positive association with adverse events and outcomes especially in young patients [76], angioplasties [77], and coronary artery bypass [78] that has been reported, negative associations have also been found [79].

On the other hand, one prospective study evaluated the association of aPLs with CAD severity and adverse outcomes in patients with acute coronary syndrome [76]. The authors found that aPLs (anti-β2GPI and anti-oxLDL/β2GPI antibodies) occurred in patients with acute coronary syndromes and were strongly associated with the severity of CAD and adverse outcomes. Anti-β2GPI antibodies were found to be a significant risk factor for MI in young premenopausal women independent of other risk factors [80]. After adjusting for traditional risk factors, IgM anti-β2GPI was a stronger risk factor for MI than IgG.

The association of aCL and aβ_2GPI antibodies with the risk of recurrent cardiac events in postinfarction patients was assessed in a large trial [74]. High IgG and low IgM aCL antibody titers were independent risk factors, conferring a 3-fold higher risk of recurrent cardiac events. No significant association of the aβ2GPI antibodies with recurrent cardiac events was found.

Lupus anticoagulant (LA) has also been related to myocardial infarction. The odds ratio for myocardial infarction in patients testing positive for LA was 5.3 and increased to 21.6 in women who used oral contraceptives and 33.7 in those who smoked [79]. Neither aCL nor aβ2GPI antibodies affected the risk of myocardial infarction [79].

Because of the nature of the myocardial damage in APS patients (mainly due to microvessel involvement rather than conventional CAD), the condition might go unrecognized. Thus, the real prevalence of myocardial ischemia is not known. In one study, the prevalence of unrecognized myocardial scarring detected by cardiac magnetic resonance was surprisingly high [81]. Despite the low pretest probability for coronary artery disease and myocardial ischemia, late gadolinium enhancement (LGE) displayed a typical pattern of myocardial ischemia in 11 % of the patients with APS as opposed to 3.7 % in control subjects. The levels of aβ2GPI antibodies had a tendency to correlate with the presence of myocardial ischemia detected by LGE.

The discrepancy in the reported data comes from the differences in the study design, differing definitions of aPL positivity, and differences in the cohorts of patients studied. In fact, most studies searched for aPLs in myocardial infarction survivors rather than vice versa. Most studies searched for aCL correlation with myocardial ischemia; however, true high-risk APS patients are those with aβ2GPI positivity in a triple laboratory positivity setting [82]. However, overall, there seems to be an increased risk of myocardial infarction and recurrent events in patients with aPLs and that APS patients have an increased risk of developing ischemic heart disease.

11.3.5 Abnormalities of Ventricular Function

Limited data are available regarding abnormalities of ventricular function in APS. The prevalence of systolic and diastolic dysfunction in APS has been examined in very small studies. From the available data, there seems to be a distinction in ventricular function involvement in patients with primary and secondary APS. Patients with primary APS appear to have more diastolic dysfunction, while patients with SLE and associated APS have more systolic dysfunction [37, 83]. This might be related to the physiopathology of the diseases; SLE probably has a higher autoimmune burden and thus affects systolic function by other mechanisms rather than only autoimmune involvement of the myocardium [83]. However, APS itself seems to contribute to increased biventricular impairment than SLE itself. Thus, it seems that SLE may lead to subclinical systolic dysfunction, whereas the presence of APS (primary or secondary) possibly contributes to diastolic dysfunction [37]. Another peculiarity of primary APS seems to be the organic selectivity. In one cross-sectional study of patients with SLE and APS [38], the parameters of right ventricular diastolic function were more pronounced than the impairment of the respective left ventricular parameters in APS patients (systemic hypertension and valvular disease patients were excluded). Echocardiographic parameters reflecting diastolic dysfunction were associated with high titers of aCL, APS, disease duration, and pulmonary hypertension. There was gradation of severity, with more severe impairment in patients with primary APS followed by the group with secondary APS. One proposed explanation was that microvascular disease might have more effect on the right ventricle, which has a substantially smaller mass than the left ventricle. Furthermore, other factors such as pulmonary hypertension, frequently associated with APS (see below the dedicated section), may also explain the predominantly right ventricular diastolic impairment. In that context, pulmonary hypertension and primary APS were the strongest independent predictors of a prolonged duration time.

The effect of aPLs (in the absence of other confounding factors) in left ventricular size and function remains uncertain, due to the small number of patients studied. In a prospective study of 18 primary APS patients without clinically evident cardiac disease, the authors report a prolonged isovolumetric relaxation time, abnormal left ventricle early filling pattern, and decreased myocardial lengthening rate compared with age- and sex-matched healthy controls [35]. Others confirmed the impaired diastolic filling in primary APS versus age- and sex-matched healthy controls [84]. There are other reports showing that aPLs are not associated with significant abnormalities of myocardial structure, systolic function, or hemodynamics [61].

Available studies describe left ventricular diastolic dysfunction in patients with APS, in the absence of systolic dysfunction or other cardiac disease. The clinical relevance of these findings remains uncertain.

11.3.6 Cardiac Thromboembolism

Spontaneous intracardiac thrombus formation is a possibility in patients with APS. Thrombus formation can occur in all cardiac chambers, with a predilection for the right ones. It may occur spontaneously on native valves or mural endocardium or can be induced by manipulations such as placement of catheters or prosthetic valves. As discussed above, the mechanism of thrombus formation remains unclear.

Thrombi may be found on the right or left chambers of the heart. Some suggest the right side chambers are favored. In a study of 40 primary APS patients, thrombus formation was reported more frequently on the right side of the heart, contrary to valve involvement, which is mostly on the left [43]. Moreover, spontaneous echo contrast was reported in 11 % of the patients. Primary APS patients are at high risk of developing intracardiac thrombi even in the absence of predisposing factors such as atrial fibrillation and evidence of structural or functional abnormalities known to promote local stasis [59]. Thrombi were detected by transesophageal echocardiography in 16 % of the primary APS patients [59]. It was encountered more frequently in the right heart chambers, and interestingly, in one patient, thrombus was located in the left atrial appendage.

The finding of intracardiac masses in the absence of factors predisposing to thrombosis poses a clinical, diagnostic, and therapeutic challenge. The main differential diagnosis is between thrombus and intracardiac tumors such as myxoma [85]. The distinction should be made on the characteristics of the finding: myxomas are usually solitary, not calcified, and attach near the fossa ovalis of the interatrial septum, invasion of the underlying cardiac structure, eventual vascularization of the mass, and presence of calcifications. TEE should be performed for diagnosis and follow-up of embolic sources in patients with APS. Despite the high diagnostic power of TEE, sometimes, other imaging techniques, such as cardiac MRI, might be necessary in the diagnostic path [86].

11.3.7 Pulmonary Hypertension

Pulmonary hypertension is one of the feared complications of pulmonary embolism. It has been described with a prevalence of 1.8–3.5 % in patients with secondary and primary APS, respectively [87]. Although in one study, the incidence was 16 % [38]. It can be due to recurrent pulmonary embolism [88] from the lower limb veins, right heart chambers (as described above), or in situ thrombosis [89]. Pulmonary hypertension is a progressive disease and over time, it may become severe (Fig. 11.4) and cause right ventricular dilation, isolated tricuspid valve insufficiency, and right heart failure.

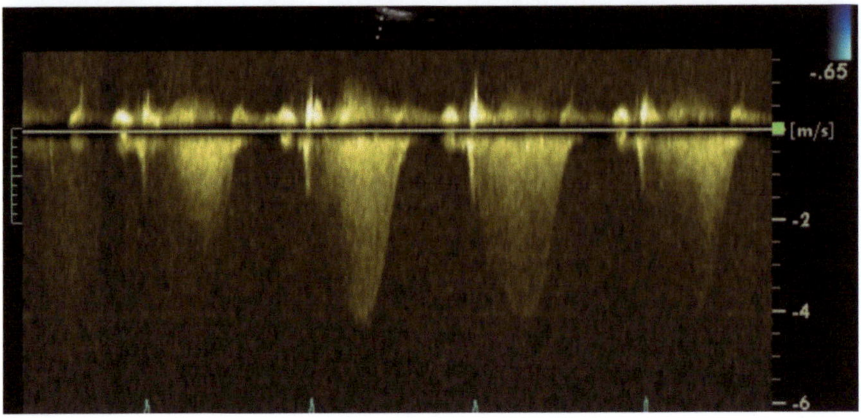

Fig. 11.4 Progressive severe CTEPH secondary to pulmonary embolism, in a patient with primary APS

A relatively high prevalence (10–20 %) of aPLs in patients with chronic thromboembolic pulmonary hypertension (CTEPH) has been observed [90]. However, not all authors have confirmed this association [91]. It is likely that aPLs might have a role in the development of CTEPH after pulmonary thromboembolism [92, 93] and, thus, testing for these antibodies should be part of the evaluation in such patients. How this could translate in a therapeutic tool is undetermined. Regardless of the etiology, CTEPH in APS patients is a severe condition, with a high mortality, and, generally, has a fatal outcome.

11.4 Treatment

The clinical presentation of heart involvement in APS includes a spectrum of conditions ranging from subclinical to overt disease. The mainstay of the therapy in APS remains anticoagulation. This section will focus on the therapeutic management of the cardiac conditions in APS.

11.4.1 Valvular Involvement

Valvular abnormalities in APS are among the best expression of the clinical spectrum of the disease: ranging from generally asymptomatic to overt disease that requires surgical intervention.

Anticoagulant therapy, the cornerstone therapy for the secondary prevention of thromboembolism in APS, did not prove to be beneficial in the regression of the vegetations in a primary APS cohort followed up by TEE for 1 year [57]. Despite therapy, valve lesions not only persisted unchanged but new lesions appeared during follow-up. Even when the follow-up was extended to 5 years, the results did not change [94]. Again, despite therapy with oral anticoagulants and aspirin, lesions did not improve or even progressed; new valve lesions also appeared.

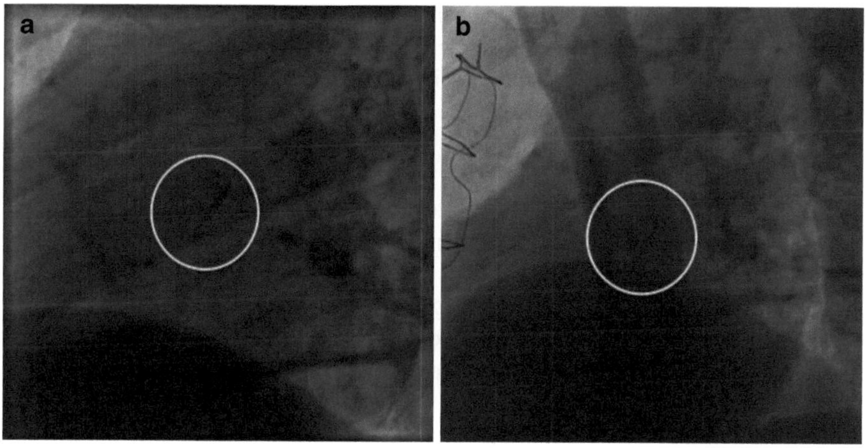

Fig. 11.5 (**a**) Fluoroscopy showing a thrombotic complication on an aortic mechanic prosthesis (*circle*). One of the leaflets is blocked by the thrombi, while the other moves freely. (**b**) Both leaflets are mobile after continuous heparin infusion (*circle*)

In a prospective TEE study, the investigators followed up primary APS patients for 5 years [43] and found that anticoagulants or antiplatelets were ineffective in the treatment and prevention of recurrences in valvular involvement; in fact, valvular involvement was unchanged (64 %) while new cardiac abnormalities were observed in 36 % patients. Long-term anticoagulation should be reserved to symptomatic patients with valvulopathy [95] and to reduce the risk of thromboembolic complications, not for the treatment of the valvular lesion itself.

The rationale for the use of corticosteroid therapy for the treatment of valve lesions in primary APS is not backed by either pathophysiologic or clinical data. Corticosteroids may reduce the inflammatory response but have no effect on the basic mechanisms of the disease. Their use may accelerate healing of valve vegetations, leading to scarring and deformity of the valves, thereby most likely leading to valve dysfunction [50]. Thus, despite consensus on the use of corticosteroid therapy for the treatment of valvular lesions in SLE, their use for the treatment of valvular lesions in primary APS is not recommended [50, 96]. The use of immunosuppressive or anti-inflammatory treatment in the setting of valvular lesions in PAPS is not backed by systematic studies, and thus their use is not recommended.

About 4–6 % of patients progress to severe valvular regurgitation necessitating replacement surgery [8]. Heart valve surgery in patients with APS is associated with considerable morbidity and mortality [97, 98]. The choice of the surgical procedure (repair vs. substitution), and the type of the valve (mechanical valve vs. a bioprosthesis), is extremely important. Despite the theoretical tendency toward a better outcome with mechanical valves, the use of tissue valves should not be sidelined [97, 98]. Due to the hypercoagulable state in APS, mechanical valves might develop thrombosis despite anticoagulation (Fig. 11.5), while tissue valves might have a minimized risk of such complications. On the other hand, there is some risk of immunologic deterioration of tissue heart valves. The choice of the type of valve remains an undecided question due to lacking long-term results [97].

Prophylaxis for infective endocarditis in patients with primary or secondary APS and valvular lesions is not recommended [99].

11.4.2 Cardiovascular disease: Accelerated Atherosclerosis, Ischemic Heart Disease, and Ventricular Dysfunction

As with other patients, treatment strategies in primary and secondary APS with cardiovascular disease (CVD) that include an aggressive control of all traditional risk factors including hyperlipidemia, hypertension, smoking, obesity, and diabetes mellitus should be performed by using both drug treatment and changes in lifestyle [95]. There is no difference in the general therapeutic strategies with CVD in the general population. Therapeutic options in CVD associated with APS include anti-platelet agents and anticoagulants, ACE inhibitors, β-blocking agents, and statins. Specific medications might be beneficial and these include folic acid, B vitamins, and, possibly, hydroxychloroquine [95].

Anticoagulation is usually prescribed in patients with a thrombotic coronary occlusion. Aspirin efficacy for the prevention of recurrent thrombosis in APS is poor. Based on two prospective studies [100, 101], an INR range of 2–3 appears safe and effective for the prevention of recurrent thrombosis in APS patients.

Ideally, young patients with STEMI should undergo primary angioplasty but might also be feasible in reestablishing coronary artery blood flow [102]. Available data on the short- and long-term outcome come from reports, some of which from more than a decade ago and, due to the advances in the field, are less relevant for the contemporary PCI. Other studies did not define and focus specifically on APS patients but rather searched retrospectively for antibodies. There are sparse reports on the success [103, 104] and failure [105, 106] of coronary artery stenting in APS. The long-term outcomes of patients with APS who undergo PCI were assessed more recently in a study of 380 PCI procedures, 19 of which performed on APS patients [107]. The investigators report worse long-term clinical outcomes in patients with APS who undergo PCI; this outcome was driven by higher rates of revascularization than other patients undergoing PCI. Importantly, despite the known propensity for thrombotic complications in patients with APS, no differences in the rates of MI or death between the APS and the control groups were observed. One of the reasons was deemed the anticoagulation therapy before and after the PCI, in addition to antiplatelet therapy [107]. However, treatment of these patients before and after PCI poses several therapeutic dilemmas, such as the duration of dual antiplatelet therapy in addition to anticoagulation, which might lead to increased bleeding risk [108], and the choice of bare metal versus drug-eluting stents, balancing the risks of thrombosis and restenosis versus bleeding [107].

Aspirin has been used for a long time to prevent CVD and reduce mortality in the general population. In the setting of APS, aspirin treatment has not been shown to add any benefit over warfarin alone; the use of aspirin may not be necessary in warfarin-treated patients [28].

Statin therapy significantly reduces the risk of CVD through beneficial effects on lipid profile, but also through pleiotropic effects on improving endothelial function, enhancing the stability of atherosclerotic plaques, decreasing oxidative stress and inflammation, and inhibiting the thrombogenic response [109]. Statins may also influence an aβ2GPI-induced proadhesive and proinflammatory endothelial phenotype [110].

Hydroxychloroquine might exert a protective effect, including benefit on lupus activity, hyperlipidemia, antiplatelet, and *desludging* effects [111]. It has even been reported to exert antiatherogenic properties [112]. However, despite these potential benefits, its effects on cardiovascular disease related to APS need to be clinically confirmed [28].

Corticosteroid use in APS-related ischemic heart disease is more harmful than useful and is not recommended.

In case of CAD, if coronary artery bypass grafting becomes necessary, the high risk of postoperative clinical events, despite aggressive anticoagulation and lack of significant preoperative comorbidities [78, 58], should be weighted against the benefits of the intervention. The perioperative management of these patients is tricky and there is no optimal method for assuring adequate perioperative anticoagulation. Due to the high risk of serious thrombotic or bleeding complications, the perioperative strategies should be carefully assessed and periods without anticoagulation kept to an absolute minimum [51, 58].

Ventricular dysfunction in APS has not been specifically addressed in terms of therapy; thus, standard pharmacologic approaches should be used [95].

11.4.3 Cardiac Embolism

Intracardiac thrombosis is a potentially life-threatening but treatable manifestation of APS. Thrombi have been treated with aggressive anticoagulation (prolonged heparin administration or thrombolysis) or surgical excision. It is unknown which option is the best therapeutic approach. Lifelong oral anticoagulation treatment (with an INR range of 2–3 in case vitamin K antagonists are used) should follow in order to prevent recurrences. Thrombus formation can cause pulmonary and systemic embolic events. In case of high risk for embolization, early surgical removal of the thrombus and adequate maintenance anticoagulation therapy might be needed for the treatment and prevention of recurrent intracardiac thrombotic events [113]. The high risk of intervention in these patients strongly supports an initial conservative approach.

11.4.4 Pulmonary Hypertension

Lifelong anticoagulation therapy is the cornerstone of the chronic pulmonary hypertension in patients with APS. In addition, if pulmonary hypertension is secondary to recurrent thromboembolism, the placement of an inferior vena cava filter may be recommended [90]. With the lack of data from dedicated trials, CTEPH should be treated like in the general population [114]. Patients should undergo vasodilator challenge to lead the choice of the therapeutic agent. Unfortunately, only 30 % of the patients respond to this test [90]. Calcium channel blockers should be used as the frontline therapy in responders. As the disease progresses and the frontline agents become inefficient, other agents such as prostacyclins, endothelin receptor antagonists, and phosphodiesterase type 5 inhibitors may be used alone or in combination.

In extreme cases of very serious disease in patients refractory to noninvasive therapeutic approaches, surgery can be taken into consideration. The surgical approaches include thromboendarterectomy or atrial septectomy. Transplantation is characterized by a high risk of failure due to the risk of renal failure because of immunosuppression [115].

The mortality in CTEPH in APS patients remains high and, in general, the outcome [90]. Women with pulmonary hypertension need to be aware of the high risk of maternal mortality associated with pregnancy [51].

References

1. Miyakis S, Lockshin MD, Atsumi T, Branch DW, Brey RL, Cervera R et al (2006) International consensus statement on an update of the classification criteria for definite antiphospholipid syndrome (APS). J Thromb Haemost 4(2):295–306. doi:10.1111/j.1538-7836.2006.01753.x
2. Shoenfeld Y, Gerli R, Doria A, Matsuura E, Cerinic MM, Ronda N et al (2005) Accelerated atherosclerosis in autoimmune rheumatic diseases. Circulation 112(21):3337–3347. doi:10.1161/CIRCULATIONAHA.104.507996
3. de Laat HB, Derksen RH, Urbanus RT, Roest M, de Groot PG (2004) beta2-glycoprotein I-dependent lupus anticoagulant highly correlates with thrombosis in the antiphospholipid syndrome. Blood 104(12):3598–3602. doi:10.1182/blood-2004-03-1107
4. Tripodi A, de Groot PG, Pengo V (2011) Antiphospholipid syndrome: laboratory detection, mechanisms of action and treatment. J Intern Med 270(2):110–122. doi:10.1111/j.1365-2796.2011.02362.x
5. Jara LJ, Medina G, Vera-Lastra O, Amigo MC (2006) Accelerated atherosclerosis, immune response and autoimmune rheumatic diseases. Autoimmun Rev 5(3):195–201. doi:10.1016/j.autrev.2005.06.005
6. Cervera R (2000) Recent advances in antiphospholipid antibody-related valvulopathies. J Autoimmun 15(2):123–125. doi:10.1006/jaut.2000.0405
7. Blank M, Shani A, Goldberg I, Kopolovic J, Amigo MC, Magrini L et al (2004) Libman-Sacks endocarditis associated with antiphospholipid syndrome and infection. Thromb Res 114(5–6):589–592. doi:10.1016/j.thromres.2004.06.039
8. Nesher G, Ilany J, Rosenmann D, Abraham AS (1997) Valvular dysfunction in antiphospholipid syndrome: prevalence, clinical features, and treatment. Semin Arthritis Rheum 27(1):27–35
9. Lev S, Shoenfeld Y (2002) Cardiac valvulopathy in the antiphospholipid syndrome. Clin Rev Allergy Immunol 23(3):341–348. doi:10.1385/CRIAI:23:3:341
10. Ziporen L, Goldberg I, Arad M, Hojnik M, Ordi-Ros J, Afek A et al (1996) Libman-Sacks endocarditis in the antiphospholipid syndrome: immunopathologic findings in deformed heart valves. Lupus 5(3):196–205
11. Amital H, Langevitz P, Levy Y, Afek A, Goldberg I, Pras M et al (1999) Valvular deposition of antiphospholipid antibodies in the antiphospholipid syndrome: a clue to the origin of the disease. Clin Exp Rheumatol 17(1):99–102
12. Afek A, Shoenfeld Y, Manor R, Goldberg I, Ziporen L, George J et al (1999) Increased endothelial cell expression of alpha3beta1 integrin in cardiac valvulopathy in the primary (Hughes) and secondary antiphospholipid syndrome. Lupus 8(7):502–507

13. Meroni PL, Borghi MO, Raschi E, Tedesco F (2011) Pathogenesis of antiphospholipid syndrome: understanding the antibodies. Nat Rev Rheumatol 7(6):330–339. doi:10.1038/nrrheum.2011.52
14. Garcia-Torres R, Amigo MC, de la Rosa A, Moron A, Reyes PA (1996) Valvular heart disease in primary antiphospholipid syndrome (PAPS): clinical and morphological findings. Lupus 5(1):56–61
15. Silbiger JJ (2009) The cardiac manifestations of antiphospholipid syndrome and their echocardiographic recognition. J Am Soc Echocardiogr 22(10):1100–1108; quiz 95. doi:10.1016/j.echo.2009.06.023
16. Cervera R, Boffa MC, Khamashta MA, Hughes GR (2009) The Euro-Phospholipid project: epidemiology of the antiphospholipid syndrome in Europe. Lupus 18(10):889–893. doi:10.1177/0961203309106832
17. Mackworth-Young CG (2004) Antiphospholipid syndrome: multiple mechanisms. Clin Exp Immunol 136(3):393–401. doi:10.1111/j.1365-2249.2004.02497.x
18. Shoenfeld Y, Harats D, George J (1998) Atherosclerosis and the antiphospholipid syndrome: a link unravelled? Lupus 7(Suppl 2):S140–S143
19. Jara LJ, Medina G, Vera-Lastra O, Shoenfeld Y (2003) Atherosclerosis and antiphospholipid syndrome. Clin Rev Allergy Immunol 25(1):79–88. doi:10.1385/CRIAI:25:1:79
20. Matsuura E, Lopez LR (2004) Are oxidized LDL/beta2-glycoprotein I complexes pathogenic antigens in autoimmune-mediated atherosclerosis? Clin Dev Immunol 11(2):103–111
21. Matsuura E, Kobayashi K, Inoue K, Lopez LR, Shoenfeld Y (2005) Oxidized LDL/beta2-glycoprotein I complexes: new aspects in atherosclerosis. Lupus 14(9):736–741
22. Rhew EY, Ramsey-Goldman R (2006) Premature atherosclerotic disease in systemic lupus erythematosus–role of inflammatory mechanisms. Autoimmun Rev 5(2):101–105. doi:10.1016/j.autrev.2005.08.008
23. Kobayashi K, Matsuura E, Liu Q, Furukawa J, Kaihara K, Inagaki J et al (2001) A specific ligand for beta(2)-glycoprotein I mediates autoantibody-dependent uptake of oxidized low density lipoprotein by macrophages. J Lipid Res 42(5):697–709
24. Kobayashi K, Kishi M, Atsumi T, Bertolaccini ML, Makino H, Sakairi N et al (2003) Circulating oxidized LDL forms complexes with beta2-glycoprotein I: implication as an atherogenic autoantigen. J Lipid Res 44(4):716–726. doi:10.1194/jlr.M200329-JLR200
25. Lopez D, Kobayashi K, Merrill JT, Matsuura E, Lopez LR (2003) IgG autoantibodies against beta2-glycoprotein I complexed with a lipid ligand derived from oxidized low-density lipoprotein are associated with arterial thrombosis in antiphospholipid syndrome. Clin Dev Immunol 10(2–4):203–211
26. Afek A, George J, Shoenfeld Y, Gilburd B, Levy Y, Shaish A et al (1999) Enhancement of atherosclerosis in beta-2-glycoprotein I-immunized apolipoprotein E-deficient mice. Pathobiology 67(1):19–25
27. Rattazzi M, Faggin E, Bertipaglia B, Pauletto P (2005) Innate immunity and atherogenesis. Lupus 14(9):747–751
28. Soltesz P, Szekanecz Z, Kiss E, Shoenfeld Y (2007) Cardiac manifestations in antiphospholipid syndrome. Autoimmun Rev 6(6):379–386. doi:10.1016/j.autrev.2007.01.003
29. Lauwerys BR, Lambert M, Vanoverschelde JL, Cosyns JP, Houssiau FA (2001) Myocardial microangiopathy associated with antiphospholipid antibodies. Lupus 10(2):123–125
30. Azeem T, Vassallo M, Samani NJ (2000) Images in cardiology. Endomyocardial fibrosis associated with antiphospholipid syndrome. Heart 84(2):156
31. Murphy JJ, Leach IH (1989) Findings at necropsy in the heart of a patient with anticardiolipin syndrome. Br Heart J 62(1):61–64
32. Greisman SG, Thayaparan RS, Godwin TA, Lockshin MD (1991) Occlusive vasculopathy in systemic lupus erythematosus. Association with anticardiolipin antibody. Arch Intern Med 151(2):389–392
33. Al-Kiyumi WA, Venugopalan P (2003) Antiphospholipid syndrome presenting as dilated cardiomyopathy in an 11-year-old boy. Acta Cardiol 58(4):359–361

34. Kaplan SD, Chartash EK, Pizzarello RA, Furie RA (1992) Cardiac manifestations of the antiphospholipid syndrome. Am Heart J 124(5):1331–1338
35. Coudray N, de Zuttere D, Bletry O, Piette JC, Wechsler B, Godeau P et al (1995) M mode and Doppler echocardiographic assessment of left ventricular diastolic function in primary antiphospholipid syndrome. Br Heart J 74(5):531–535
36. Bidani AK, Roberts JL, Schwartz MM, Lewis EJ (1980) Immunopathology of cardiac lesions in fatal systemic lupus erythematosus. Am J Med 69(6):849–858
37. Paran D, Caspi D, Levartovsky D, Elkayam O, Kaufman I, Litinsky I et al (2007) Cardiac dysfunction in patients with systemic lupus erythematosus and antiphospholipid syndrome. Ann Rheum Dis 66(4):506–510. doi:10.1136/ard.2005.044073
38. Tektonidou MG, Ioannidis JP, Moyssakis I, Boki KA, Vassiliou V, Vlachoyiannopoulos PG et al (2001) Right ventricular diastolic dysfunction in patients with anticardiolipin antibodies and antiphospholipid syndrome. Ann Rheum Dis 60(1):43–48
39. Nihoyannopoulos P, Gomez PM, Joshi J, Loizou S, Walport MJ, Oakley CM (1990) Cardiac abnormalities in systemic lupus erythematosus Association with raised anticardiolipin antibodies. Circulation 82(2):369–375
40. Leung WH, Wong KL, Lau CP, Wong CK, Liu HW (1990) Association between antiphospholipid antibodies and cardiac abnormalities in patients with systemic lupus erythematosus. Am J Med 89(4):411–419
41. Aguilar JA, Summerson C (2000) Intracardiac thrombus in antiphospholipid antibody syndrome. J Am Soc Echocardiogr 13(9):873–875
42. Coppock MA, Safford RE, Danielson GK (1988) Intracardiac thrombosis, phospholipid antibodies, and two-chambered right ventricle. Br Heart J 60(5):455–458
43. Turiel M, Muzzupappa S, Gottardi B, Crema C, Sarzi-Puttini P, Rossi E (2000) Evaluation of cardiac abnormalities and embolic sources in primary antiphospholipid syndrome by transesophageal echocardiography. Lupus 9(6):406–412
44. Rastegar R, Harnick DJ, Weidemann P, Fuster V, Coller B, Badimon JJ et al (2003) Spontaneous echo contrast videodensity is flow-related and is dependent on the relative concentrations of fibrinogen and red blood cells. J Am Coll Cardiol 41(4):603–610
45. Lang IM (2004) Chronic thromboembolic pulmonary hypertension–not so rare after all. N Engl J Med 350(22):2236–2238. doi:10.1056/NEJMp048088
46. Atsumi T, Khamashta MA, Haworth RS, Brooks G, Amengual O, Ichikawa K et al (1998) Arterial disease and thrombosis in the antiphospholipid syndrome: a pathogenic role for endothelin 1. Arthritis Rheum 41(5):800–807. doi:10.1002/1529-0131(199805)41:5<800::AID-ART5>3.0.CO;2-J
47. Roldan CA (2008) Valvular and coronary heart disease in systemic inflammatory diseases: Systemic Disorders in heart disease. Heart 94(8):1089–1101. doi:10.1136/hrt.2007.132787
48. Long BR, Leya F (2008) The role of antiphospholipid syndrome in cardiovascular disease. Hematol Oncol Clin N Am 22(1):79–94, vi–vii. doi:10.1016/j.hoc.2007.10.002
49. Cervera R (2004) Coronary and valvular syndromes and antiphospholipid antibodies. Thromb Res 114(5–6):501–507. doi:10.1016/j.thromres.2004.06.026
50. Hojnik M, George J, Ziporen L, Shoenfeld Y (1996) Heart valve involvement (Libman-Sacks endocarditis) in the antiphospholipid syndrome. Circulation 93(8):1579–1587
51. Tenedios F, Erkan D, Lockshin MD (2006) Cardiac manifestations in the antiphospholipid syndrome. Rheum Dis Clin North Am 32(3):491–507. doi:10.1016/j.rdc.2006.05.008
52. Qaddoura F, Connolly H, Grogan M, Orszulak TA, Schaff HV, Chandrasekaran K et al (2005) Valve morphology in antiphospholipid antibody syndrome: echocardiographic features. Echocardiography 22(3):255–259. doi:10.1111/j.0742-2822.2005.04021.x
53. Brenner B, Blumenfeld Z, Markiewicz W, Reisner SA (1991) Cardiac involvement in patients with primary antiphospholipid syndrome. J Am Coll Cardiol 18(4):931–936
54. Galve E, Ordi J, Barquinero J, Evangelista A, Vilardell M, Soler-Soler J (1992) Valvular heart disease in the primary antiphospholipid syndrome. Ann Intern Med 116(4):293–298
55. O'Neill D, Magaldi J, Dobkins D, Greco T (1995) Dissolution of intracardiac mass lesions in the primary antiphospholipid antibody syndrome. Arch Intern Med 155(3):325–327
56. Agirbasli MA, Hansen DE, Byrd BF 3rd (1997) Resolution of vegetations with anticoagulation after myocardial infarction in primary antiphospholipid syndrome. J Am Soc Echocardiogr 10(8):877–880

57. Espinola-Zavaleta N, Vargas-Barron J, Colmenares-Galvis T, Cruz-Cruz F, Romero-Cardenas A, Keirns C et al (1999) Echocardiographic evaluation of patients with primary antiphospholipid syndrome. Am Heart J 137(5):973–978
58. Koniari I, Siminelakis SN, Baikoussis NG, Papadopoulos G, Goudevenos J, Apostolakis E (2010) Antiphospholipid syndrome; its implication in cardiovascular diseases: a review. J Cardiothorac Surg 5:101. doi:10.1186/1749-8090-5-101
59. Erdogan D, Goren MT, Diz-Kucukkaya R, Inanc M (2005) Assessment of cardiac structure and left atrial appendage functions in primary antiphospholipid syndrome: a transesophageal echocardiographic study. Stroke 36(3):592–596. doi:10.1161/01.STR.0000154858.27353.df
60. Krause I, Lev S, Fraser A, Blank M, Lorber M, Stojanovich L et al (2005) Close association between valvar heart disease and central nervous system manifestations in the antiphospholipid syndrome. Ann Rheum Dis 64(10):1490–1493. doi:10.1136/ard.2004.032813
61. Farzaneh-Far A, Roman MJ, Lockshin MD, Devereux RB, Paget SA, Crow MK et al (2006) Relationship of antiphospholipid antibodies to cardiovascular manifestations of systemic lupus erythematosus. Arthritis Rheum 54(12):3918–3925. doi:10.1002/art.22265
62. Roldan CA, Shively BK, Lau CC, Gurule FT, Smith EA, Crawford MH (1992) Systemic lupus erythematosus valve disease by transesophageal echocardiography and the role of antiphospholipid antibodies. J Am Coll Cardiol 20(5):1127–1134
63. Kupferwasser LI, Hafner G, Mohr-Kahaly S, Erbel R, Meyer J, Darius H (1999) The presence of infection-related antiphospholipid antibodies in infective endocarditis determines a major risk factor for embolic events. J Am Coll Cardiol 33(5):1365–1371
64. Habib G, Badano L, Tribouilloy C, Vilacosta I, Zamorano JL, Galderisi M et al (2010) Recommendations for the practice of echocardiography in infective endocarditis. Eur J Echocardiogr 11(2):202–219. doi:10.1093/ejechocard/jeq004
65. Marijon E, Celermajer DS, Tafflet M, El-Haou S, Jani DN, Ferreira B et al (2009) Rheumatic heart disease screening by echocardiography: the inadequacy of World Health Organization criteria for optimizing the diagnosis of subclinical disease. Circulation 120(8):663–668. doi:10.1161/CIRCULATIONAHA.109.849190
66. Klarich KW, Enriquez-Sarano M, Gura GM, Edwards WD, Tajik AJ, Seward JB (1997) Papillary fibroelastoma: echocardiographic characteristics for diagnosis and pathologic correlation. J Am Coll Cardiol 30(3):784–790
67. Jimenez S, Garcia-Criado MA, Tassies D, Reverter JC, Cervera R, Gilabert MR et al (2005) Preclinical vascular disease in systemic lupus erythematosus and primary antiphospholipid syndrome. Rheumatology 44(6):756–761. doi:10.1093/rheumatology/keh581
68. Medina G, Casaos D, Jara LJ, Vera-Lastra O, Fuentes M, Barile L et al (2003) Increased carotid artery intima-media thickness may be associated with stroke in primary antiphospholipid syndrome. Ann Rheum Dis 62(7):607–610
69. Ames PR, Margarita A, Sokoll KB, Weston M, Brancaccio V (2005) Premature atherosclerosis in primary antiphospholipid syndrome: preliminary data. Ann Rheum Dis 64(2):315–317. doi:10.1136/ard.2004.023952
70. Grobbee DE, Bots ML (1994) Carotid artery intima-media thickness as an indicator of generalized atherosclerosis. J Intern Med 236(5):567–573
71. Der H, Kerekes G, Veres K, Szodoray P, Toth J, Lakos G et al (2007) Impaired endothelial function and increased carotid intima-media thickness in association with elevated von Willebrand antigen level in primary antiphospholipid syndrome. Lupus 16(7):497–503. doi:10.1177/0961203307080224
72. Cervera R, Piette JC, Font J, Khamashta MA, Shoenfeld Y, Camps MT et al (2002) Antiphospholipid syndrome: clinical and immunologic manifestations and patterns of disease expression in a cohort of 1,000 patients. Arthritis Rheum 46(4):1019–1027
73. Brey RL, Abbott RD, Curb JD, Sharp DS, Ross GW, Stallworth CL et al (2001) beta(2)-Glycoprotein 1-dependent anticardiolipin antibodies and risk of ischemic stroke and myocardial infarction: the honolulu heart program. Stroke 32(8):1701–1706
74. Bili A, Moss AJ, Francis CW, Zareba W, Watelet LF, Sanz I (2000) Anticardiolipin antibodies and recurrent coronary events: a prospective study of 1150 patients. Thrombogenic Factors, and Recurrent Coronary Events Investigators. Circulation 102(11):1258–1263

75. Iverson GM, von Muhlen CA, Staub HL, Lassen AJ, Binder W, Norman GL (2006) Patients with atherosclerotic syndrome, negative in anti-cardiolipin assays, make IgA autoantibodies that preferentially target domain 4 of beta2-GPI. J Autoimmun 27(4):266–271. doi:10.1016/j.jaut.2006.09.007
76. Greco TP, Conti-Kelly AM, Greco T Jr, Doyle R, Matsuura E, Anthony JR et al (2009) Newer antiphospholipid antibodies predict adverse outcomes in patients with acute coronary syndrome. Am J Clin Pathol 132(4):613–620. doi:10.1309/AJCP2FJUT2YZGITK
77. Niessner A, Hornykewycz S, Graf S, Nikfardjam M, Speidl WS, Probst P et al (2004) Preexisting anticardiolipin antibodies and development of restenosis after coronary balloon angioplasty: predictive value for a complicated course? Blood Coagul Fibrinolysis 15(4):311–316
78. Hegde VA, Vivas Y, Shah H, Haybron D, Srinivasan V, Dua A et al (2007) Cardiovascular surgical outcomes in patients with the antiphospholipid syndrome–a case-series. Heart Lung Circ 16(6):423–427. doi:10.1016/j.hlc.2007.03.010
79. Urbanus RT, Siegerink B, Roest M, Rosendaal FR, de Groot PG, Algra A (2009) Antiphospholipid antibodies and risk of myocardial infarction and ischaemic stroke in young women in the RATIO study: a case-control study. Lancet Neurol 8(11):998–1005. doi:10.1016/S1474-4422(09)70239-X
80. Meroni PL, Peyvandi F, Foco L, Bernardinelli L, Fetiveau R, Mannucci PM et al (2007) Anti-beta 2 glycoprotein I antibodies and the risk of myocardial infarction in young premenopausal women. J Thromb Haemost 5(12):2421–2428. doi:10.1111/j.1538-7836.2007.02763.x
81. Sacre K, Brihaye B, Hyafil F, Serfaty JM, Escoubet B, Zennaro MC et al (2010) Asymptomatic myocardial ischemic disease in antiphospholipid syndrome: a controlled cardiac magnetic resonance imaging study. Arthritis Rheum 62(7):2093–2100. doi:10.1002/art.27488
82. Pengo V, Ruffatti A, Legnani C, Testa S, Fierro T, Marongiu F et al (2011) Incidence of a first thromboembolic event in asymptomatic carriers of high-risk antiphospholipid antibody profile: a multicenter prospective study. Blood 118(17):4714–4718. doi:10.1182/blood-2011-03-340232
83. Laskin CA, Clark CA, Spitzer KA (2005) Antiphospholipid syndrome in systemic lupus erythematosus: is the whole greater than the sum of its parts? Rheum Dis Clin N Am 31(2):255–272, vi. doi:10.1016/j.rdc.2005.01.011
84. Hasnie AM, Stoddard MF, Gleason CB, Wagner SG, Longaker RA, Pierangeli S et al (1995) Diastolic dysfunction is a feature of the antiphospholipid syndrome. Am Heart J 129(5):1009–1013
85. Esteban E, Blanes A, Moreno MT, Canovas SJ, Montero JA, Sotillo JF (2002) Right atrial myxoma in a patient with antiphospholipid antibodies. Rev Esp Cardiol 55(9):999–1002
86. Erkan D, Erel H, Yazici Y, Prince MR (2002) The role of cardiac magnetic resonance imaging in antiphospholipid syndrome. J Rheumatol 29(12):2658–2659
87. Vianna JL, Khamashta MA, Ordi-Ros J, Font J, Cervera R, Lopez-Soto A et al (1994) Comparison of the primary and secondary antiphospholipid syndrome: a European Multicenter Study of 114 patients. Am J Med 96(1):3–9
88. Brucato A, Baudo F, Barberis M, Redaelli R, Casadei G, Allegri F et al (1994) Pulmonary hypertension secondary to thrombosis of the pulmonary vessels in a patient with the primary antiphospholipid syndrome. J Rheumatol 21(5):942–944
89. Chaouat A, Weitzenblum E, Higenbottam T (1996) The role of thrombosis in severe pulmonary hypertension. Eur Respir J 9(2):356–363
90. Espinosa G, Cervera R, Font J, Asherson RA (2002) The lung in the antiphospholipid syndrome. Ann Rheum Dis 61(3):195–198
91. Miyata M, Suzuki K, Sakuma F, Watanabe H, Kaise S, Nishimaki T et al (1993) Anticardiolipin antibodies are associated with pulmonary hypertension in patients with mixed connective tissue disease or systemic lupus erythematosus. Int Arch Allergy Immunol 100(4):351–354
92. Nagai H, Yasuma K, Katsuki T, Shimakura A, Usuda K, Nakamura Y et al (1997) Primary antiphospholipid syndrome and pulmonary hypertension with prolonged survival. A case report. Angiology 48(2):183–187
93. Font J, Lopez-Soto A, Cervera R, Balasch J, Pallares L, Navarro M et al (1991) The 'primary' antiphospholipid syndrome: antiphospholipid antibody pattern and clinical features of a series of 23 patients. Autoimmunity 9(1):69–75

94. Zavaleta NE, Montes RM, Soto ME, Vanzzini NA, Amigo MC (2004) Primary antiphospholipid syndrome: a 5-year transesophageal echocardiographic followup study. J Rheumatol 31(12): 2402–2407
95. Lockshin M, Tenedios F, Petri M, McCarty G, Forastiero R, Krilis S et al (2003) Cardiac disease in the antiphospholipid syndrome: recommendations for treatment. Committee consensus report. Lupus 12(7):518–523
96. Shahian DM, Labib SB, Schneebaum AB (1995) Etiology and management of chronic valve disease in antiphospholipid antibody syndrome and systemic lupus erythematosus. J Card Surg 10(2):133–139
97. Gorki H, Malinovski V, Stanbridge RD (2008) The antiphospholipid syndrome and heart valve surgery. Eur J Cardiothorac Surg 33(2):168–181. doi:10.1016/j.ejcts.2007.11.004
98. Colli A, Mestres CA, Espinosa G, Plasin MA, Pomar JL, Font J et al (2010) Heart valve surgery in patients with the antiphospholipid syndrome: analysis of a series of nine cases. Eur J Cardiothorac Surg 37(1):154–158. doi:10.1016/j.ejcts.2009.06.046
99. Habib G, Hoen B, Tornos P, Thuny F, Prendergast B, Vilacosta I et al (2009) Guidelines on the prevention, diagnosis, and treatment of infective endocarditis (new version 2009): the Task Force on the Prevention, Diagnosis, and Treatment of Infective Endocarditis of the European Society of Cardiology (ESC). Endorsed by the European Society of Clinical Microbiology and Infectious Diseases (ESCMID) and the International Society of Chemotherapy (ISC) for Infection and Cancer. Eur Heart J 30(19):2369–2413
100. Crowther MA, Ginsberg JS, Julian J, Denburg J, Hirsh J, Douketis J et al (2003) A comparison of two intensities of warfarin for the prevention of recurrent thrombosis in patients with the antiphospholipid antibody syndrome. N Engl J Med 349(12):1133–1138. doi:10.1056/NEJMoa035241
101. Finazzi G, Marchioli R, Brancaccio V, Schinco P, Wisloff F, Musial J et al (2005) A randomized clinical trial of high-intensity warfarin vs. conventional antithrombotic therapy for the prevention of recurrent thrombosis in patients with the antiphospholipid syndrome (WAPS). J Thromb Haemost 3(5):848–853. doi:10.1111/j.1538-7836.2005.01340.x
102. Takeuchi S, Obayashi T, Toyama J (1998) Primary antiphospholipid syndrome with acute myocardial infarction recanalised by PTCA. Heart 79(1):96–98
103. Biceroglu S, Ildizli Demirbas M, Karaca M, Yalcin M, Yilmaz H (2010) Acute thrombotic occlusion of right coronary and left circumflex coronary arteries in a patient with antiphospholipid syndrome: successful stent implantation. Case Rep Med 2010:198594. doi:10.1155/2010/198594
104. Jankowski M, Dudek D, Dubiel JS, Musial J (1998) Successful coronary stent implantation in a patient with primary antiphospholipid syndrome. Blood Coagul Fibrinolysis 9(8):753–756
105. Su HM, Lee KT, Chu CS, Sheu SH, Lai WT (2003) Acute thrombosis after elective direct intracoronary stenting in primary antiphospholipid syndrome: a case report. Kaohsiung J Med Sci 19(4):177–182. doi:10.1016/S1607-551X(09)70468-1
106. Weissman A, Coplan NL (2006) Antiphospholipid antibody syndrome and acute stent thrombosis. Rev Cardiovasc Med 7(4):244–246
107. Perl L, Netzer A, Rechavia E, Bental T, Assali A, Codner P et al (2012) Long-term outcome of patients with antiphospholipid syndrome who undergo percutaneous coronary intervention. Cardiology 122(2):76–82. doi:10.1159/000338347
108. Denas G, Padayattil Jose S, Gresele P, Erba N, Testa S, De Micheli V et al (2013) Major bleeding in patients undergoing PCI and triple or dual antithrombotic therapy: a parallel-cohort study. J Thromb Thrombolysis 35(2):178–184. doi:10.1007/s11239-012-0790-y
109. Liao JK, Laufs U (2005) Pleiotropic effects of statins. Annu Rev Pharmacol Toxicol 45:89–118. doi:10.1146/annurev.pharmtox.45.120403.095748
110. Meroni PL, Borghi MO, Raschi E, Ventura D, Sarzi Puttini PC, Atzeni F et al (2004) Inflammatory response and the endothelium. Thromb Res 114(5–6):329–334. doi:10.1016/j.thromres.2004.06.045
111. Petri M (2000) Hopkins Lupus Cohort 1999 update. Rheum Dis Clin North Am 26(2):199–213, v
112. Bruce IN (2005) Cardiovascular disease in lupus patients: should all patients be treated with statins and aspirin? Best Pract Res Clin Rheumatol 19(5):823–838. doi:10.1016/j.berh.2005.05.001

113. Ye ZX, Yu WC, Hsueh CM, Leu HB, Chen JW, Lin SJ (2005) Antiphospholipid syndrome presenting as intracardiac thrombus with pulmonary embolism. Circ J 69(10):1290–1292
114. Galie N, Hoeper MM, Humbert M, Torbicki A, Vachiery JL, Barbera JA et al (2009) Guidelines for the diagnosis and treatment of pulmonary hypertension: the Task Force for the Diagnosis and Treatment of Pulmonary Hypertension of the European Society of Cardiology (ESC) and the European Respiratory Society (ERS), endorsed by the International Society of Heart and Lung Transplantation (ISHLT). Eur Heart J 30(20):2493–2537. doi:10.1093/eurheartj/ehp297
115. Pengo V, Biasiolo A, Marson P, De Silvestro G, Agostini C, Livi U (1996) Immunosuppressive treatment in a heart transplantation candidate with antiphospholipid syndrome. Clin Rheumatol 15(5):504–507

Skin Involvement in Antiphospholipid Syndrome

12

Angelo Valerio Marzano, Silvia Alberti Violetti, Riccardo Lazzari, and Emilio Berti

12.1 Introduction

Since the first description of antiphospholipid syndrome (APS) [1], a number of dermatological manifestations have been described (Table 12.1) [2–5]. The skin involvement is frequently the presenting feature of the syndrome and, although none of the cutaneous lesions is pathognomonic for APS, some of them may be helpful for its diagnosis [2–5]. The cutaneous manifestations of APS range from mild symptoms like livedo reticularis to life-threatening conditions such as widespread skin necrosis. Livedo reticularis represents the skin sign most frequently seen in APS and is significantly associated with ischemic arterial events [2, 3]; on the other hand, anetoderma, malignant atrophic papulosis, ulcerations resembling pyoderma gangrenosum, and widespread necrosis are conditions regarded as rarely occurring during the course of APS [2].

12.2 Livedo Reticularis

Livedo reticularis (LR) is the most frequently associated cutaneous manifestation in patients with APS, seen as the presenting sign in up to 40 % of patients and observed in up to 70 % of patients who suffer from APS secondary to systemic

A.V. Marzano, MD (✉) • S.Alberti Violetti, MD • R. Lazzari, MD
Dipartimento di Fisiopatologia Medico-Chirurgica e dei Trapianti,
Università degli Studi di Milano, Milan, Italy

Unità Operativa di Dermatologia, IRCCS Fondazione Ca' Granda,
Ospedale Maggiore Policlinico, Via Pace 9, Milan 20122, Italy
e-mail: angelovalerio.marzano@policlinico.mi.it

E. Berti, MD
Università degli Studi di Milano-Bicocca,
Unità Operativa di Dermatologia, IRCCS Fondazione Ca' Granda,
Ospedale Maggiore Policlinico, Milan, Italy

© Springer International Publishing Switzerland 2015

P.L. Meroni (ed.), *Antiphospholipid Antibody Syndrome: From Bench to Bedside*,
Rare Diseases of the Immune System, DOI 10.1007/978-3-319-11044-8_12

Table 12.1 Dermatologic manifestations associated with the antiphospholipid syndrome

Livedo reticularis
Skin ulcerations
Postphlebitic/Postthrombotic
Livedoid vasculopathy-like
Pyoderma gangrenosum-like
Digital gangrene
Pseudovasculitic manifestations
Purpura
Palmar/plantar erythema and/or cyanosis
Papules/nodules
Malignant atrophic papulosis-like
Extensive cutaneous necrosis
Subungual splinter hemorrhages
Anetoderma
Thrombocytopenic purpura

lupus erythematosus (SLE) [6]. LR is a mottled red or bluish discoloration of the skin with a net-like pattern induced by a vascular disturbance with stagnation of blood in dilated superficial capillaries and venules [2]. It is due to reduced blood flow and lowered oxygen tension at the peripheries of the skin segments. The vascular units in the skin are arranged in inverted cones, supplied by a central arteriole coming perpendicularly from vessels in the fascia: the clinical feature of LR results from deposits of deoxygenated blood at the junction between cones [3]. In the English literature, the term *cutis marmorata* is used for physiological livedo, characterized by regular, unbroken, symmetrical circles, mainly localized on the limbs of children or young women. It is usually vasomotor with variations depending on temperature. LR refers to all other livedos; the so-called livedo racemosa is characterized by an irregular pattern with broken large branches and is localized not only on the limbs but also on the trunk and buttocks. Histopathology of LR is usually not conclusive because it does not show thrombosis [2, 6]; however, vascular proliferation or endarteritis obliterans of arterioles has been reported [3]. The pathophysiology is unclear but it may be related to interaction of antiphospholipid antibodies (aPLs) with endothelial cells, leading to endothelial dysfunction and arterial thrombosis [7]. Frances et al. [2] found that LR is more frequently associated with arterial events than venous thrombosis in patients with APS, proposing this skin sign as a useful marker for the arterial subset of APS. No treatment has proven to be effective for LR, which may spread or appear despite anticoagulant or antiplatelet therapies. Considering the high prevalence of arterial thrombosis in patients with LR in the context of APS, it is important to reduce other risk factors such as smoking or oral contraceptives containing estrogen [6].

12.3 Idiopathic Livedo Reticularis with Cerebrovascular Accidents (Sneddon's Syndrome)

Sneddon's syndrome is a rare disorder of uncertain pathophysiology, described by Sneddon in 1965 [8]. It is clinically characterized by the association of LR with cerebrovascular accidents, consisting of strokes or transient ischemic attacks. It affects young or middle-aged women, before the age of 45 years. LR, typically occurring on the trunk and buttocks, but also on the extremities and face, may precede the onset of cerebral manifestations by years [7]. Cutaneous manifestations other than LR include acrocyanosis, Raynaud's phenomenon, and, less frequently, skin necrosis. In Sneddon's syndrome, skin biopsy is usually nondiagnostic, because no specific histopathological changes are detected in the majority of cases [4]. However, Zelger et al. [9], studying a large series of LR skin specimens taken from Sneddon's syndrome patients, found that only small- to medium-sized arteries at the dermal-subcutis edge are involved in a stage-specific pattern. Early lesions are characterized by a lymphohistiocytic endotheliitis with partial or complete occlusion of vascular lumen. In intermediate phase lesions, histology shows proliferating subendothelial cells and dilated capillaries in the adventitia of the occluded vessel, evolving in fibrosis and shrinkage of vessels in the late phase. Two distinct subsets of Sneddon's syndrome have been categorized: one is aPL related with preferential arteriolar involvement and the other is regarded as a primary non-aPL-related small artery disease, primarily affecting the brain and skin vessels [7]. The relationship between Sneddon's syndrome and APS is under debate. The reported prevalence of aPLs in Sneddon's syndrome ranges from 0 to 85 % and some authors have suggested that the positivity of aPLs may identify a subgroup of primary APS [10].

Chronic anticoagulation with warfarin is warranted for patients with Sneddon's syndrome, although this treatment is not effective for livedo; low-dose antiplatelet therapy with aspirin is frequently used, although its efficacy is not proven [11].

12.4 Skin Ulcerations

Skin ulcerations are a well-known feature in patients with lupus anticoagulant positivity; in a European study on 1,000 patients with APS, the frequency of leg ulcers was 5.5 % and they were the presenting manifestation in 3.9 % of cases [12]. In SLE, 87 % of patients with leg ulcers are anticardiolipin antibody-positive [2]. Different types of skin ulcerations, whose clinical features and pathophysiological aspects are described below, may occur during the course of APS [2–5]

12.4.1 Postphlebitic or Postthrombotic Ulcers

Postphlebitic or postthrombotic ulcers usually manifest in patients with recurrent phlebitis or deep venous thrombosis of the lower extremities. The typical presentation is astasis dermatitis with erythema and edema.

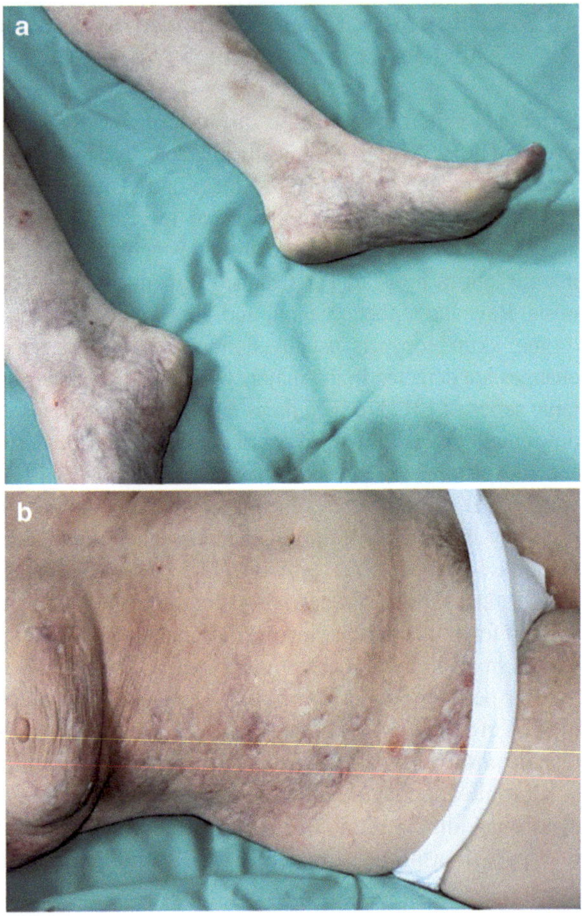

Fig. 12.1 (**a**) Mottled bluish discoloration of the skin on the lower extremities in a patient with livedoid vasculopathy. (**b**) Typical porcelain white scars defined as atrophie blanche

12.4.2 Atrophie Blanche

Atrophie blanche was first described in 1929 by Milian in young to middle-aged woman showing 3–8 mm painful lesions around the malleoli that rapidly progress to punched-out ulcers; these ulcers heal with a porcelain white scar surrounded by telangiectasias, which is termed *atrophie blanche*. The association with aPLs, particularly in SLE, is frequent [6]. Nowadays, atrophie blanche is not regarded as a distinct entity but as a limited form of livedoid vasculopathy.

12.4.3 Livedoid Vasculopathy

In livedoid vasculopathy (LV), the ulcerations described above usually involve lower extremities (Fig. 12.1a) and resolve leaving the characteristic scars of atrophie blanche (Fig. 12.1b); a rare widespread cutaneous presentation has also been reported [13, 14]. LV may be associated with infections or systemic autoimmune diseases, including SLE and APS, of which it is often the sole manifestation [15], but sometimes no

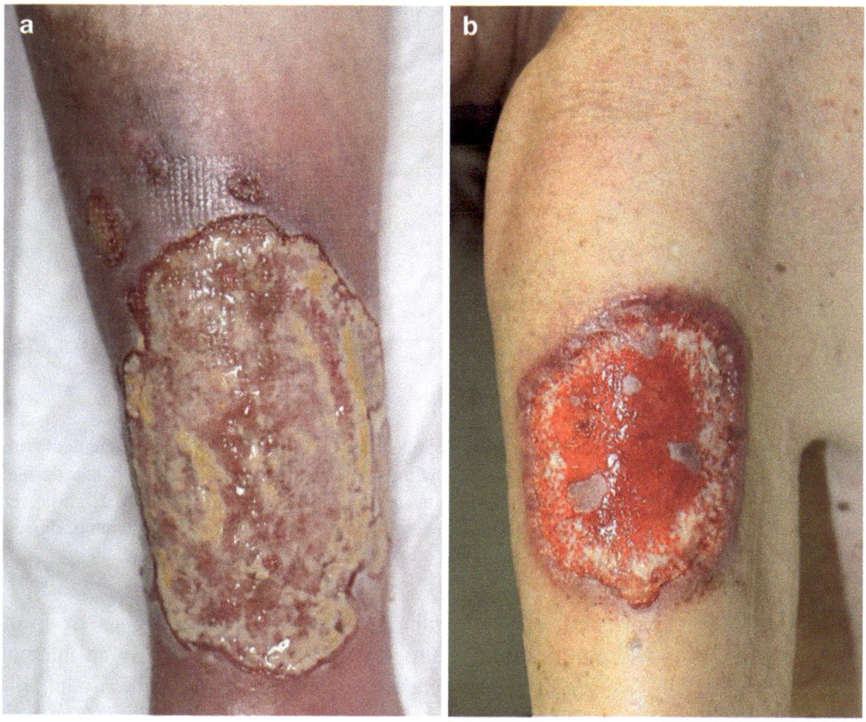

Fig. 12.2 (**a**) Ulcerations clinically resembling pyoderma gangrenosum (PG) in a patient with antiphospholipid syndrome. (**b**) A typical PG ulcer with the characteristic violaceous undermined border

underlying disorder can be detected. The latter, "idiopathic" form of LV is at present considered to be a noninflammatory thrombotic disease due to occlusion of dermal small vessels [16, 17] that may occur in patients with coagulation abnormalities [18–21]. Histologically, LV shows segmental hyalinization, endothelial proliferation, and thrombosis of the upper and mid-dermal small vessels associated with a mild, mainly perivascular, lymphocytic infiltrate. In cases associated with autoimmune disorders, immune-mediated mechanisms are considered to be responsible for vascular damage, leading to a true small vessel vasculitic process. Antiplatelet treatment, such as low dose aspirin, represents the first-line therapy; pentoxifylline, prostacyclin, and anticoagulant agents have also been reported, the last ones particularly for highly relapsing and widespread cases. Immunosuppressive agents, most notably systemic corticosteroids and cyclosporin, are reserved for refractory cases or for cases in which vasculitic changes are seen on skin histology [14].

12.4.4 Pyoderma Gangrenosum-Like Ulcers

A few cases of ulcerations clinically resembling pyoderma gangrenosum (PG) have been reported in association with primary or SLE-related APS (Fig. 12.2a) [22–24]. The lesion differs from typical PG ulcers (Fig. 12.2b) in lacking violaceous undermined borders and involving also sites other than the legs. PG is a rare skin disease nowadays

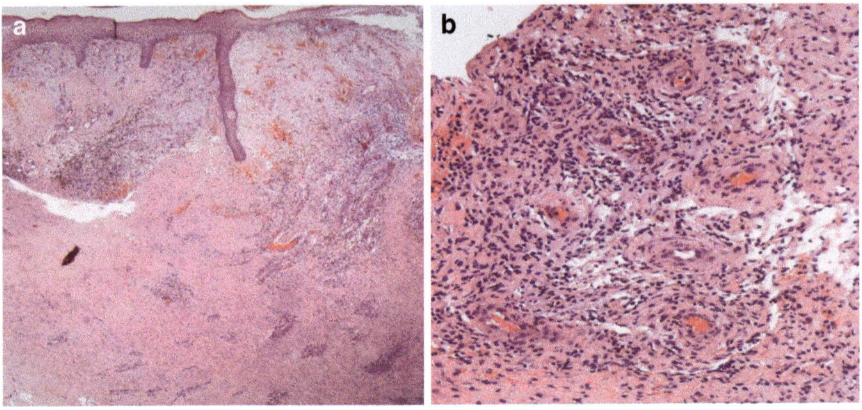

Fig. 12.3 Skin biopsy specimens taken from a pyoderma gangrenosum-like ulcer in a patient with antiphospholipid syndrome. (**a**) Histology showing epidermal ulceration and a dense dermal inflammatory infiltrate (haematoxylin-eosin stain; original magnification, X20). (**b**) High-power view showing the mixed, mainly lymphohistiocytic infiltrate, with thrombotic occlusion of dilated dermal small vessels (haematoxylin-eosin stain; original magnification, X200)

classified within the spectrum of neutrophilic dermatoses, a heterogeneous group of forms caused by the accumulation of neutrophils in the skin and, rarely, in internal organs [25, 26]. PG is associated with an underlying disease, most commonly inflammatory bowel diseases, rheumatoid arthritis, and hematological malignancies, in around 40 % of cases [27, 28] and is regarded as autoinflammatory in origin [29, 30]. The typical histology of PG is characterized by a mainly neutrophilic dermal inflammatory infiltrate, but it is often not specific; in PG-like APS ulcers, thrombotic changes may be present (Fig. 12.3). The treatment for PG-like APS ulcerations is the same used for PG: topical corticosteroids or tacrolimus for localized cases [31]; systemic corticosteroids alone or in combination with immunosuppressants, notably cyclosporin, for more extensive presentations; and tumor necrosis factor-α antagonists for refractory forms [32].

12.5 Digital Gangrene

Cutaneous gangrene has been reported to occur in 19 % of APS patients [33]. The prevalence of digital gangrene (Fig. 12.4a) is 3.3–7.5 %, and in 2.5 % of the cases, it is the presenting feature [3, 6]. Gangrene, which may be preceded by distal erythema, cyanotic macules, or pseudo-cellulitis, is caused by occlusion, or sometimes stenosis, of large- or medium-sized vessels. Regarding treatment, anticoagulation therapy is required [2, 7].

12.6 Pseudovasculitis Manifestations

Cutaneous pseudovasculitic lesions represent a group of manifestations that simulate cutaneous vasculitis [2], whose clinical features are typically polymorphic [14]; these pseudovasculitic lesions include: (i) Purpura, frequently necrotic, sometimes

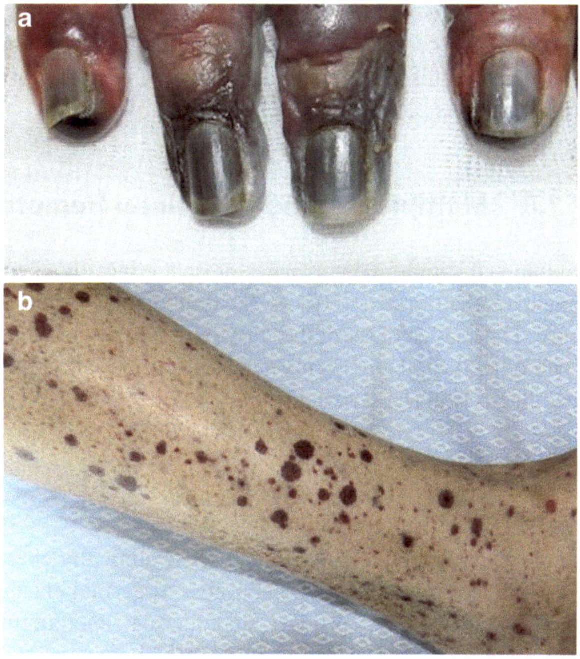

Fig. 12.4 (**a**) Digital gangrene. (**b**) Purpuric lesions on the legs

evolving in livedoid vasculitis-like ulcers; (ii) small palmar and plantar, erythematous or cyanotic lesions; (iii) papules and nodules on the limbs, ears, neck, and thighs, histologically characterized by thrombotic vessels or vessels containing organized thrombi in the dermis and/or in the subcutaneous tissue [34]. This group includes also lesions mimicking malignant atrophic papulosis. Malignant atrophic papulosis or Degos' disease is a rare vasculopathic disorder causing occlusion of small- and medium-sized arteries [35]. The skin manifestations are usually the presenting feature, followed by gastrointestinal tract and central nervous system involvement, possibly leading to a fatal evolution. Ocular, cardiovascular and pulmonary changes are also reported [35]. Cutaneous lesions begin as pink or red, dome-shaped papules, 2–5 mm in size, which become necrotic and umbilicated with a central white scar and an edematous telangiectatic border [35]. The pathogenesis of Degos' disease is still unclear, although viral, autoimmune, and coagulation abnormalities have been suggested to play a role [7].

12.7 Extensive Cutaneous Necrosis

Widespread cutaneous necrosis represents a rare manifestation of APS, which is reported in about 2 % of patients with APS [3, 12] and is secondary to diffuse microvascular thrombosis. Its onset is often acute with extensive painful purpura followed by a black necrotic plaque with an active purpuric border. Bullae and necrotic-ulcerative lesions may also develop in affected areas. Unlike warfarin-induced skin necrosis, it may relapse despite warfarin withdrawal. Histology from initial purpuric lesions reveals diffuse skin vessel thrombosis. Treatment is conservative with local antiseptic therapy in combination with serial debridement of the necrotic eschar. Long-term systemic anticoagulation therapy minimizes thrombotic recurrences. Administration of high-dose systemic corticosteroids may reduce concurrent vasculitis [2, 36].

12.8 Multiple Subungual Splinter Hemorrhages

Subungual splinter hemorrhages present clinically as tiny, linear longitudinally oriented, reddish-brown to black, distal subungual lesions, failing to blanch under pressure. The sudden onset of these lesions on multiple fingers is significantly associated with other thrombotic events involving various sites, particularly the brain and adrenal glands [2]. The prevalence of this skin sign in APS patients is 0.7 % [12].

12.9 Anetoderma

Anetoderma is a rare cutaneous disease clinically characterized by localized areas of wrinkled or flaccid skin due to loss of dermal elastic tissue [37–40]. In its idiopathic form, named primary anetoderma, anetoderma is frequently associated with autoimmune disorders, such as SLE, cutaneous lupus erythematosus [41], and APS. The correlation of aPLs with anetoderma was reported by Stephansson and Niemi [42], who, reviewing a group of patients affected by SLE with or without aPLs, observed that 15 % of those with positive aPLs developed anetoderma, while none of those without these antibodies developed such skin condition. In the study by Cervera et al. [12], the prevalence of anetoderma in APS patients was 2 %. The secondary form of anetoderma may be caused by a number of conditions, including infections (e.g., Lyme borreliosis, human immunodeficiency virus), intake of some drugs (e.g., penicillamine), or malignant disorders (e.g., cutaneous B-cell lymphoma) [2, 43]. Anetoderma is also classified into the Jadassohn-Pellizzari type, in which there are preceding inflammatory lesions, and the Schweninger-Buzzi type, with no preceding inflammatory lesions. Histology of anetoderma lesions shows focal loss of elastic fibers with perivascular and periadnexal inflammatory infiltrates as well as microthrombi. The etiopathogenesis of this disease remains unclear. Regarding the pathophysiological role of aPLs in anetoderma associated with APS, it has been hypothesized that microthromboses in the dermal vessels may account for the development of local ischemia, leading to degeneration of elastic tissue [5, 42, 44]. Conversely, the destruction of elastic fibers may also be immunologically mediated: it has been suggested that aPLs bind directly to the elastic fibers because of the presence of an antigen epitope that is phospholipid related, possibly apolipoprotein H [44]. Some investigators proposed that hypoxia-reoxygenation caused by microthrombi enhances expression of some metalloproteinases, leading to the destruction of the elastic fibers [45]. Another hypothesis is the possible presence of a common epitope between elastic fibers and ß2-glycoprotein I [7, 43].

12.10 Thrombocytopenic Purpura

Thrombocytopenic purpura (Fig. 12.4b) is a rare manifestation of APS, occurring in 3.4 % of APS patients and being the presenting feature in 1.5 % of cases. Mucosa bleeding is often associated [2].

Conclusions

The dermatological manifestations of APS may be the presenting features of the disease. This syndrome is associated with many and protean cutaneous manifestations such as LV, skin ulcerations that may mimic PG, digital gangrene, pseudovasculitic manifestations, anetoderma, and the rare and life-threatening condition of widespread necrosis. The awareness of the skin manifestations related to APS as well as their histopathological pattern may facilitate early diagnosis of this condition and the institution of specific treatment.

References

1. Hughes GRV (1984) Connective tissue disease and the skin. The Prosser-White oration. 1983. Clin Exp Dermatol 9:535–544
2. Frances C (2010) Dermatological manifestations of Hughes' antiphospholipid antibody syndrome. Lupus 9:1071–1077
3. Francès C, Niang S, Laffitte E et al (2005) Dermatologic manifestations of the antiphospholipid syndrome: two hundred consecutive cases. Arthritis Rheum 52:1785–1793
4. Francès C, Piette JC (2000) The mystery of Sneddon syndrome: relationship with antiphospholipid syndrome and systemic lupus erythematosus. J Autoimmun 15:139–143
5. Gibson GE, Su WPD, Pittelkow MR (1997) Antiphospholipid syndrome and the skin. J Am Acad Dermatol 36:970–982
6. Uthman IW, Khamashta MA (2006) Livedo racemosa: a striking dermatological sign for the antiphospholipid syndrome. J Rheumatol 33:2379–2382
7. Weinstein S, Piette W (2008) Cutaneous manifestations of antiphospholipid antibody syndrome. Hematol Oncol Clin North Am 22:67–77
8. Sneddon I (1965) Cerebrovascular lesions and livedo reticularis. Br J Dermatol 77:180–185
9. Zelger B, Sepp N, Stockhammer G et al (1993) Sneddon's syndrome. A long-term follow-up of 21 patients. Arch Dermatol 129:437–447
10. Caldas CA, de Carvalho JF (2011) Primary antiphospholipid syndrome with and without Sneddon's syndrome. Rheumatol Int 31:197–200
11. Erkan D, Harrison MJ, Levy R et al (2007) Aspirin for primary thrombosis prevention in the antiphospholipid syndrome: a randomized, double-blind, placebo-controlled trial in asymptomatic antiphospholipid antibody-positive individuals. Arthritis Rheum 56:2382–2391
12. Cervera R, Piette JC, Font J et al (2002) Antiphospholipid syndrome: clinical and immunologic manifestations and patterns of disease expression in a cohort of 1,000 patients. Arthritis Rheum 46:1019–1027
13. Marzano AV, Vanotti M, Alessi E (2003) Widespread livedoid vasculopathy. Acta Derm Venereol 83:457–460
14. Marzano AV, Vezzoli P, Berti E (2013) Skin involvement in cutaneous and systemic vasculitis. Autoimmun Rev 12:467–476
15. Acland KM, Darvay A, Wakelin SH et al (1999) Livedoid vasculitis: a manifestation of the antiphospholipid syndrome? Br J Dermatol 140:131–135

16. Jorizzo JL (1998) Livedoid vasculopathy: what is it? Arch Dermatol 134:491–493
17. Papi M, Didona B, De Pità O et al (1998) Livedo vasculopathy vs small vessel cutaneous vasculitis: cytokine and platelet P-selectin studies. Arch Dermatol 134:447–452
18. Calamia KT, Balabanova M, Perniciaro C et al (2002) Livedo (livedoid) vasculitis and the factor V Leiden mutation: additional evidence for abnormal coagulation. J Am Acad Dermatol 46:133–137
19. Hegemann B, Helmbold P, Marsch WC (2002) Livedoid vasculitis with ulcerations: the role of antithrombin III deficiency and its therapeutic consequences. Arch Dermatol 138:841–842
20. Boyvat A, Kundakçi N, Babikir MO et al (2000) Livedoid vasculopathy associated with heterozygous protein C deficiency. Br J Dermatol 143:840–842
21. Cocuroccia B, Tonanzi T, Menaguale G et al (2002) Livedoid vasculopathy and skin ulcers in patients with inherited thrombophilia. Eur J Dermatol 12:360–363
22. Canãs CA, Durán CE, Bravo JC et al (2010) Leg ulcers in the antiphospholipid syndrome may be considered as a form of pyoderma gangrenosum and they respond favorably to treatment with immunosuppression and anticoagulation. Rheumatol Int 30(9):1253–1257
23. Schmid MH, Hary C, Marstaller B et al (1998) Pyoderma gangrenosum associated with the secondary antiphospholipid syndrome. Eur J Dermatol 8:45–47
24. Hod T, Lazarov A, Edelstein E et al (2009) A huge pyoderma gangrenosum-like lesion as a presenting sign of antiphospholipid antibody syndrome. J Rheumatol 36:1557–1559
25. Wallach D, Vignon-Pennamen MD (2006) From acute febrile neutrophilic dermatosis to neutrophilic disease: forty years of clinical research. J Am Acad Dermatol 55:1066–1071
26. Marzano AV, Cugno M, Trevisan V et al (2010) Role of inflammatory cells, cytokines and matrix metalloproteinases in neutrophil-mediated skin diseases. Clin Exp Immunol 162:100–107
27. Marzano AV, Trevisan V, Lazzari R et al (2011) Pyoderma gangrenosum: study of 21 patients and proposal of a 'clinicotherapeutic' classification. J Dermatolog Treat 22:254–260
28. Marzano AV, Borghi A, Stadnicki A et al (2014) Cutaneous manifestations in patients with inflammatory bowel diseases: pathophysiology, clinical features, and therapy. Inflamm Bowel Dis 20:213–227
29. Marzano AV, Ishak RS, Saibeni S et al (2013) Autoinflammatory skin disorders in inflammatory bowel diseases, pyoderma gangrenosum and Sweet's syndrome: a comprehensive review and disease classification criteria. Clin Rev Allergy Immunol 45:202–210
30. Marzano AV, Fanoni D, Antiga E et al (2014) Expression of cytokines, chemokines and other effector molecules in two prototypic autoinflammatory skin diseases, pyoderma gangrenosum and sweet's syndrome. Clin Exp Immunol 178:48–56
31. Marzano AV, Trevisan V, Lazzari R et al (2010) Topical tacrolimus for the treatment of localized, idiopathic, newly diagnosed pyoderma gangrenosum. J Dermatolog Treat 21:140–143
32. Marzano AV, Tourlaki A, Alessi E et al (2008) Widespread idiopathic pyoderma gangrenosum evolved from ulcerative to vegetative type: a 10-year history with a recent response to infliximab. Clin Exp Dermatol 33:156–159
33. Alegre VA, Gastineau DA, Winkelmann RK (1989) Skin lesions associated with circulating lupus anticoagulant. Br J Dermatol 120:419–429
34. Ishikawa O, Takahashi A, Tamura A et al (1999) Cutaneous papules and nodules in the diagnosis of the antiphospholipid syndrome. Br J Dermatol 140:725–729
35. Theodoridis A, Makrantonaki E, Zouboulis CC (2013) Malignant atrophic papulosis (Köhlmeier-Degos disease) – a review. Orphanet J Rare Dis 8:10
36. Dutton JW, Vosburg RW, McClellan WT (2013) Widespread cutaneous necrosis and antiphospholipid antibody syndrome: discussion of a rare case. Plast Reconstr Surg 131(6):941e–942e
37. Jadassohn J (1892) Ueber eine eigenartige form von "atrophia maculosa cutis". Arch Derm Syph 1(Suppl 1):S342–S358
38. Venencie PY, Winkelmann RK, Moore BA (1984) Ultrastructural findings in the skin lesions of patients with anetoderma. Acta Derm Venereol 64:112–120
39. Venencie PY, Winkelmann RK (1984) Histopathologic findings in anetoderma. Arch Dermatol 120:1040–1044
40. Venencie PY, Winkelmann RK (1985) Monoclonal antibody studies in the skin lesions of patients with anetoderma. Arch Dermatol 121:747–749

41. Marzano A, Vanotti M, Alessi E (2004) Anetodermic lupus panniculitis and antiphospholipid antibodies: report of three cases. Acta Derm Venereol 84:385–388
42. Stephansson EA, Niemi KM (1995) Antiphospholipid antibodies and anetoderma: are they associated? Dermatology 191:204–209
43. Eungdamrong J, Fischer M, Patel R et al (2012) Anetoderma secondary to antiphospholipid antibodies. Dermatol Online J 18:26
44. Romaní J, Pérez F, Llobet M et al (2001) Anetoderma associated with antiphospholipid antibodies: case report and review of the literature. J Eur Acad Dermatol Venereol 15:175–178
45. Sparsa A, Piette JC, Wechsler B et al (2003) Anetoderma and its prothrombotic abnormalities. J Am Acad Dermatol 49:1008–1012

Additional Organs Involved in Antiphospholipid Syndrome: Eye, Ear-Nose-Throat, Lung, Gastroenteric System, Endocrine Glands

13

Maria De Santis, Angela Ceribelli, and Carlo Selmi

13.1 General Terms

Antiphospholipid (PL) syndrome (APS) is a multiorgan disease and as such, albeit in rare cases, its manifestations can be found in the eye, ear-nose-throat district, lung, gastrointestinal system, and endocrine glands. In these cases, particularly when they represent the first manifestation, the diagnosis can be challenging. Moreover, due to the frequent association of APS and systemic lupus erythematosus (SLE), it is often difficult to establish if a clinic manifestation is primarily related to APS, SLE, or both. In the present chapter we will review the available reports, mostly represented by single cases or small series, of these additional less obvious organs involved in APS (Fig. 13.1).

13.2 Eye Involvement in APS

While the eye involvement is uncommon in APS, ocular structures are more commonly affected in SLE and this is generally associated with a disease flare or central nervous system involvement. In SLE the main ophthalmological manifestations include hemorrhage, retinal cotton wool spots, microangiopathy, and vasoocclusion based on immune complex-mediated vasculopathy and complement activation [1]. Eye involvement has been described in young women with anti-PL as optic neuritis

M. De Santis • A. Ceribelli • C. Selmi (✉)
Division of Rheumatology and Clinical Immunology, Humanitas Clinical and Research Center, Rozzano, Milan, Italy

BIOMETRA Department, University of Milan, Milan, Italy
e-mail: carlo.selmi@unimi.it

© Springer International Publishing Switzerland 2015

P.L. Meroni (ed.), *Antiphospholipid Antibody Syndrome: From Bench to Bedside*, Rare Diseases of the Immune System, DOI 10.1007/978-3-319-11044-8_13

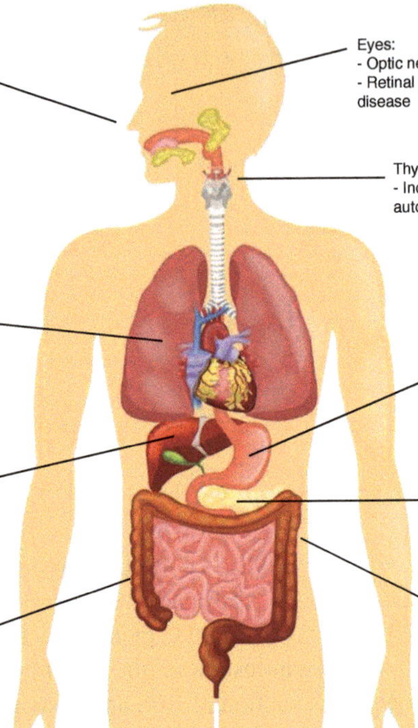

Fig. 13.1 The potential involvement of the eye, ear-nose-throat, lung, gastrointestinal system, and endocrine glands in APS is illustrated

or retinal or choroidal vasoocclusive disease [2–4]. The few reported cases show unilateral or bilateral pattern, and they generally have an acute onset. In some patients, these manifestations in APS were secondary to SLE, while in other cases they were associated to the presence of lupus anticoagulant (LAC) and were the first manifestation of APS. This is important in particular for the early identification of young patients with thrombotic eye disease with still unknown diagnosis of APS. Another interesting aspect is that other coagulation abnormalities can be associated to thrombotic eye involvement, especially when ischemic optic neuropathy is diagnosed [5]. This implies that not only anti-PL can be responsible for the ischemic process (in particular LAC), but also deficiency of anticoagulant protein C, protein S, and antithrombin may be present [5]. In all cases, the presence of an ocular thrombotic disease requires to initiate an anticoagulant therapy to improve the prognosis of these patients.

13.3 Ear-Nose-Throat and Pulmonary Involvement in APS

The involvement of the ear-nose-throat district in APS is considered rare, and in fact no cases of hearing loss or cochleovestibular involvement directly associated with APS have been reported [6]. On the contrary in SLE patients, a significant percentage of patients has hearing or vestibular dysfunctions [7]. However, one case report describes the unusual association between relapsing polychondritis (RPC) and APS [8]. RPC is the immune-mediated inflammation of cartilaginous structures of ears, nose, eyes and joints, and in about one third of cases, RPC is associated with other connective tissue diseases. Among these, a case report suggests that RPC could be a preclinical condition for APS, even if no other literature supports this link between the two diseases [8].

The upper airways are not commonly involved in APS, except for a few anecdotic reports [9, 10]. In particular, some cases of epistaxis were described in association to severe thrombocytopenia in APS. Regarding the lower airways, a few cases of pulmonary hemorrhage and acute interstitial pneumonia have been reported in particular during the "catastrophic APS" [9, 10]. This condition is defined as a life-threatening multiple organ thrombosis, due to micro thrombosis, but also large vein and artery involvement, in which there is a high risk of unusual organ involvement [11]. After kidney involvement, pulmonary complications are second in frequency (66 %) in catastrophic APS with development of acute respiratory distress syndrome and pulmonary emboli as main manifestations, followed by pulmonary hemorrhage, microthrombi, pulmonary edema, and infiltrates. Dyspnea is a common presenting symptom in catastrophic APS, so this rare variant should be immediately considered for APS patients rapidly worsening in their pulmonary function to avoid life-threatening consequences [12]. Pulmonary arterial hypertension (PAH) due to APS chronic thromboembolism can be a complication of primary APS or APS secondary to SLE. This latter case was described in an observational study of three patients who developed PAH during pregnancy that caused the death of two patients after delivery. Thus, the high mortality rate must be considered especially when this APS complication develops during pregnancy [12]. Chronic thromboembolic PAH usually requires surgical treatment, as in the forms due to other thrombotic conditions, through pulmonary thromboendarterectomy. In some cases PAH is due to pulmonary microvascular abnormalities similar to those identified in idiopathic pulmonary hypertension and may also benefit from pharmacotherapy of pulmonary hypertension. However, also in these cases anticoagulation is the first step of patient management because of the high risk of recurrent embolization and local in situ thrombosis [13].

13.4 Gastrointestinal Involvement in APS

Gastrointestinal involvement is uncommon also in SLE patients and when it is not associated with anti-PL-induced thrombotic events, it is due to vasculitis [14]. Gastrointestinal mucosal ulcerations have been described during thrombotic microangiopathy and disseminated intravascular coagulopathy due to APS [14, 15]. These features may represent the onset of catastrophic APS that predominantly affects and occludes small vessels of intra-abdominal organs such as bowel, liver, and pancreas [16]. Other isolated thromboembolic events involving the gastroenteric tract have been reported in APS patients [17], including portal vein thrombosis [18],

Table 13.1 Signs and symptoms of Budd-Chiari syndrome

Clinical presentation	Signs and symptoms
Acute and subacute type	Rapid abdominal pain
	Hepatomegaly
	Ascites
	Jaundice
	Kidney failure
Chronic type (most common)	Progressive ascites
	No jaundice
	50 % kidney failure
Fulminant type (unusual)	Liver decompensation
	Hepatomegaly
	Ascites
	Jaundice
	Kidney failure

Budd-Chiari syndrome [19], and mesenteric thrombosis [20]. Budd-Chiari syndrome may manifest in different ways and these are illustrated in Table 13.1.

13.5 Endocrine Gland Involvement in APS

While almost all endocrine glands can be affected in SLE patients, in APS there are a few reports of endocrine alterations associated with the disease. Adrenal insufficiency is considered the most common endocrine manifestation in APS patients [21]. Primary adrenal insufficiency due to bilateral adrenal hemorrhage and infarction was described in a case series of 16 patients affected by APS. This complication may be irreversible in most cases, but the study shows that the adrenal function could be recovered in a few cases and measurement of cortisol levels in the early morning could be used for follow-up of adrenal function [22]. APS should be considered in any patient with adrenal insufficiency even in the absence of other thrombotic manifestations.

Autoimmune thyroid disease can be associated with increased titers of anti-PL antibodies, in particular of anticardiolipin antibodies, in patients affected by autoimmune thyroid diseases, even if not in the context of APS [23]. Hypopituitarism and Sheehan syndrome are increasingly being reported in association with anti-PL, but no complete report or observational studies have been published so far. It is also advisable to assess anti-PL in the sera of patients presenting with pituitary insufficiency [21]. Data regarding the prevalence and significance of anti-PL in diabetic patients remains uncertain, but an increased incidence of anti-PL (anticardiolipin, anti-phosphatidylserine, and anti-phosphatidylethanolamine) in type I and II diabetic patients has been reported. In particular, the incidence of IgA isotype to phosphatidylethanolamine was higher than other isotypes to other phospholipids; moreover, the anti-phosphatidylethanolamine antibodies were associated to proliferative retinopathy in diabetic patients [24]. Subsequently, the presence of anti-phosphatidylinositol and anti-phosphatidylcholine in diabetic sera has been found and appears to be associated with macroangiopathic complications [25]. Finally, only a few cases of ovarian and testicular derangements have been reported [5]. Further studies are needed to clarify the relationship between anti-PL and thyroid disorders and diabetes mellitus.

References

1. Nag TC, Wadhwa S (2006) Vascular changes of the retina and choroid in systemic lupus erythematosus: pathology and pathogenesis. Curr Neurovasc Res 3:159–168
2. Im CY, Kim SS, Kim HK (2002) Bilateral optic neuritis as first manifestation of systemic lupus erythematosus. Korean J Ophthalmol 16:52–58
3. Snyers B, Lambert M, Hardy JP (1990) Retinal and choroidal vaso-occlusive disease in systemic lupus erythematosus associated with antiphospholipid antibodies. Retina 10:255–260
4. Acheson JF, Gregson RM, Merry P, Schulenburg WE (1991) Vaso-occlusive retinopathy in the primary anti-phospholipid antibody syndrome. Eye 5(Pt 1):48–55
5. Acheson JF, Sanders MD (1994) Coagulation abnormalities in ischaemic optic neuropathy. Eye 8(Pt 1):89–92
6. Kobayashi S, Fujishiro N, Sugiyama K (1992) Systemic lupus erythematosus with sensorineural hearing loss and improvement after plasmapheresis using the double filtration method. Intern Med 31:778–781
7. Batuecas-Caletrio A, del Pino-Montes J, Cordero-Civantos C, Calle-Cabanillas MI, Lopez-Escamez JA (2013) Hearing and vestibular disorders in patients with systemic lupus erythematosus. Lupus 22:437–442
8. Sciascia S, Bazzan M, Baldovino S, Vaccarino A, Rossi D, Russo A, Roccatello D (2011) Antiphospholipid syndrome and relapsing polychondritis: an unusual association. Lupus 20:1336–1337
9. Magro CM, Pope-Harman A, Moh P, Ross P Jr (2002) Primary anti-phospholipid antibody syndrome caused by isolated anti-phosphatidylethanolamine antibodies presenting as cryptogenic fibrosing alveolitis with recurrent pulmonary hemorrhage after single-lung transplantation. J Heart Lung Transplant 21:1232–1236
10. Kobayashi S, Inokuma S (2009) Intrapulmonary hemorrhage in collagen-vascular diseases includes a spectrum of underlying conditions. Intern Med 48:891–897
11. Asherson RA (2005) The catastrophic antiphospholipid (asherson's) syndrome in 2004–a review. Autoimmun Rev 4:48–54
12. McMillan E, Martin WL, Waugh J, Rushton I, Lewis M, Clutton-Brock T, Townend JN, Kilby MD, Gordon C (2002) Management of pregnancy in women with pulmonary hypertension secondary to sle and anti-phospholipid syndrome. Lupus 11:392–398
13. Mirrakhimov AE, Hill NS (2014) Primary antiphospholipid syndrome and pulmonary hypertension. Curr Pharm Des 20:545–551
14. Johnsen SJ, Valborgland T, Gudlaugsson E, Bostad L, Omdal R (2010) Thrombotic microangiopathy and the antiphospholipid syndrome. Lupus 19:1569–1572
15. Stinson J, Tomkin G, McDonald G, Jackson F, Harrison M, Murray A, Feighery C, Jackson J (1990) Recurrent disseminated intravascular coagulation and fulminant intra hepatic thrombosis in a patient with the anti-phospholipid syndrome. Am J Hematol 35:281–282
16. Asherson RA (2005) Multiorgan failure and antiphospholipid antibodies: the catastrophic antiphospholipid (asherson's) syndrome. Immunobiology 210:727–733
17. Witt M, Zecher D, Anders HJ (2006) Gastrointestinal manifestations associated with systemic lupus erythematosus. Eur J Med Res 11:253–260
18. Pati HP, Srivastava A, Sahni P (2003) Extra hepatic portal vein thrombosis in a child associated with lupus anticoagulant. J Trop Pediatr 49:191–192

19. Mackworth-Young CG, Melia WM, Harris EN, Gharavi AE, Sivathondan Y, Derue G, Sherlock S, Hughes GR (1986) The budd-chiari syndrome. Possible pathogenetic role of anti-phospholipid antibodies. J Hepatol 3:83–86
20. Kim HW, Hong TH, Moon MH, Jo KH (2010) Postoperative acute superior mesenteric venous thrombosis after cardiac surgery in a patient with anti-phospholipid syndrome. Eur J Cardiothorac Surg 37:1230
21. Mehdi AA, Salti I, Uthman I (2011) Antiphospholipid syndrome: endocrinologic manifestations and organ involvement. Semin Thromb Hemost 37:49–57
22. Ramon I, Mathian A, Bachelot A, Hervier B, Haroche J, Boutin-LeThi Huong D, Costedoat-Chalumeau N, Wechsler B, Karmali R, Velkeniers B, Touraine P, Coussieu C, Bennani A, Renard-Penna R, Grenier PA, Wahl D, Piette JC, Amoura Z (2013) Primary adrenal insufficiency due to bilateral adrenal hemorrhage-adrenal infarction in the antiphospholipid syndrome: long-term outcome of 16 patients. J Clin Endocrinol Metabol 98:3179–3189
23. Paggi A, Caccavo D, Ferri GM, Di Prima MA, Amoroso A, Vaccaro F, Bonomo L, Afeltra A (1994) Anti-cardiolipin antibodies in autoimmune thyroid diseases. Clin Endocrinol (Oxf) 40:329–333
24. Gargiulo P, Goldberg J, Romani B, Schiaffini R, Ciampalini P, Faulk WP, McIntyre JA (1999) Qualitative and quantitative studies of autoantibodies to phospholipids in diabetes mellitus. Clin Exp Immunol 118:30–34
25. Gin H, Vergnot V, Diakou V, Perret AM, Poix J, Cassagne C, Maneta-Peyret L (2002) Antiphospholipid antibodies in diabetes mellitus. Clin Chem Lab Med 40:604–608

Differential Diagnosis

14

Domenico Prisco, Giacomo Emmi, Elena Silvestri, Lucia Ciucciarelli, Elena Niccolai, Mario Milco D'Elios, Danilo Squatrito, and Lorenzo Emmi

14.1 Introduction

The antiphospholipid antibody syndrome (APS) is a systemic, acquired, immune-mediated systemic disease characterized by episodes of thrombosis (venous, arterial, or of the microcirculation) and/or pregnancy morbidities, associated with the persistent presence of circulating autoantibodies directed to molecular complexes consisting of phospholipids and proteins (confirmed at least in two occasions 12 weeks apart). APS should always be considered as a potential diagnosis for young patients presenting with a history of thrombotic events, especially when they occur without any obvious external trigger or any inherited thrombophilic mutation

D. Prisco (✉)
SOD Patologia Medica, Center for Autoimmune Systemic Diseases – Behçet Center and Lupus Clinic – AOU Careggi, Florence, Italy

Department of Experimental and Clinical Medicine, University of Florence, V.le L.go G. Brambilla 3, Florence, 50134, Italy
e-mail: priscod@aou-careggi.toscana.it

L. Emmi
SOD Patologia Medica, Center for Autoimmune Systemic Diseases – Behçet Center and Lupus Clinic – AOU Careggi, AOU Careggi Hospital, V.le L.go G. Brambilla 3, Florence, 50134, Italy
e-mail: lorenzoemmi@yahoo.it

G. Emmi • E. Silvestri • L. Ciucciarelli • E. Niccolai • M.M. D'Elios • D. Squatrito
Department of Experimental and Clinical Medicine, University of Florence, V.le L.go G. Brambilla 3, Florence, 50134, Italy
e-mail: giacomaci@yahoo.it; benedetta.s@tin.it; lucia.ciucciarelli@libero.it; elena.niccolai@unifi.it; mariomilco.delios@unifi.it; d.squatrito@yahoo.it;

© Springer International Publishing Switzerland 2015

P.L. Meroni (ed.), *Antiphospholipid Antibody Syndrome: From Bench to Bedside*, Rare Diseases of the Immune System, DOI 10.1007/978-3-319-11044-8_14

(even if 2006 criteria do not exclude APS patients with other inherited or acquired pro-thrombotic conditions) or for women with recurrent pregnancy losses or later fetal deaths. Many other disorders are able to mimic APS, so a broad range of alternative diagnoses should be investigated and ruled out during clinical workup. In 2006, new classification criteria were formulated to allow a well-defined and shared picture of the syndrome [1]. According to these criteria, it is possible to identify the following conditions:

1. *Positivity of antiphospholipid antibodies (aPL) associated with usual clinical manifestations*
   - (Athero)thrombotic events in typical sites (in particular deep vein thrombosis of the upper and lower limbs, pulmonary embolism, stroke, and myocardial infarction) or typical disorders of pregnancy
2. *Positivity of aPL associated with unusual clinical manifestations*
   - (Athero)thrombotic events in atypical sites (particularly liver, mesenteric, renal and adrenal vessels, and cerebral venous sinus thrombosis)
3. *Positivity of aPL associated with non-criterial clinical manifestations (but possibly associated with APS during follow-up) or incomplete clinical manifestations (especially of pregnancy)*
   - A large spectrum of nonthrombotic cardiac and pulmonary involvement and osteoarticular, ocular, and hematological manifestations (see below)
   - Pregnancy disorders suggestive, but not completely fulfilling Miyakis criteria (e.g., 2 consecutive abortions before the 10th week of gestation or 3 or more nonconsecutive abortions before the 10th week)

In the first type of situations, diagnosis is relatively simple in some cases of primary APS when clinical presentation includes only acute thrombosis or pregnancy loss. However, in more complex cases special attention deserves the exclusion of certain conditions, in particular microangiopathic syndromes or systemic lupus erythematosus (SLE). In the second group the diagnosis of APS may be more complex due to nonspecific clinical manifestations; in this case, different clinical conditions must be considered before diagnosis of APS is done (e.g., an acute abdominal pain due to visceral thrombosis). In the third case the patient presents with non-criterial clinical features, due to conditions potentially associated with APS, which deserve a careful follow-up to detect early clinical criteria and to establish appropriate therapy.

A "seronegative" form of the syndrome has been described and recently revised, but we will not consider this entity in this chapter.

In this chapter we will consider these three possibilities, focusing on clinical signs and on the main aspects of the differential diagnosis. For a schematic representation of the text, see Fig. 14.1.

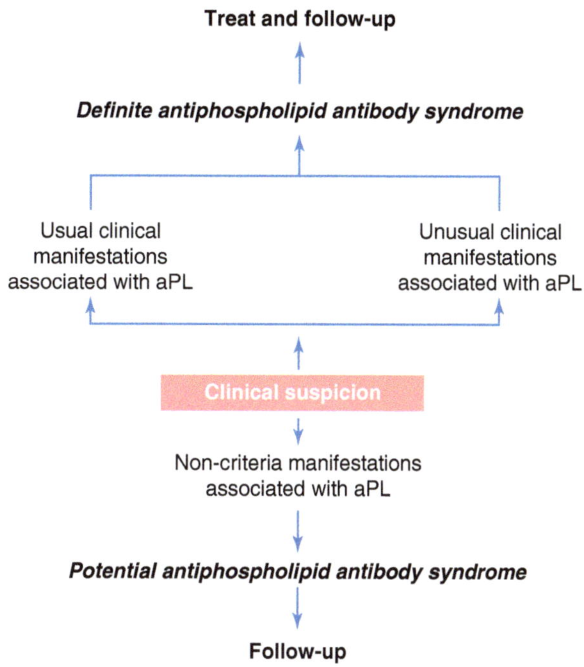

Fig. 14.1 Clinical suspicion for definite and non-criterial APS

Table 14.1 Main differential diagnosis

SLE
Behçet's syndrome
Demyelinating diseases (multiple sclerosis, Devic's syndrome)
Microangiopathic syndromes (TTP/HUS, HELLP)[a]
Heparin-induced thrombocytopenia (HIT)
Disseminated intravascular coagulation (DIC)
Hyperviscosity syndromes
Sneddon's syndrome, Susac's syndrome, Degos disease, Moyamoya syndrome (very rare)

[a]*TTP* thrombotic thrombocytopenic purpura, *HUS* hemolytic uremic syndrome, *HELLP* hemolysis, elevated liver enzymes, and low platelets

14.2 Definite APS with Usual Clinical Manifestations

The clinical picture of APS is protean and very variable in the single patient, as thrombotic events can involve both arterial and venous vessels of any size and anatomical district and sometimes APS diagnosis requires a broad number of medical conditions to be ruled out (Table 14.1).

14.2.1 Systemic Lupus Erythematosus

A particular liaison exists between APS and SLE; the 2006 International consensus conference for the first time pointed out that the definition of secondary APS is not necessary and appropriate, since SLE and APS may represent a different spectrum of the same disease [1]. In clinical practice, we often challenge the following three scenarios:

1. Patients who fulfill the international criteria for both SLE and APS. In this case, the two entities coexist.
2. Patients with APS who also present some features of SLE, such as autoimmune hemolytic anemia, mild reduction of complement, and antinuclear antibodies (ANA) at borderline titer without any further specificity. These subjects can be considered as APS patients which likely will evolve into SLE in the future; in this case the early introduction of hydroxychloroquine therapy has been recommended [2].
3. Patients with APS and renal involvement; in this case a significant titer of circulating ANA, the presence of other autoantibody specificities (such as antibodies anti-native DNA, anti-Sm, or anti-C1q), complement consumption, and above all the suggestive histological findings from renal biopsy are all crucial to distinguish SLE renal involvement from APS.

Whenever APS primarily involve the central nervous system (CNS), the main clinical challenge is the differential diagnosis with neuro-SLE, since both the conditions share similar neurological symptoms and MR findings [3]. The detection of a significant titer of specific circulating autoantibodies (e.g., anti-ribosomal P) and low complement levels should be suggestive of SLE. However, many patients with neuro-SLE show also circulating aPL; therefore, ischemic lesions seen on brain MR could be either the result of APS microthrombosis or alternatively of SLE inflammation. The discrimination between the two conditions could be very challenging for clinicians; however, this step is crucial since in the first case anticoagulants are the mainstay of therapy, while in the other SLE requires the use of high-dose steroids usually combined with immunosuppressants drugs [4].

14.2.2 Behçet's Syndrome

Neuro-Behçet (NB) represents an important differential diagnosis for APS with predominant cerebral involvement. Of note both diseases can be responsible for cerebral venous sinus thrombosis and parenchymal lesions [5]. NB brain inflammatory lesions are typically located deeply at the level of basal ganglia and brainstem, while APS usually involves the subcortical and periventricular white matter areas. Differential diagnosis between the two conditions is crucial because in NB immunosuppressive treatment is required [6]. Moreover, a particular subset of Behçet patients is indeed very prone to vascular thrombosis that in these cases could represent the main clinical manifestation, further complicating the differential diagnosis with APS. Due to their primary inflammatory vascular origin, the thrombotic events in Behçet syndrome are usually better responsive to corticosteroid or immunosuppressive drugs than to anticoagulation [7]. Noteworthy the inappropriate use of anticoagulants in Behçet could be very dangerous when these drugs are used in patients with clinically occult pulmonary artery aneurisms, since the risk of rupture is very high in this setting [8]. Oral aphthosis is the most frequent clinical sign in Behçet; however, it lacks specificity due to its high frequency in the general and otherwise healthy population. Moreover, about 5 % percent of Behçet patients lack oral aphtosis. The same considerations are valid for HLA- B51 antigen, often wrongly used as a Behçet diagnostic biomarker, due to its high prevalence in Behçet patients, but aphtosis can also be found in approximately 30 % of unaffected people. HLA-B51 screening test and other laboratory investigations are not included in the classification criteria, since the diagnosis/classification of Behçet currently relies only on clinical findings [9]. Moreover, aPL could be present at low titer in Behçet patients. However, recurrent oral and genital (bipolar) aphthosis and uveitis when present are pathognomonic for Behcet's disease and point to the correct diagnosis.

14.2.3 Demyelinating Diseases (Multiple Sclerosis and Neuromyelitis Optica)

Multiple sclerosis (MS) lesions can be hardly differentiated from neuro-APS on brain MR, since their radiologic morphology and location could be similar in the two conditions [10]. A further complication is represented by the not unusual finding of ANA and aPL positivity in MS patients, although often at very low titer. Lesions involving the periventricular and *corpus callosum* areas are more suggestive of SM than APS; moreover, the detection of oligoclonal bands from cephalospinal fluid further supports the diagnosis of demyelinating disease [11]. Neuromyelitis optica (NMO), previously named Devic's syndrome, is a recently recognized disease, now considered a separate disorder from MS, since it recognizes a different inflammatory pathway. The presence of aquaporin-4 (anti-NMO) antibodies is considered the main pathogenetic player and a very useful diagnostic tool at the same time. The diagnosis of NMO should be suspected in patients who present with optic neuritis, usually more severe than in MS, and/or with longitudinally extended transverse myelitis, defined as a spinal inflammatory lesion involving at least three consecutive vertebrae. In this scenario testing patients for anti-NMO antibodies is strongly recommended [12]. NMO can coexist with SLE and APS in the same patient and this overlap created some degree of confusion in the past. Indeed, some neurological symptoms have been ascribed to SLE/APS rather than to NMO. This is the case, for example, of transverse myelitis frequently reported as an APS complication (among non-criteria clinical clues) but often with no data available on anti-NMO status. Recognizing NMO typical ocular/spinal pattern is hence considered fundamental for further investigating the presence of circulating anti-NMO, since this lead to the correct treatment with plasmapheresis or eventually with other immunosuppressive approach [13].

14.2.4 Microangiopathic Syndromes

Catastrophic antiphospholipid syndrome (CAPS), thrombotic thrombocytopenic purpura (TTP), hemolytic uremic syndrome (HUS), and hemolysis, elevated liver enzymes, and low platelets (HELLP) syndrome all belong to the group of thrombotic microangiopathy syndromes; these disorders are histologically characterized by small vessel occlusion with hyaline thrombi and fibrin deposition, various degree of platelet consumption, intravascular hemolysis with red cells fragmentation producing schistocytes, and clinical/laboratoristic findings of organ dysfunction. Since aPL have been not infrequently detected in such conditions and since conversely APS does not uncommonly show some degree of microangiopathic involvement, the term MAPS (microangiopathic antiphospholipid syndrome) has been proposed as an "umbrella" to include many conditions [14, 15].

Thrombotic Thrombocytopenic Purpura

TTP, also named Moschowitz syndrome, is clinically characterized by severe neurological involvement, fever, thrombocytopenia, microangiopathic hemolytic anemia, and more rarely kidney dysfunction. Useful tools to diagnose this condition are the presence of schistocytes, elevated levels of circulating ultra large von Willebrand factor (ULVWF) multimers, and, in acquired autoimmune type, the detection of antibodies against the metalloproteinase-disintegrin ADAMTS13 [16]. Differential diagnosis could be hard since aPL have been occasionally reported in TTP patients; diagnostic clues helping in differential diagnosis are the rarity of severe episodes of thrombocytopenia in APS, while the occurrence of hemolytic anemia, the presence of schistocytes on peripheral blood smear, the elevated LDH levels, and the detection of ULVWF further support the diagnosis of TTP.

Hemolytic Uremic Syndrome

HUS is a disorder characterized by thrombocytopenia and microangiopathic anemia with microvascular thrombosis, tissue ischemia with necrosis, and renal failure. It has been distinguished into diarrhea-associated HUS, the most frequent and usually linked to Shiga-like toxin-producing bacteria (STEC-HUS), and diarrhea-nonassociated or atypical HUS. The latter constitutes only 5–10 % of HUS in children, but the majority of HUS in adults. Despite its rarity, atypical HUS is endowed with a very intriguing pathogenesis, since it can be triggered by genetical defect or by the presence of circulating proteins affecting the complement system [17, 18]. Clinical features suggesting HUS are the rapid onset of renal failure and the presence of microangiopathic anemia associated with thrombocytopenia; in the typical presentation the temporal occurrence of a previous episode of diarrhea as well as the absence of aPL further supports the diagnosis.

Clinical/laboratory findings	CAPS	TTF/HUS	HELLP	DIC	HIT
Previous history	PAPS/SLE	Malignancy/ non	Pregnancy	Infection/ malignancy	Heparin exposure
Thrombosis	Small/large vessels	Small vessels	Small vessels	Small vessels	Large/Small vessels
Fibrinogen	Normal/ high	Normal/ high	Normal/ high	Low	Normal
Haemolytic anemia	+/–	+	+	+/–	–
Schistocytes	+	++	+/–	+/–	+/–
Thrombocytopenia	+	++	++	++	++
aPL	++	–	+/–	–	–
Antibodies	aPL	Anti ADAMTS13		–	ANTI HEPARIN-PF4

Fig.14.2 Differential diagnosis between microangiopathies, DIC, and HIT

Hemolysis Elevated Liver Enzymes and Low Platelets

HELLP syndrome can complicate pregnancy, even in pregnant women with history of APS or aPL positivity. This condition is more common in multiparous women; 70 % of cases occur between the 27th and the 37th week of gestation, while in the remaining 30 % diagnosis is made during the *postpartum* period. The HELLP syndrome is characterized by upper right quadrant abdominal pain, nausea, vomiting, generalized edema, signs of hemolysis, elevated liver enzymes, severe thrombocytopenia, and renal dysfunction; noteworthy, severe hypertension is not usually found in HELLP syndrome, and this can help distinguish it from preeclampsia, even if the two conditions can coexist in 70–80 % of cases [19]. This scenario is even more complicated considering that some APS patients can experience HELLP syndrome during pregnancy, indicating that probably circulating aPL can affect the occurrence of HELLP in predisposed women [20].

For the main causes of recurrent miscarriage, see Fig. 14.2.

14.2.5 Heparin-Induced Thrombocytopenia

Another condition that must be considered in the differential diagnosis of APS is heparin-induced thrombocytopenia (HIT), clinically characterized by thrombocytopenia and thrombotic events and histologically by multiple thrombotic occlusions of small vessels [21]. This entity should be suspected early during heparin treatment and always considered as potentially fatal. Two forms of HIT have been described: type I HIT, not immune-mediated, has a favorable prognosis since it is not associated with thrombotic events; type II HIT, with an underlying immunological mechanism, is associated with microthrombosis involving multiple anatomical sites. Type I HIT occurs in approximately 10 % of patients undergoing both unfractionated heparin (UH) or low molecular weight heparin (LMWH) treatment and is thought to be caused by direct platelet activation from heparin. It occurs very early usually within the first 4/5 days of therapy and resolves without treatment and without any complication. Type II HIT is conversely a dreaded complication, potentially involving 1–5 % of patients undergoing heparin therapy. Approximately 50 % of patients with type II HIT may experience thrombotic events affecting both the arterial and the venous vascular district. The risk of mortality in such cases is estimated to be about 20–30 %. The likelihood of developing type II HIT is considered to be between 10 and 40 times higher when unfractionated heparin is used compared to LMWH. It should be suspected when the platelet count falls by about 50 % compared to baseline after 5–15 days from the beginning of heparin therapy. Type II HIT can present in three ways: (a) production of specific antiplatelet antibodies without thrombocytopenia; (b) antibodies associated with thrombocytopenia but not with thrombotic complications; and (c) antibodies, thrombocytopenia, and thrombosis. The pathogenesis of HIT has been recently better defined and the complex heparin-platelet factor 4 (PF4) identified as the major immunological target of antibody response. During the early phase heparin binds to PF4, generating the heparin-PF4 complex toward which IgG antibodies are produced. In HIT the heparin-PF4-IgG complex is also able to activate platelets via FcγRIIa receptor, causing microthrombosis and thrombocytopenia. The resulting platelet activation is also associated with serotonin release and thrombin generation. HIT laboratory diagnosis, based on detection of antibodies to heparin-PF4 complex, can be made mainly using the following two methods: a serotonin release assay (SRA), characterized by low sensitivity but very specific for HIT, or alternatively an ELISA test, more sensitive than the previous one, but less specific for HIT; neither of the above cited tests anyways represents the gold standard and the diagnosis is currently based on probability according to a compatible clinical scenario [22].

Finally HIT management is very problematic and consists of both the immediate discontinuation of heparin and the beginning of an alternative anticoagulation strategy with (a) direct thrombin inhibitors, (b) heparinoids, and (c) pentasaccharides. The differential diagnosis with APS can be difficult because both can be associated with low platelet count and thrombosis, even if thrombocytopenia is generally more severe in HIT than in APS. Obviously previous heparin exposure, the precise timing of thrombocytopenia insorgence, and the absence of circulating aPL are all points to make a correct diagnosis.

14.2.6 Disseminated Intravascular Coagulation

Disseminated intravascular coagulation (DIC) is a serious disorder, secondary to infections, surgery, chronic inflammatory diseases, different obstetrical diseases, and solid and hematological malignancies. It is characterized by disseminated microvascular thrombosis, consumptive coagulopathy, and hemorrhagic diathesis,

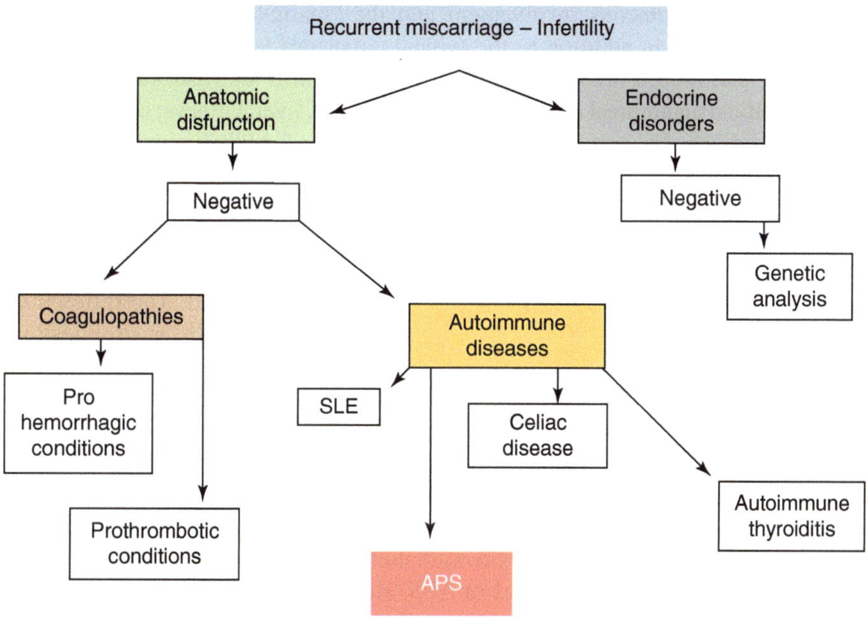

Fig. 14.3 Main causes of recurrent miscarriage

which can eventually lead to multiple organ failure. Laboratory features of DIC are thrombocytopenia, prolonged clotting times, reduced plasma fibrinogen, and increased levels of fibrin degradation products. Interestingly, DIC could both mimic and complicate APS, especially in its catastrophic form; indeed, CAPS is a condition with widespread intravascular thrombosis resulting in multiorgan failure. More frequently DIC presents thrombotic and hemorrhagic complications at the same time [23]

For differential diagnosis between microangiopathies, HIT, and DIC, see Fig. 14.3.

14.2.7 Hyperviscosity Syndromes

Patients with hyperviscosity syndrome (e.g., in multiple myeloma or Waldenstrom's macroglobulinemia) may present cerebral ischemia and transitory ocular problems, such as *amaurosis fugax*, and sometimes a differential diagnosis with APS may be needed.

14.2.8 Other Clinical Clues

The malignant atrophic papulosis (MAP), also known as Köhlmeier-Degos disease, needs to be differentiated from APS. It exists in two variants: the "benign" type with only cutaneous involvement and the "malignant" type with internal organ involvement in addition to the typical cutaneous lesions. These latter systemic type can indeed involve not only the skin but also the gastrointestinal tract or other critical anatomical districts such as eye, heart, liver, kidneys, and CNS. The differential diagnosis is especially with neuro-APS or CAPS. Typical skin lesions are erythematous papules that evolve into atrophic scars with a porcelain white center, histopathologically indistinguishable from certain cutaneous lesions of SLE. Gastrointestinal involvement is present in approximately 60 % of patients and is the most common cause of death, while the CNS involvement is characterized by single or multiple infarcts in the brain and spinal cord. The differential diagnosis is based on (a) the presence of typical skin lesions, (b) gastrointestinal symptoms, and (c) the absence of aPL [24].

Susac's syndrome (SS) is a noteworthy autoimmune disease caused by microangiopathy damage affecting the precapillary arterioles of the brain, retina, and inner ear. It is clinically characterized by the following triad: encephalopathy with typical radiological features on MR, branch retinal artery occlusions on fluorescein angiography, and neurosensorial hearing loss. Even if brain MR showing *corpus callosum* is very suggestive of SS, symptoms and clinical signs can also mimic vascular neurological presentations of APS. However, in this case the research of aPL is usually negative; moreover, SS requires treatment with immunosuppressive drugs [25].

Sneddon's syndrome, a disorder characterized by the occurrence of cerebrovascular disease associated with livedo reticularis, is another condition that sometimes can give some problems of differential diagnosis with APS. For more detail about this entity, see the paragraph "non-criteria clinical clues."

14.3 Definite APS with Unusual Clinical Manifestations

As mentioned above, APS must be also taken into consideration when arterial or venous thrombosis is present in atypical sites or recurs during appropriate anticoagulant treatment.

14.3.1 Kidney Manifestations

Kidney manifestations – renal involvement is definitely less frequent and less recognized in APS than in SLE. From a pathological point of view, it differs mainly for its primary vascular involvement with only secondary glomerular damage [26, 27]. The most well-known renal complications are renal vein thrombosis, clinically characterized by nephrotic syndrome (nephrotic syndrome, however, can in turn be complicated by renal vein thrombosis), renal infarction, and kidney microangiopathy. The latter mainly involve the afferent arterioles and it is histologically characterized by thrombotic microangiopathy with fibrin deposition and microthrombi causing secondary glomerular dysfunction, interstitial fibrosis, and tubular atrophy;

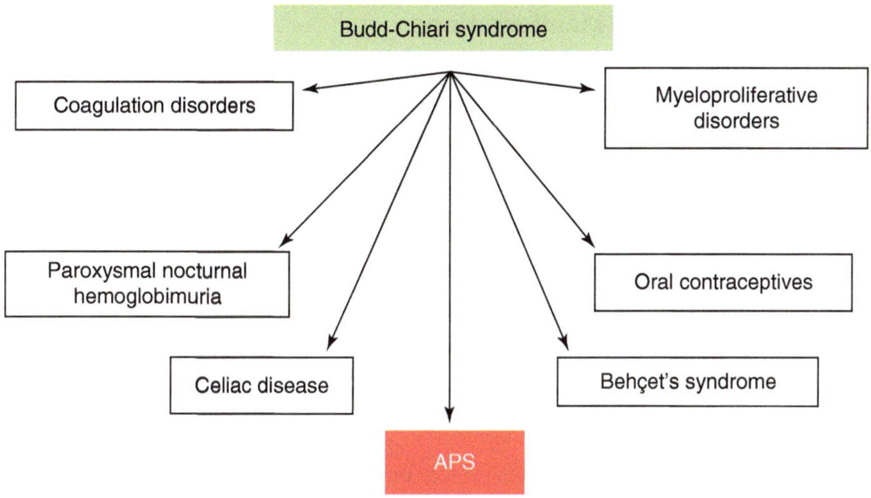

Fig. 14.4 Different causes of Budd-Chiari syndrome

it clinically manifests itself with hypertension and laboratory signs of renal failure. The criteria for the diagnosis of APS-associated nephropathy include the presence of aPL and typical histopathologic finding of thrombotic microangiopathy, involving both arterioles and glomerular capillaries [28]. In patients with SLE and aPL, a biopsy procedure is strongly recommended to differentiate inflammatory from thrombotic lesions, since the two conditions require different therapeutic approaches. Noteworthy, the presence of damage secondary to APS on kidney histology severely affects the prognosis of patients with lupus nephritis. Long-term warfarin therapy has been recommended for such patients [29].

14.3.2 Gastrointestinal Manifestations

Gastrointestinal manifestations – these manifestations are mainly represented by arterial thrombosis or alternatively to venous involvement in different anatomical sites such as sovraepatic (Budd-Chiari syndrome), portal, mesenteric (with risk of intestinal ischemia), and more rarely of the splenic veins [30] (see also Fig. 14.4). Vasculitis with prevalent involvement of gastrointestinal tract, in particular Schonlein-Henoch and polyarteritis nodosa, should be differentiated from APS. However, differently from vasculitides, APS is not usually associated with increased inflammatory markers. The involvement of the intra-abdominal district is even more frequent during CAPS course and this entity should be always suspected in patients who present with severe and multiorgan ischemic dysfunction rapidly developing, often in less than 1 week [31].

14.3.3 Neurological Manifestations

Neurological manifestations – cerebral venous thrombosis, as opposed to cerebral ischemic events, are rare manifestations of APS, but must always be considered [32].

14.3.4 Endocrinological Manifestations

Endocrinological manifestations – adrenal insufficiency secondary to acute vascular infarction is a rare but well-known manifestation of APS [33].

14.4 Non-criteria Clinical Clues

The differential diagnosis becomes rather complex for the so called "non-criteria," the clinical clues that do not allow a diagnosis of definite APS according to Myakis criteria; however, these clinical signs strongly suggest the suspicion of underlying APS or the possibility of evolution over time toward it. These patients represent a significant proportion of subjects to be evaluated prospectively in order to detect early symptoms of definite disease.

14.4.1 Nonthrombotic Cardiac and Pulmonary Manifestations

Nonthrombotic cardiac and pulmonary manifestations – echocardiographic studies demonstrated a spectrum of heart valves abnormalities, especially of the mitral valve, ranging from mild valve thickening to the typical nonbacterial thrombotic lesions (Libman-Sacks endocarditis) [34]. Isolated case reports of cardiomyopathy in APS patients have also been published; however, a convincing pathogenetic relationship with circulating aPL has not been clearly demonstrated [35]. Pulmonary nonthrombotic manifestations are quite rare in APS patients and are mainly represented by intra-alveolar hemorrhage, acute respiratory distress syndrome (ARDS), and fibrosing alveolitis [36, 37].

14.4.2 Cutaneous Manifestations

Cutaneous manifestations – these are mainly represented by *livedo*, acrocyanosis, and peripheral ulcers [38, 39]. *Livedo* in particular represents one of the most commonly reported cutaneous manifestation in patients with APS. Histologically *livedo* is characterized by partial or complete lumen occlusion of small or medium caliber arteries located in the dermo-hypodermis level, with no evidence of perivascular inflammatory infiltrates. The skin inspection reveals reticulated, purple, red, or bluish lesions which are persistent and more evident with cold exposure but usually not reversible by heating. Lower limbs are more frequently involved than upper limbs

Table 14.2 Main cutaneous manifestations in APS patients

Livedo racemosa
Digital necrosis
Splinter hemorrhages
Postphlebitic ulcers
Pseudo-vasculitic lesions
Primary anetoderma

and trunk. The lesion is defined as *livedo reticularis* when its borders are circular and continuous, while on the other hand, *livedo racemosa* is characterized by irregular and interrupted borders. Interestingly only *livedo racemosa* is associated with pathological conditions and in particular with APS, while *livedo reticularis* is considered a benign condition and is more commonly encountered during clinical practice. For this reason the term *livedo reticularis*, currently included also into the APS non-criteria features, could be indeed considered a misnomer and should be ideally changed with the more accurate dermatologic definition of *livedo racemosa* [40]. Some diagnostic difficulties arise in the differential diagnosis between APS and Sneddon's syndrome, since both can be marked by the presence of *livedo* and cerebrovascular accidents. Sneddon's syndrome patients usually present also with high blood pressure; moreover, circulating aPL are rarely detected in such condition. The extent of *livedo*, usually very pronounced, and the absence of circulating aPL represent important clues for diagnosing Sneddon's syndrome. In selected circumstances a skin biopsy can show the typical histological findings of endothelial cells proliferation and occlusion of the small cutaneous vessels [41]. For the main cutaneous manifestation, see Table 14.2.

14.4.3 Ocular Manifestations

Ocular manifestations – *Amaurosis fugax* is certainly the most frequent ophthalmologic sign, usually not associated with any pathological fundoscopic findings, and it may represent a manifestation of cerebrovascular disease (in particular transient ischemic attack). On the other hand, APS may be responsible for severe ocular events, such as artery or vein thrombosis, retinal vascular occlusive retinopathy, and ischemic optic neuropathy, the latter also occurring in other autoimmune diseases such as giant cell arteritis (GCA). However, unlike other inflammatory or immune-rheumatological condition, APS is not usually associated with an elevation of inflammatory markers and this is particularly important in differentiating the diseases from GCA in patients with rapidly progressive and severe visual impairment. Moreover, consider APS in the differential diagnosis workup is critical, for example, in the correct diagnosis of young patients presenting with ocular vaso-occlusive disease without any traditional thromboembolic risk factors or obvious causes [42, 43].

14.4.4 Hematological Manifestations

Hematological manifestations – these may be present in APS patients with thrombocytopenia, autoimmune hemolytic anemia, and Evans syndrome. It is noteworthy that thrombocytopenia was previously included into the APS classification criteria, while currently is considered a non-criterial APS complication. When SLE and APS coexist in the same patient, it is challenging to distinguish which one of the two conditions determines low circulating platelets. However, APS-associated thrombocytopenia is generally considered less severe and rarely requires aggressive treatment, and it is not usually associated with the developing of hemorrhagic complications. The current criteria of APS-associated thrombocytopenia consist of coexistence of aPL positivity with thrombocytopenia <100,000/mm^3 confirmed in two different samples. Mild thrombocytopenia is indeed found in 30–40 % of patients and this close relation justifies why aPL screening is strongly recommended in every patients with idiopathic thrombocytopenia [44]. Clinical conditions to be excluded in the differential diagnosis are in particular pseudo-thrombocytopenia, TTP, DIC, and HIT. Finally, Evans syndrome, a hematological condition characterized by the association of thrombocytopenia and hemolytic anemia, was also reported to be associated with APS [45].

14.4.5 Musculoskeletal Manifestations

Musculoskeletal manifestations – APS patients may rarely suffer from arthralgia and arthritis, which, if present, could be the first symptoms of an associated connective tissue disease. Aseptic bone necrosis, especially of the femoral head, is rare but it has been reported in patients with APS in both its classical and catastrophic variant [46]. If a patient with APS at any time reports pain of the lower limbs worsened under load and improved at rest, it is mandatory to perform an MR scan in order to rule out this complication. The pathogenesis of osteonecrosis is not yet completely understood; however, it is believed that microthrombosis or vasculopathy is involved more than classical ischemia from medium arterial vessel occlusion [47].

References

1. Miyakis S, Lockshin MD, Atsumi T et al (2006) International consensus statement on an update of the classification criteria for definite antiphospholipid syndrome (APS). J Thromb Haemost 4(2):295–306
2. Petri M (2011) Use of hydroxychloroquine to prevent thrombosis in systemic lupus erythematosus and in antiphospholipid antibody-positive patients. Curr Rheumatol Rep 13(1):77–80
3. Sanna G, D'Cruz D, Cuadrado MJ (2006) Cerebral manifestations in the antiphospholipid (Hughes) syndrome. Rheum Dis Clin North Am 32(3):465–490
4. Fanouriakis A, Boumpas DT, Bertsias GK (2013) Pathogenesis and treatment of CNS lupus. Curr Opin Rheumatol 25(5):577–583
5. Stam J (2005) Thrombosis of the cerebral veins and sinuses. N Engl J Med 352(17): 1791–1798

6. Al-Araji A, Kidd DP (2009) Neuro-Behçet's disease: epidemiology, clinical characteristics, and management. Lancet Neurol 8(2):192–204
7. Silvestri E, Emmi G, Prisco D (2014) Anti-TNF-α agents in vascular Behçet's disease. Expert Rev Cardiovasc Ther 12(4):415–416
8. Hatemi G, Silman A, Bang D, EULAR Expert Committee (2008) EULAR recommendations for the management of Behçet disease. Ann Rheum Dis 67(12):1656–1662
9. Yazici H, Yazici Y (2014) Criteria for Behçet's disease with reflections on all disease criteria. J Autoimmun 48–49:104–107
10. Cuadrado MJ, Khamashta MA, Ballesteros A et al (2000) Can neurologic manifestations of Hughes (antiphospholipid) syndrome be distinguished from multiple sclerosis? Analysis of 27 patients and review of the literature. Medicine (Baltimore) 79(1):57–68
11. Link H, Huang YM (2006) Oligoclonal bands in multiple sclerosis cerebrospinal fluid: an update on methodology and clinical usefulness. J Neuroimmunol 180(1–2):17–28
12. Papadopoulos MC, Verkman AS (2012) Aquaporin 4 and neuromyelitis optica. Lancet Neurol 11(6):535–544
13. Squatrito D, Colagrande S, Emmi L (2010) Devic's syndrome and primary APS: a new immunological overlap. Lupus 19(11):1337–1339
14. Asherson RA, Cervera R (2008) Microvascular and microangiopathic antiphospholipid-associated syndromes ("MAPS"): semantic or antisemantic? Autoimmun Rev 7(3):164–167
15. Merrill JT, Asherson RA (2006) Catastrophic antiphospholipid syndrome. Nat Clin Pract Rheumatol 2(2):81–89
16. Shenkman B, Einav Y (2014) Thrombotic thrombocytopenic purpura and other thrombotic microangiopathic hemolytic anemias: diagnosis and classification. Autoimmun Rev 13(4–5): 584–586
17. Mele C, Remuzzi G, Noris M (2014) Hemolytic uremic syndrome. Semin Immunopathol. doi:10.1007/s00281-014-0416-x
18. Noris M, Mescia F, Remuzzi G (2012) STEC-HUS, atypical HUS and TTP are all diseases of complement activation. Nat Rev Nephrol 8(11):622–633
19. Abildgaard U, Heimdal K (2013) Pathogenesis of the syndrome of hemolysis, elevated liver enzymes, and low platelet count (HELLP): a review. Eur J Obstet Gynecol Reprod Biol 166(2):117–123
20. Appenzeller S, Souza FH, Wagner Silva de Souza A et al (2011) HELLP syndrome and its relationship with antiphospholipid syndrome and antiphospholipid antibodies. Semin Arthritis Rheum 41(3):517–523
21. Chong BH, Isaacs A (2009) Heparin-induced thrombocytopenia: what clinicians need to know. Thromb Haemost 101(2):279–283
22. Prechel M, Walenga JM (2008) The laboratory diagnosis and clinical management of patients with heparin-induced thrombocytopenia: an update. Semin Thromb Hemost 34(1):86–96
23. Taylor FB Jr, Toh CH et al (2001) Towards definition, clinical and laboratory criteria, and a scoring system for disseminated intravascular coagulation. Thromb Haemost 86(5): 1327–1330
24. Theodoridis A, Makrantonaki E, Zouboulis CC (2013) Malignant atrophic papulosis (Köhlmeier-Degos disease) – a review. Orphanet J Rare Dis 8:10
25. García-Carrasco M, Mendoza-Pinto C, Cervera R (2014) Diagnosis and classification of Susac syndrome. Autoimmun Rev 13(4–5):347–350
26. Pons-Estel GJ, Cervera R (2014) Renal involvement in antiphospholipid syndrome. Curr Rheumatol Rep 16(2):397
27. Sciascia S, Cuadrado MJ, Khamashta M et al (2014) Renal involvement in antiphospholipid syndrome. Nat Rev Nephrol 10(5):279–289
28. Tektonidou MG (2009) Renal involvement in the antiphospholipid syndrome (APS)-APS nephropathy. Clin Rev Allergy Immunol 36(2–3):131–140
29. Tektonidou MG, Sotsiou F, Nakopoulou L et al (2004) Antiphospholipid syndrome nephropathy in patients with systemic lupus erythematosus and antiphospholipid antibodies: prevalence, clinical associations, and long-term outcome. Arthritis Rheum 50(8):2569–2579

30. Uthman I, Khamashta M (2007) The abdominal manifestations of the antiphospholipid syndrome. Rheumatology (Oxford) 46(11):1641–1647
31. Cervera R, Bucciarelli S, Plasín MA et al (2009) Catastrophic antiphospholipid syndrome (CAPS): descriptive analysis of a series of 280 patients from the "CAPS Registry". J Autoimmun 32(3–4):240
32. Gillis D, Wong RC (2012) Rarer clinical associations of antiphospholipid antibodies. Semin Thromb Hemost 38(4):328–332
33. Mehdi AA, Salti I, Uthman I (2011) Antiphospholipid syndrome: endocrinologic manifestations and organ involvement. Semin Thromb Hemost 37(1):49–57
34. Tenedios F, Erkan D, Lockshin MD (2005) Cardiac involvement in the antiphospholipid syndrome. Lupus 14(9):691–696
35. Vaccaro F, Caccavo D, Roumpedaki E et al (2008) Dilated cardiomyopathy due to thrombotic microangiopathy as the only manifestation of antiphospholipid syndrome: a case report. Int J Immunopathol Pharmacol 21(1):237–241
36. Kanakis MA, Kapsimali V, Vaiopoulos AG et al (2013) The lung in the spectrum of antiphospholipid syndrome. Clin Exp Rheumatol 31(3):452–457
37. Barnini T, Silvestri E, Emmi G et al (2012) Pulmonary fibrosis and lymphocytic alveolitis associated with triple antiphospholipid antibody positivity: a diagnostic puzzle. Clin Exp Rheumatol 30(5):806
38. Frances C (2010) Dermatological manifestations of Hughes' antiphospholipid antibody syndrome. Lupus 19(9):1071–1077
39. Asherson RA, Francès C, Iaccarino L et al (2006) The antiphospholipid antibody syndrome: diagnosis, skin manifestations and current therapy. Clin Exp Rheumatol 24(1 Suppl 40):S46–S51
40. Dean SM (2011) Livedo reticularis and related disorders. Curr Treat Options Cardiovasc Med 13(2):179–191
41. El Benaye J, Hsaini Y, Zoobo T et al (2013) Sneddon's syndrome. Presse Med 42(2):138–144
42. Suvajac G, Stojanovich L, Milenkovich S (2007) Ocular manifestations in antiphospholipid syndrome. Autoimmun Rev 6(6):409–414
43. Utz VM, Tang J (2011) Ocular manifestations of the antiphospholipid syndrome. Br J Ophthalmol 95(4):454–459
44. Provan D, Stasi R, Newland AC et al (2010) International consensus report on the investigation and management of primary immune thrombocytopenia. Blood 115(2):168–186
45. Rückert A, Glimm H, Lübbert M et al (2008) Successful treatment of life-threatening Evans syndrome due to antiphospholipid antibody syndrome by rituximab-based regimen: a case with long-term follow-up. Lupus 17(8):757–760
46. Rueda JC, Duque MA, Mantilla RD et al (2009) Osteonecrosis and antiphospholipid syndrome. J Clin Rheumatol 15(3):130–132
47. Asherson RA, Cervera R, Shepshelovich D et al (2006) Nonthrombotic manifestations of the antiphospholipid syndrome: away from thrombosis? J Rheumatol 33(6):1038–1044

Treatment of Thrombosis in Antiphospholipid Syndrome

15

Simon Braham, Paolo Bucciarelli, and Marco Moia

15.1 Introduction

Antiphospholipid syndrome (APS) is an acquired cause of venous thromboembolism (VTE), i.e., deep vein thrombosis and/or pulmonary embolism in patients with systemic lupus erythematosus or other autoimmune diseases, as well as in the general population. Antiphospholipid antibodies (aPLs), particularly lupus anticoagulant, are important thrombotic risk factors [1]. Growing evidence demonstrates that aPLs, particularly antibodies specific for β_2 glycoprotein I, are not merely a marker of thrombophilia but are pathogenic, directly contributing to hypercoagulability. Current management of VTE in patients with APS does not substantially differ from that in the general population of patients with VTE and without APS. However, a more problematic monitoring of the anticoagulant treatment, both in the acute and in the long-term management, and the high risk of recurrences makes the treatment of VTE in patients with APS more challenging and deserves some special considerations. The intensity and duration of anticoagulation with vitamin K antagonists (VKA) for longer-term secondary prophylaxis are therefore important issues.

The treatment of acute VTE in patients with APS is the same as for other patients with VTE. In the acute phase of VTE, anticoagulation with unfractionated heparin (UH) or low-molecular-weight heparin (LMWH), or fondaparinux, followed by VKA (i.e., warfarin, acenocoumarol, or phenprocoumon) is still the standard of care [2].

New oral anticoagulants, i.e., the direct inhibitor of coagulation factor IIa dabigatran etexilate and the direct inhibitors of factor Xa rivaroxaban, apixaban, or edoxaban, may

S. Braham • P. Bucciarelli • M. Moia (✉)
Fondazione IRCCS Ca' Granda Ospedale Maggiore Policlinico Milano, Angelo Bianchi Bonomi Hemophilia and Thrombosis Centre, Via F. Sforza 35, Milan 20122, Italy
e-mail: simon.braham@gmail.com; bucciarelli@policlinico.mi.it; moia@policlinico.mi.it

© Springer International Publishing Switzerland 2015

P.L. Meroni (ed.), *Antiphospholipid Antibody Syndrome: From Bench to Bedside*, Rare Diseases of the Immune System, DOI 10.1007/978-3-319-11044-8_15

be useful alternatives, but their efficacy and safety in patients with APS have still to be proven in proper studies. The main characteristics of these new drugs and their possible advantages and limits are addressed in the second part of this chapter.

15.2 Treatment of Acute VTE

15.2.1 Parenteral Anticoagulation

The vast majority of patients with APS and diagnosis of VTE should immediately receive parenteral anticoagulation, i.e., therapeutic doses of subcutaneous LMWH or fondaparinux or intravenous UH. Only patients with acute PE associated with hypotension (systolic blood pressure < 90 mmHg) who do not have a high bleeding risk should be systemically administered thrombolytic therapy, followed by heparins/fondaparinux. From studies in patients with VTE, LMWH or fondaparinux (administered at fixed, body-weight-adjusted, therapeutic doses) were at least as effective and safer than intravenous monitored UH [2]. Moreover, they have a lower incidence of side effects such as heparin-induced thrombocytopenia (HIT) and osteoporosis. The advantage of LMWH and fondaparinux over UH may be even more relevant in those patients with LA who have baseline prolonged activated partial thromboplastin time (aPTT), which makes UH monitoring cumbersome and unreliable.

The therapeutic doses of LMWH range from 125 to 200 anti-FXa units/die depending on the different molecule. Fondaparinux is administered at a single daily dose of 5.0 mg for body weight < 50 kg, of 7.5 mg for body weight between 50 and 100 kg, and of 10 mg for body weight > 100 kg. LMWH and fondaparinux are both cleared by the kidney. Renal insufficiency increases plasma levels of these drugs, thus increasing the risk of bleeding. In case of severe renal insufficiency (i.e., creatinine clearance < 30 mL/min), the use of LMWH or fondaparinux at therapeutic doses is generally contraindicated. LMWH doses could be empirically reduced or monitored by a chromogenic assay of anti Xa activity in patient's plasma. However, since this laboratory test is not frequently available, patients with severe renal insufficiency are preferably treated with UH. When intravenous UH is chosen, an initial IV bolus (80 U/kg or 5,000 U) should be administered, followed by continuous infusion (initially at a dose of 18 U/kg/h or 1,300 U/h) with dose adjustment to achieve and maintain an aPTT prolongation that corresponds to plasma heparin levels of 0.3–0.7 IU/mL anti Xa activity. With the more commonly used reagents, this corresponds to an aPTT ratio from 1.5 to 2.5 times the baseline values. However, in patients with LA and baseline prolonged aPTT ratio, this hypothetical equivalence may be unreliable and therefore intravenous UH may result to being very difficult to manage even by experienced physicians.

15.2.2 Oral Anticoagulation

VKA act by inhibiting the vitamin K-dependent liver synthesis of four coagulation factors (II, VII, IX, and X) and two natural anticoagulant proteins (protein C and protein S).

Hence, they are indirect inhibitors requiring few days to achieve their therapeutic effect. They should be started as soon as possible after parenteral anticoagulation, in order to reduce the time of administration of heparin/fondaparinux. As well known, VKA are ineffective as antithrombotic drugs during the very first days of administration, so that it is mandatory to continue the administration of the parenteral active anticoagulant drug for at least 5 days after the first dose of VKA. The parenteral anticoagulant drug can subsequently withdrawn provided that the International Normalized Ratio (INR), the test of choice for VKA monitoring derived from the prothrombin time, is >2.0 for at least two consecutive days. Several drugs as well as some dietary constituents and alcohol intake may interact with VKA and interfere with their anticoagulant intensity. Hence, a constant VKA monitoring with INR is required (at least every 4–6 weeks), preferably in specialized centers.

15.2.3 Regimen, Control, and Duration

Retrospective studies of APS patients suggested that high-intensity treatment with an INR ≥3.0 was more effective than less intensive regimens [3]. However, two more recent randomized controlled trials found that high-intensity treatment (INR 3.1–4.0) is no better than moderate intensity (INR 2.0–3.0) [4, 5]. Since a moderate intensity treatment requires less frequent laboratory controls and has a lower risk of hemorrhage, this is now, in most cases, the standard of care. A higher target INR (>3.0) is suggested, on the basis of expert opinion, in case of recurrent VTE despite an INR in the therapeutic range [6]. It should be pointed out that most available retrospective and prospective studies included both patients with VTE and arterial thrombosis, so that it is not known if these different clinical manifestations of thrombotic APS may benefit from different treatment regimens.

INR results can be unreliable in a subset of patients with APS. In 6.5–10 % of patients with lupus anticoagulant, the antiphospholipid antibodies (aPLs) may prolong the prothrombin time assay leading to an unreliable INR value [7–9]. The reagents used to test the prothrombin time and to derive INR values may have different sensitivity to aPLs. A coagulation assay that is not affected by aPLs, for example, a chromogenic factor II activity assay, may be used to overcome this problem [10]. Therefore, in selected patients with APS, INR should be checked simultaneously to a chromogenic assay of factor II. This procedure may apply to patients with baseline prolonged prothrombin time, or with unexplained very unstable INR values, or with recurrent thrombosis and INR values apparently within the therapeutic interval. For INR within the therapeutic values, the chromogenic factor II level should range approximately from 15 to 25 %, while for factor II plasma levels above 30 %, the degree of anticoagulation is inadequate. In such patients, different reagents for INR determination should be tested and/or the INR therapeutic target individually chosen according with this procedure [10, 11].

The duration of anticoagulation for secondary prophylaxis of VTE in APS is also an important issue, which is closely related to the risk of recurrence. The risk of recurrent VTE in APS patients off anticoagulation is generally high. Previous

Table 15.1 Risk of VTE recurrence in patients with APS

High-risk patients	Low-risk patients
Lupus anticoagulant presence	Isolated intermittently positive aCL or aβ_2GPI at low titers
aCL at medium–high titers	Previous single venous thrombosis
Double or triple positivity (LA, aCL, aβ2GPI)	Removable risk factor
Presence of SLE	
Presence of hereditary thrombophilia	
Presence of coexistent cardiovascular risk factors	
Previous arterial thrombosis	
Recurrent thrombosis (arterial, venous, or both) during anticoagulation therapy	

LA lupus anticoagulant, *aCL* anticardiolipin, *aβ_2GPI* anti-β_2 glycoprotein I, *SLE* systemic lupus erythematosus

reports found an incidence from 10 to 29 % per year [12] or of 50 % at 2 years and 78 % at 8 years [13]. Patients with APS can be divided in two categories: "high"-risk and "low"-risk patients (Table 15.1). Long-term anticoagulation is generally recommended in patients with APS and after a first unprovoked thrombotic event. Conversely, data about the optimal duration of anticoagulant treatment in patients with APS after a single thrombotic event provoked by a removable risk factor are lacking. Therefore, the duration of treatment should be individually planned. The acceptance and the cooperation of a patient are essential for such a demanding treatment as lifelong anticoagulation. For this reason, patients should always be involved in the decisions about long-term management of VTE, with adequate information about the presumed risk of recurrence without anticoagulation and on the risks and the burden of lifelong anticoagulation.

15.2.4 Other Treatments

Immunosuppressive drugs, such as corticosteroids and rituximab, are neither thought to be necessary in the acute phase of VTE in APS nor effective in preventing recurrent VTE associated with aPLs, except for resistant APS [14–16], and in the case of catastrophic APS. Combined VKA and acetylsalicylic acid (ASA) have been proposed in patients with APS and arterial events [17]. However, since the evidence of an increased efficacy of this association is lacking and the increased risk of bleeding is proven, a careful assessment of the patients' bleeding risk should be performed before starting this regimen. Statins, hydroxychloroquine, or LMWH has also been suggested in patients with recurrent thrombosis during VKA, provided that any possible attempt to optimize the quality of VKA treatment, in order to obtain a good time in therapeutic range, has been made (Table 15.2).

Table 15.2 Secondary thromboprophylaxis regimens for patients with established APS

Patients with definite APS and first venous event	Anticoagulant therapy with VKA to a target INR of 2.5 (range 2.0–3.0) indefinitely.
	Duration of treatment can be limited to about 6 months in patients with low-risk aPL profile and provoked VTE
Patients with definite APS and arterial events	Anticoagulant therapy with VKA to a target INR of 3.0 (range 2.5–3.5) or VKA to a target INR of 2.5 combined with antiplatelet treatment (i.e., ASA 100 mg). Check the patient's bleeding risk before starting the combined VKA-ASA regimen
Patients with recurrent refractory thrombosis	Consider statins, hydroxychloroquine, or LMWH in refractory cases

APS antiphospholipid syndrome, *VKA* vitamin K antagonist, *ASA* acetylsalicylic acid, *INR* international normalized ratio, *LMWH* low-molecular-weight heparin

15.3 New Oral Anticoagulant Drugs

The limitation and, in some cases, the difficulty to correctly manage VKA therapy have driven the search for new oral anticoagulant drugs (NOA). To date, three NOA have been licensed by FDA and EMA for the prevention of VTE in patients undergoing major elective orthopedic surgery and of stroke and systemic embolism in patients with atrial fibrillation: the direct inhibitor of coagulation factor IIa dabigatran etexilate and the direct inhibitors of factor Xa rivaroxaban and apixaban [18]. Other NOA are currently under investigation (edoxaban, betrixaban, others) and will probably be available in a few years. Rivaroxaban has already been licensed also for patients with VTE, both for the acute treatment and for the secondary prophylaxis. These agents represent a major advance as, unlike VKA, they do not interact with diet and alcohol intake and have few reported drug interactions affecting anticoagulant intensity. Furthermore, laboratory monitoring is not routinely required due to their predictable anticoagulant effects. Table 15.3 summarizes the main pharmacological characteristics of NOA already available in Europe for clinical use.

The efficacy and safety of NOA in the prevention of stroke or systemic embolization in patients with non-valvular atrial fibrillation have been demonstrated in large phase III clinical trials, all showing that these drugs are as effective as warfarin, with a similar incidence of major bleeding [19–21]. Of particular relevance is the lower incidence of intracranial hemorrhage in patients taking NOA than in those taking VKA. Conversely, the rate of GI bleeding is higher in the former group than in the latter.

Currently, rivaroxaban is the only NOA which is licensed for the treatment of VTE (both deep vein thrombosis and pulmonary embolism) in adults, following the results of the EINSTEIN-DVT and EINSTEIN-PE studies [22, 23], while both dabigatran and apixaban are under review for the treatment of acute VTE. Unfortunately, to date the safety and efficacy of NOA in children have not been established yet, so that they can be used in adult patients only. NOA are potentially teratogenic and must not be used in pregnancy and during breastfeeding, and women with childbearing potential must be warned about this problem.

Table 15.3 Pharmacological characteristics of NOA

	Rivaroxaban	Dabigatran	Apixaban
Target	Factor Xa	Factor IIa	Factor Xa
Pro-drug	No	Yes	No
Bioavailability	>80 %	6 %	>50 %
Plasma protein binding	92–95 %	34–35 %	87 %
Time to peak	3 h	2 h	3 h
Half-life[a]	9 h	14–17 h	9–14 h
Dosing	Fixed dose o.d.	Fixed dose b.i.d.	Fixed dose b.i.d.
Routine drug monitoring	No	No	No
Excretion	66 % renal	80 % renal	25 % renal
	33 % fecal		55 % fecal

o.d. once daily, *b.i.d.* twice daily
[a]with normal creatinine clearance

As for all NOA, which are direct coagulation inhibitors, rivaroxaban can be started directly after the diagnosis of VTE, without bridging with heparins or fondaparinux. The initial dosage is 15 mg b.i.d for 3 weeks, followed by 20 mg o.d., and the tablets should be taken during meal.

15.3.1 Role of NOA in Patients with APS

Due to their better profile in comparison with VKA (no need of routine laboratory monitoring, no reported interactions with food or alcohol, few reported drug interactions), NOA are expected to result in improved quality of life in VTE patients with APS who require an indefinite period of anticoagulation [24]. Because aPLs interfere with a number of hemostatic mechanisms, a possible influence of these antibodies on the anticoagulant effect of NOA cannot be excluded. Therefore, the efficacy and safety of NOA in the treatment of VTE patients with APS might be different from those in VTE patients without APS. Despite aPL status was not documented in the available clinical trials, it is very likely that patients with APS were included in the study populations in phase III clinical trials of rivaroxaban (and other NOA) versus VKA for the treatment of VTE. Nevertheless, the results of ongoing prospective "ad hoc" trials of NOA in patients with APS, such as the RAPS (Rivaroxaban in AntiPhospholipid Syndrome) [25], are urgently needed. Until these results are not available, the use of rivaroxaban (and in future the other NOA) seems to be justified in selected patients with APS and scanty VKA management or with VTE recurrence during VKA treatment.

15.3.2 Cautions and Contraindications with NOA

Despite the fact that therapy with NOA does not require routine laboratory monitoring, NOA administration, as with other anticoagulants, should be implemented within a structured setting, where an experienced staff provides patients with clear information about the anticoagulant treatment and the risk and management of bleeding.

Renal impairment may necessitate dose reduction or avoidance of NOA. Dose adjustment of rivaroxaban is not required in case of mild renal impairment (creatinine clearance 50–80 mL/min), while a reduction of the dose from 20 mg o.d. to 15 mg o.d. should be considered for moderate renal impairment (creatinine clearance 30–49 mL/min). Rivaroxaban should be used with caution when creatinine clearance is between 15 and 29 mL/min and is not recommended in patients with severe renal impairment (creatinine clearance <15 mL/min). The recommendations in case of renal disease are more strict for dabigatran (contraindicated for creatinine clearance <30 mL/min) because it is predominantly excreted by the kidneys and less for apixaban (only a 25 % renal excretion). Periodic monitoring of renal function is particularly recommended in elderly patients or in situations potentially leading to renal impairment, such as infections and dehydration. Liver impairment is not a contraindication for rivaroxaban use, except in case of severe hepatic disease associated with coagulopathy and clinically relevant bleeding risk.

Laboratory tests in patients on NOA are desirable only in specific clinical settings, including patients at extremes of body weight, with renal impairment, and with poor compliance; in case of hemorrhagic or thrombotic complications; and when surgery or other interventions are required [26]. The diluted thrombin time or the ecarin thrombin time are the most sensitive tests for dabigatran, while a modified prothrombin time or an anti-factor Xa assay are the most suitable tests for monitoring rivaroxaban [27]. However, the experience with such tests, particularly in patients with APS, is very limited and requires a support by experts in blood coagulation.

References

1. Galli M, Borrelli G, Jacobsen EM, Marfisi RM, Finazzi G, Marchioli R, Wisloff F, Marziali S, Morboeuf O, Barbui T (2007) Clinical significance of different antiphospholipid antibodies in the WAPS (warfarin in the antiphospholipid syndrome) study. Blood 110:1178–1183
2. Kearon C, Akl EA, Comerota AJ, Prandoni P, Bounameaux H, Goldhaber SZ, Nelson ME, Wells PS, Gould MK, Dentali F, Crowther M, Kahn SR (2012) Antithrombotic therapy for VTE disease. Antithrombotic therapy and prevention of thrombosis, 9th ed: American College of Chest Physicians evidence-based clinical practice guidelines. Chest 141:419S–494S
3. Khamashta MA, Cuadrado MJ, Mujic F, Taub NA, Hunt BJ, Hughes GRV (1995) The management of thrombosis in the antiphospholipid-antibody syndrome. N Engl J Med 332:993–997
4. Crowther MA, Ginsberg JS, Julian J, Denburg J, Hirsh J, Douketis J, Laskin C, Fortin P, Anderson D, Kearon C, Clarke A, Geerts W, Forgie M, Green D, Costantini L, Yacura W, Wilson S, Gent M, Kovacs MJ (2003) A comparison of two intensities of warfarin for the prevention of recurrent thrombosis in patients with the antiphospholipid antibody syndrome. N Engl J Med 349:1133–1138
5. Finazzi G, Marchioli R, Brancaccio V, Schinco P, Wisloff F, Musial J, Baudo F, Berrettini M, Testa S, D'Angelo A, Tognoni G, Barbui T (2005) A randomized clinical trial of high-intensity warfarin vs. conventional antithrombotic therapy for the prevention of recurrent thrombosis in patients with the antiphospholipid syndrome (WAPS). J Thromb Haemost 3:848–853

6. Ruiz-Irastorza G, Hunt BJ, Khamashta MA (2007) A systematic review of secondary thromboprophylaxis in patients with antiphospholipid antibodies. Arthritis Care Res 57: 1487–1495
7. Moll S, Ortel TL (1997) Monitoring warfarin therapy in patients with lupus anticoagulants. Ann Intern Med 127:177–185
8. Sanfelippo MJ, Sennet J, McMahon EJ (2000) Falsely elevated INRs in warfarin-treated patients with the lupus anticoagulant. WMJ 99:62–64
9. Rosborough TK, Shepherd MF (2004) Unreliability of international normalized ratio for monitoring warfarin therapy in patients with lupus anticoagulant. Pharmacotherapy 24:838–842
10. Kasthuri RS, Roubey RA (2007) Warfarin and the antiphospholipid syndrome: does one size fit all? Arthritis Rheum 57:1346–1347
11. Tripodi A, Chantarangkul V, Clerici M, Negri B, Galli M, Mannucci PM (2001) Laboratory control of oral anticoagulant treatment by the INR system in patients with the antiphospholipid syndrome and lupus anticoagulant. Results of a collaborative study involving nine commercial thromboplastins. Br J Haematol 115:672–678
12. Galli M, Barbui T (2003) Antiphospholipid antibodies and thrombosis: strength of association. Hematol J 4:180–186
13. Derksen RHWM, De Groot PG, Kater L, Nieuwenhuis HK (1993) Patients with antiphospholipid antibodies and venous thrombosis should receive long term anticoagulant treatment. Ann Rheum Dis 52:689–692
14. Rubenstein E, Arkfeld DG, Metyas S, Shinada S, Ehresmann S, Liebman HA (2006) Rituximab treatment for resistant antiphospholipid syndrome. J Rheumatol 33:355–357
15. Chalam KV, Gupta SK, Agarwal S (2007) Rituximab effectively reverses papilledema associated with cerebral venous sinus thrombosis in antiphospholipid antibody syndrome. Eur J Ophthalmol 17:867–870
16. Adamson R, Sangle S, Kaul A, Hughes GR, D'Cruz DP (2008) Clinical improvement in antiphospholipid syndrome after rituximab therapy. J Clin Rheumatol 14:359–360
17. Cuadrado MJ, Bertolaccini ML, Seed PT, Tektonidou MG, Aguirre A, Mico L, Gordon C, Ruiz-Irastorza G, Egurbide MV, Gil A, Espinosa G, Houssiau F, Rahman A, Martin H, McHugh N, Galindo M, Akil M, Amigo MC, Murru V, Khamashta MA (2014) Low-dose aspirin vs low-dose aspirin plus low-intensity warfarin in thromboprophylaxis: a prospective, multicentre, randomized, open, controlled trial in patients positive for antiphospholipid antibodies (ALIWAPAS). Rheumatology 53:275–284
18. Garcia D, Libby E, Crowther MA (2010) The new oral anticoagulants. Blood 115:15–20
19. Connolly SJ, Ezekowitz MD, Yusuf S et al RE-LY Steering Committee and Investigators (2009) Dabigatran versus warfarin in patients with atrial fibrillation. N Engl J Med 361:1139–1151
20. Patel MR, Mahaffey KW, Gar J, Pan G, Singe DE, Hacke W et al ROCKET-AF Investigators (2011) Rivaroxaban versus warfarin in nonvalvular atrial fibrillation. N Engl J Med 365:883–891
21. Granger CB, Alexander JH, McMurray JJ et al for the ARISTOTLE Committee and Investigators (2011) Apixaban versus warfarin in patients with atrial fibrillation. N Engl J Med 365:981–992
22. Bauersachs R, Berkowitz SD, Brenner B et al EINSTEIN Investigators (2010) Oral rivaroxaban for symptomatic venous thromboembolism. N Engl J Med 363:2499–2510
23. Büller HR, Prins MH, Lensing AW et al EINSTEIN-PE Investigators (2012) Oral rivaroxaban for the treatment of symptomatic pulmonary embolism. N Engl J Med 366:1287–1297
24. Arachchillage DJ, Cohen H (2013) Use of new oral anticoagulants in antiphospholipid syndrome. Curr Rheumatol Rep 15:331–339
25. RAPS trial details available at: http://isrctn.org/ IRSCTN68222801
26. Garcia D, Barrett YC, Ramacciotti E, Weitz JI (2013) Laboratory assessment of the anticoagulant effects of the next generation of oral anticoagulants. J Thromb Haemost 11:245–252
27. Tripodi A (2013) The laboratory and the direct oral anticoagulants. Blood 121:4032–4035

Treatment of Pregnancy Complications 16

Barbara Acaia, Federica Rossi,
and Cecilia Beatrice Chighizola

16.1 Introduction

Obstetric manifestations enlisted in the classification criteria for the antiphospholipid syndrome (APS) comprise otherwise unexplained pregnancy loss (PrL) – either early (at least three consecutive events before the 10th gestational week) or late (one event at or after the 10th gestational week) – and/or premature birth (before the 34th gestational week) due to eclampsia, preeclampsia, or placental insufficiency, associated with the persistent positivity at medium–high titers for antiphospholipid antibodies (aPL) [1]. Additional aPL-associated complications of pregnancy, not considered in the current APS criteria, include abruptio placentae, hemolysis, elevated liver enzymes, low platelets (HELLP) syndrome, and deep venous thrombosis. A precise estimates of the frequency of aPL-related obstetric complications is still lacking; in a multicenter prospective cohort of 590 pregnant APS women and 1,580 pregnancies, early miscarriages were reported in 35.4 % of cases, fetal death in 16.9 %, premature birth in 10.6 %, preeclampsia in 9.5 %, eclampsia in 4.4 %, and abruptio placentae in 2 % [2].

Three laboratory tests are routinely used to detect serum aPL: two solid-phase assays to evaluate antibodies against β2 glycoprotein I (anti-β2GPI antibodies) and cardiolipin (aCL), and the functional assay lupus anticoagulant (LA) [1]. A given

B. Acaia (✉) • F. Rossi
U.O. Ostetricia e Ginecologia I, U.O.S. Patologia della Gravidanza, IRCCS Fondazione Ca' Granda Ospedale Maggiore Policlinico, Mangiagalli, Regina Elena,
Via della Commenda 12, Milan 20122, Italy
e-mail: barbara.acaia@gmail.com

C.B. Chighizola
Department of Clinical Sciences and Community Health, University of Milan, Milan, Italy

Istituto Auxologico Italiano, Milan, Italy

© Springer International Publishing Switzerland 2015
P.L. Meroni (ed.), *Antiphospholipid Antibody Syndrome: From Bench to Bedside*,
Rare Diseases of the Immune System, DOI 10.1007/978-3-319-11044-8_16

aPL profile confers a peculiar risk of clinical event: patients with a triple aPL positivity are at highest risk for both thrombosis and pregnancy failure; LA is the strongest predictor of clinical manifestations, increasing the risk of miscarriage by tenfold [3–5]. aPL titers and isotypes should also be considered, with IgG being clinically more meaningful compared to IgM [6]. Additional risk factors for pregnancy morbidity include low C3 and C4 at baseline and at the time of pregnancy failure, a platelet decrease greater than 20 %, a previous history of obstetric complications, and an associated autoimmune condition [7, 8].

APS generally does not provide a contraindication for pregnancy, but in case of concomitant illness – such as severe pulmonary hypertension, heart failure, and renal failure – conception should be avoided, because of the high risk of maternal morbidity and mortality. Women carrying aPL who experience a disease flare within the previous 6 months, those who developed a thrombotic event in the previous semester and those with uncontrolled hypertension should also be discouraged to remain pregnant [9].

Without any treatment, approximately 20–30 % of pregnancies in aPL-positive women will end with a successful outcome. Therefore, women with APS should be considered at high risk and managed in a joint rheumatologic-obstetric clinic throughout the whole gestation. Preconceptional and multidisciplinary counselling is necessary in order to determine the risk of maternal as well as fetal complications. The general schedule should include more frequent visits as pregnancy progresses, with regular blood pressure measurement and urinalysis [10]. Follow-up of these women should also include Doppler studies of the uteroplacental circulation to assess placental function and fetal growth and to predict the occurrence of complications such as preeclampsia and fetal distress [11, 12].

Clinical management of APS patients during pregnancy course aims at preventing obstetric recurrences and at avoiding thrombotic events. The association of low-dose aspirin (LDASA) and prophylactic doses of heparin, either synthetic unfractioned heparin (UFH) or low-molecular weight heparin (LMWH), is currently regarded as the standard of care for women with aPL-related obstetric manifestations [13]. Thanks to such combo approach, more than 70 % of pregnant APS women deliver a viable infant [10]. However, despite the advancements in the therapeutic management of obstetric APS, there still remain some critical issues, mainly due to the several limitations flawing the literature. First, some studies have included patients not fulfilling APS criteria: indeed, in most studies any type of PrL was regarded as a sufficient criterion for APS, without excluding other potential causes of pregnancy wastage. Other studies recruited women with any preterm birth because of preeclampsia, eclampsia, or placental insufficiency. However, since placenta-mediated obstetric complications are relatively common in the general population, APS classification criteria included only cases requiring delivery before 34 weeks [1]. Another critical issue of available literature is provided by the inclusion of women with transient or low-titer aPL positivity: such positivity does not display a clinical significance, being reported in other diseases and in healthy individuals. Literature is also impinged by design bias, with most studies being of retrospective nature.

To highlight evidence about the treatment of obstetric APS, three systematic reviews have been performed to date (Empson et al. 2005 [14]; Mak et al. 2010 [15]; Ziakas et al. 2010 [16]). Available evidence about the therapeutic strategies in aPL-related pregnancy complication is hereby widely discussed.

16.2 Historical Notes of Treatment of Obstetric APS

Prednisone and LDASA constituted the mainstay of early APS treatment: thanks to the combination of high-dose prednisone and LDASA, a successful outcome was obtained in 75 % of treated pregnancies.

The first case series on steroids in obstetric APS dates back to 1983, when Lubbe treated with prednisone 6 LA positive women with recurrent PrL, observing a successful outcome in five cases [17]. However, the enthusiasm about steroids was to wane rather quickly: critical issues were raised in 1989, with Lockshin observing a considerable rate of maternal and fetal morbidity in those receiving steroids, including gestational diabetes, hypertension, premature rupture of membranes, and pre-eclampsia [18].

Treatment with LDASA alone was first proposed in the management of obstetric APS in 1988 [19], since then conflicting results have been presented. Several observational studies reported pregnancy success rates as high as 79–100 % with LDASA alone [20–25], whereas in a randomized controlled trial, the rate of positive obstetric outcomes was comparable between the placebo group (84 %) and the group treated with LDASA (80 %), suggesting that LDASA is not beneficial in women with aPL and recurrent PrL [26]. This finding was further supported by Tulppala who did not observe differences in obstetric outcomes between aCL-positive women receiving LDASA or placebo [27]. On the other hand, prophylactic treatment with LDASA during pregnancy reduced the rate of miscarriages from 72 to 38 % in a retrospective study [25] and preconceptional prescription of LDASA appeared to be significantly associated with favorable neonatal outcome in a multivariate analysis [20].

The earlier reports of heparin use date back to 1990 [28]; the first randomized controlled study came in 1992, when Cowchock showed that the regimen of UFH plus LDASA was equally efficacious than prednisone plus LDASA, but associated with less morbidity [29]; this observation was later to be confirmed by many other studies [21, 30]. Furthermore, the addition of UFH to LDASA was shown to increase the rate of successful pregnancies in two early randomized controlled trials. Kutteh conducted the first prospective study in 1996; he treated 50 patients with at least three consecutive PrL and confirmed aPL positivity with either LDASA or LDASA plus UFH. UFH plus LDASA provided a significantly better pregnancy outcome than LDASA alone (rate of viable infants: 80 % versus 44 %, respectively) [31]. Accordingly, Rai showed that the combination treatment (LDASA + UFH) was superior to LDASA alone. In this randomized controlled trial, 90 pregnant women with a history of at least three miscarriages and persistent aPL were recruited; the rate of live births was 71 % among women treated with LDASA + UFH and 42 %

among those receiving LDASA alone [32]. These two studies allowed defining the optimal management of obstetric APS, an approach that has remained substantially unchanged over time.

16.3 Mechanism of Action of Antiplatelet and Anticoagulant Agents in Obstetric APS

Antiplatelets as LDASA are more effective in preventing arterial thrombosis: in the high-flow, high-shear arterial circulation, platelet adhesion and aggregation play a major role. In obstetric APS, LDASA has been shown not only to prevent placental thrombosis but also to stimulate the production of interleukin (IL) -3, a cytokine that favors placental and fetal development [33].

Conversely, anticoagulants are especially active in the low-flow, low-shear venous vasculature where fibrin-rich clot forms. Anticoagulant drugs include vitamin K antagonists (VKA), heparin, and its derivatives. However, warfarin must be avoided throughout the first trimester of pregnancy, specifically during organogenesis between the 6th and the 10th week of gestation, because of the high risk of fetal malformations. After the 12th week, warfarin increases the risk of fetal bleeding. Therefore, heparin derivatives such as UFH and LMWH are preferred. To note, heparin's activity in APS is not merely attributable to its anticoagulant action. Indeed, heparin directly interacts with β2 glycoprotein I (β2GPI), the main antigenic target of aPL. Similarly, it has been suggested that the protective effects exerted by heparin in obstetric APS may be related to its anticomplement activity, as it inhibits the activation of complement cascade induced by aPL [34]. In vitro, heparin restores the placental expression of heparin-binding epidermal growth factor-like growth factor, a molecule involved in blastocyst implantation and prevents both in vitro and in vivo aPL-inhibited endometrial angiogenesis [35–37].

16.4 Current Management of Obstetric APS

The American College of Chest Physicians recently published guidelines for the management of obstetric APS [38]:

- Women with APS without previous thrombosis:
  LDASA together with either UFH (5,000–7,000 IU sc every 12 h) or LMWH in usual prophylactic doses (i.e., enoxaparin 40 mg sc every 24 h).
- Women with APS and previous thrombosis:
  LDASA plus therapeutic UFH or LMWH in usual therapeutic doses (i.e., enoxaparin 1 mg/kg sc every 12 h).

The recommendations included in these guidelines are supported by the three available meta-analyses [14–16]. It should be noted that studies investigating the optimal management of women with obstetric APS focused mainly on the most common aPL-related clinical manifestation in pregnancy, namely, early PrL; much less evidence is available about other obstetrical complications due to aPL.

16.4.1 Treatment of Early Pregnancy Loss

The three available meta-analyses support the standard approach for obstetric APS with heparin plus LDASA: Empson considered six randomized and quasi-randomized controlled trials, concluding that LDASA plus UFH but not LMWH significantly reduced the rate of PrL compared with aspirin alone [14]. Mak analyzed five randomized controlled trials, observing a significantly higher live birth rate among women receiving heparin (either UFH or LMWH) plus LDASA compared to those on LDASA alone [15]. Ziakas evaluated five randomized controlled trials, reporting a treatment effect in favor of UFH but not LMWH [16]. Indeed, LDASA plus UFH significantly reduced PrL compared with aspirin alone, whereas LMWH combined with LDASA displayed no statistically significant effect compared to LDASA alone or to IVIg, even though the point estimates were in the direction of benefit.

The lack of a significant effect by LMWH reported by the three meta-analyses should be ascribed to the randomized controlled trial by Laskin, who in 2009 observed no difference in pregnancy success between LMWH+LDASA and LDASA alone [39]. To note, the two studies directly comparing LMWH to UFH in the management of APS pregnancies did not observe any difference in outcome [40, 41].

Heparin dosage represents a critical issue: in fact, a wide heterogeneity has been observed across the studies, with very few authors specifically addressing this point. A pharmacokinetics study identified dalteparin 5,000 U daily as the optimal dosing regimen [42]. Consistently, Kutteh suggested that lower-dose UFH (5,000 U twice daily) was as affective as higher dose (10,000 U twice daily) in the treatment of aPL-associated PrL [43]. Recently, Ruffatti reported a 97 % live-birth rate among APS women receiving prophylactic adjusted dose of LMWH, suggesting that LMWH dose adjustment as pregnancy progresses and maternal/fetal body weight increases may provide an efficacious treatment option [44].

Both UFH and LMWH display important side effects, such as heparin-induced thrombocytopenia and osteoporosis; it is therefore recommended to properly supplement pregnant women on heparin with calcium and vitamin D. Conversely, the bleeding risk seems to be rather low among pregnant women on heparin: in a series of 89 pregnancies treated with LMWH, bleeding complications were observed in 6.7 % of cases, but none was major [45].

As expected, in a meta-analysis of available studies, the association of prednisone and LDASA did not reduce the rate of PrL, but was associated with a three times greater risk of premature delivery and gestational diabetes compared to other regimens [14].

16.4.2 Treatment of Late Pregnancy Loss

The management of women with prior fetal loss follows the same indications than those for early miscarriages even if Ziakas didn't find any significant effect of therapy with heparin plus LDASA on pregnancy outcome [16].

16.4.3 Treatment of Preeclampsia, Eclampsia, and HELLP Syndrome

aPL are among the most significant risk factors for preeclampsia [46]; however, this complication is reported rather rarely in APS treatment trials. A recent meta-analysis evaluating 31 randomized trials on primary prevention of preeclampsia in high-risk individuals (not only aPL-positive) showed that antiplatelet agents were associated with a 10 % reduction in preeclampsia and prematurity rates [47]. On the other hand, in two aspirin only trials, preeclampsia rates were even a little higher among women receiving placebo compared to those treated with LDASA [31, 32].

HELLP syndrome complicates approximately 10–12 % of pregnancies with preeclampsia/eclampsia. A 2005 retrospective study of 16 cases of aPL-associated HELLP syndrome in 15 women showed that treatment with LDASA and LMWH substantially decreased the risk of HELLP in subsequent pregnancies, with all 16 pregnancies ending with a live birth [45]. Apart from this large case series, 10 case reports about women with HELLP syndrome treated with heparin have been published, leading to a live birth in 3 cases [48–54].

16.4.4 Treatment of Other Pregnancy Complications

More than 10 % of untreated APS women deliver small for gestational age infants [52], while preterm birth is reported to complicate 12–35 % of pregnancies in aPL-positive women [39]. With respect to these pregnancy complications, Empson observed that UFH maintained a treatment advantage when composite outcomes were considered (PrL or IUGR, PrL or premature delivery), while LDASA alone had no significant effect on any of the considered outcomes [14].

Even though the literature does not provide a solid evidence for the management aPL-related pregnancy complications other than early PrL, the rationale of using the same therapeutic approach lays in the observation that aPL-associated PrL, preeclampsia, eclampsia, IUGR, and HELLP syndrome are all mediated by the same pathogenic mechanisms: β2GPI-dependent aPL target placental tissues interfering with multiple physiologic pathways, leading to the inhibition of trophoblast differentiation, growth, and invasion and of endometrial endothelial cell differentiation, eventually resulting in defective placentation [55].

16.5 Management of Pregnant Women with Thrombotic APS

A history of vascular thrombosis was found to be significantly associated with a poor infant outcome together with LA and triple positivity [56]. Moreover, Bramham observed that women with previous thrombosis display a worse obstetric prognosis compared to women with APS obstetric manifestations only, with significantly higher rates of preterm delivery and small for gestational age babies [57]. Unfortunately, clinical studies have not included pregnant APS women who experienced thrombotic events. The management of these women is rather troublesome, as warfarin has a teratogenic potential; nevertheless, one study evaluated warfarin in APS pregnancies, without observing any difference with enoxaparin [58]. Currently, it is recommended to switch warfarin to heparin as soon as pregnancy is confirmed. Treatment with full antithrombotic doses of LMWH plus LDASA throughout the entire pregnancy is an accepted approach [38]. Warfarin could be exceptionally prescribed in the second trimester until close to delivery, when heparin must be resumed [13, 59, 60].

16.6 Treatment of Refractory Obstetric APS

Not all women receiving standard treatment succeed in having a live birth. The heterogeneity in pregnancy outcomes may be related to differences in the clinical features and the serologic profile. Besides aPL profile, traditional risk factors, such as advanced maternal age, increased BMI, and proinflammatory maternal diseases (i.e., metabolic syndrome), could affect pregnancy outcome.

To date, no evidence-based recommendation is available about which treatment should be instituted when first-line therapies fail. In a 2008 survey of physicians experienced in obstetric APS management, the most common therapeutic strategy in case of refractory obstetric APS consisted in increasing LMWH from a prophylactic to a therapeutic dose, even though this approach is not supported by any evidence [61]. Another strategy envisages the combination of standard treatment with one or more therapeutic tool among IVIg, prednisone, and plasma exchange.

It should be noted that to date there is no evidence of a clear beneficial effect of IVIg in obstetric APS. The first report of IVIg use in obstetric APS was that of Carreras et al. [62], followed by few more anecdotal reports [63–66] and case series [67–72] supporting the benefits of IVIg. However, a Cochrane analysis considering five studies concluded that IVIg are associated with an increased risk of PrL or premature birth compared with heparin and LDASA [14].

Prednisone might provide another therapeutic option for refractory cases because of its action on inflammatory mechanisms underlying obstetric APS. However, low-dose prednisone only can be an option. In fact, even if steroids are mostly inactivated by placental metabolism allowing just a small percentage to cross into the fetal circulation, high-dose corticosteroids are clearly associated with an increased rate of complications, as previously discussed. Indeed, a UK group recently reported a marked increase in the live-birth rate in women with refractory events (from 4 to 61 %) thanks to the addition of prednisone 10 mg daily in the first trimester [73]. The early administration allows an effect on placentation without inducing the premature rupture of membranes.

Plasma exchange is an additional therapeutic tool; the rationale behind apheretic treatments lays in the removal of aPL from bloodstream. Some authors support the safety and tolerability of plasma exchange during pregnancy [74], even though available evidence of the efficacy of this treatment in obstetric APS is merely restricted to case reports from a single center [75, 76].

16.7 Management of Pregnant Women with Secondary APS

In approximately 40 % of cases, pregnant aPL-positive patients carry an autoimmune disease, mainly systemic lupus erythematosus (SLE). These women carry a consistent obstetric risk factor, since lupus itself, and to a lesser extent other rheumatic conditions, exerts a strong impact on pregnancy course.

Women with SLE should be counselled preconceptionally, in order to schedule pregnancy during remission; in particular, the disease should have been stable for at least 6 months. Pregnancies in these patients must be strictly followed by a joint team of obstetricians and rheumatologists to precisely assess the individual risk and to modify the pharmacological treatment avoiding teratogen compounds. During pregnancy course and in the postpartum, women should be carefully monitored for any possible disease flare [9]. It should be remembered that some of the immunosuppressive drugs used to control disease activity during pregnancy are contraindicated during lactation [59].

16.8 Treatment of aPL-Positive Women Not Fulfilling APS Criteria

The optimal management of low-titer aPL-positive pregnant women is a matter of debate, as currently available evidence is inconsistent. Some studies were not supportive of a treatment benefit [77, 78], and recently aPL-positive women on LDASA were found to present a pregnancy outcome similar to controls, suggesting that in this setting, an approach with LDASA only might be sufficient [79]. On the other hand, another study reported that untreated patients with low aPL levels and APS-like obstetrical events have a poor pregnancy outcome, similar to those with full-blown APS [80]. Consistently, women with aPL positivity at low titers have been shown to be at high risk of developing severe obstetric APS, thus warranting full treatment [81].

Although there is no recommendation on how to treat women not fulfilling APS criteria, most physicians experienced in obstetric APS management prescribe

LDASA [61], since aPL-positive women display an increased risk of preeclampsia and LDASA was reported to decrease such risk [47].

16.9 Peripartum Management

Proper peripartum management of anticoagulation is crucial. In case of epidural anesthesia or analgesia, epidural anesthesia can be safely performed 12 h after the last dose of LMWH at thromboprophylactic doses, and it can be resumed 6–8 h after the procedure. LDASA does not add a significant risk for spinal hematoma, and it can be safely maintained. For induction or scheduled cesarean, UFH and prophylactic LMWH should be discontinued 12 h before admission [38].

During puerperium the thrombotic risk is very high, with a procoagulant state compensating for excessive maternal bleeding at delivery. Therefore, it is recommended to continue thromboprophylaxis with LDASA plus UFH or LMWH for 4–6 weeks after delivery in women with obstetric manifestations only [38]. In this regard, it has recently emerged that, despite treatment with LDASA, APS women with at least three early losses present a higher annual thrombotic risk as compared to women with recurrent abortions due to thrombophilic defects, women with PrL but negative thrombophilic profile, and asymptomatic aPL carriers, with a greater 12-year cumulative thrombotic incidence compared to control women [82, 83]. Therefore, these patients definitely are worth a primary thromboprophylaxis. When administered at full antithrombotic doses, LMWH should be stopped 24 h before epidural anesthesia or it should be replaced by thromboprophylactic dose 12 h *before*, and it can be resumed not earlier than 24 h afterwards. After delivery, women receiving long-term anticoagulation can be safely switched to warfarin [84, 85]. Both heparin and warfarin have been shown to be safe for breastfeeding mothers [59].

Conclusions

Antiplatelet and anticoagulant agents currently provide the cornerstone of the treatment of obstetric APS: there is consensus that the regimen combining preconceptional LDASA and heparin should be the first-line treatment for obstetric APS while IVIg, steroids, and plasma exchange should be reserved to refractory cases. Many clinical issues remain still unresolved, such as the optimal treatment of cases not responsive to conventional treatment or the management of patients not fulfilling clinical and laboratory APS criteria (e.g., women with a history of two early events or with low-titer aPL positivity). In particular, no treatment trial has ever investigated the optimal treatment of aPL women stratifying upon the different risk profile (aPL profile, associated autoimmune conditions, previous obstetrical history). Hopefully, these critical issues will be soon overcome thanks to a clear-cut evidence, even though we reckon it is not straightforward to conduct well-designed, large, multicenter trials in pregnant APS women due to ethical issues.

References

1. Miyakis S, Lockshin MD, Atsumi M et al (2006) International consensus statement on an update of the classification criteria for definite antiphospholipid syndrome (APS). J Thromb Haemost 4:295–306
2. Cervera R, Piette JC, Font J et al (2002) Antiphospholipid syndrome: clinical, and immunologic manifestations and pattern of disease expression in a color of 1000 patients. Arthritis Rheum 46:1019–1027
3. Neville C, Rauch J, Kassis J et al (2009) Antiphospholipid antibodies predict imminent vascular events independently from other risk factors in a prospective cohort. Thromb Haemost 101:100–107
4. Pengo V, Ruffatti A, Legnani C et al (2010) Clinical course of high-risk patients diagnosed with antiphospholipid syndrome. J Thromb Haemost 8:237–242
5. Rai RS, Clifford K, Cohen H et al (1995) High prospective fetal loss rate in untreated pregnancies of women with recurrent miscarriage and antiphospholipid antibodies. Hum Reprod 10:3301–3304
6. De Groot PG, Lutters B, Derksen RHWM et al (2004) Lupus anticoagulants and the risk of a first episode of deep venous thrombosis. J Thromb Haemost 3:1993–1997
7. Rai R, Regan L (1997) Obstetric complications of antiphospholipid antibodies. Curr Opin Obstet Gynecol 9:387–390
8. Ruffatti A, Del Ross T, Ciprian M et al (2009) Risk factors for a first thrombotic event in antiphospholipid antibody carriers. A multicenter, retrospective follow-up study. Ann Rheum Dis 68:397–399
9. Ruiz-Irastorza G, Khamashta MA (2011) Lupus and pregnancy: integrating clues from the bench and bedside. Eur J Clin Invest 41:672–678
10. Danza A, Ruiz-Irastorza G, Khamashta MA (2012) Antiphospholipid syndrome in obstetrics. Best Pract Res Clin Obstet Gynaecol 26:65–76
11. Le Thi Huong D, Wechsler B, Vauthier-Brouzes D et al (2006) The second trimester Doppler ultrasound examination is the best predictor of late pregnancy outcome in systemic lupus erythematosus and/or the antiphospholipid syndrome. Rheumatology (Oxford) 45:332–338
12. Cnossen JS, Morris RK, ter Riet G et al (2008) Use of uterine artery Doppler ultrasonography to predict pre-eclampsia and intrauterine growth restriction: a systematic review and bivariable meta-analysis. CMAJ 178:701–711
13. Ruiz-Irastorza G, Khamashta MA (2007) Antiphospholipid syndrome in pregnancy. Rheum Dis Clin North Am 33:287–297
14. Empson M, Lassere M, Craig J et al (2005) Prevention of recurrent miscarriage for women with antiphospholipid antibody or lupus anticoagulant. Cochrane Database Syst Rev. doi:10.1002/14651858.CD002859
15. Mak A, Cheung MW, Cheak AA et al (2010) Combination of heparin and aspirin is superior to aspirin alone in enhancing livebirths in patients with recurrent pregnancy loss and positive anti-phospholipid antibodies: a meta-analysis of randomized controlled trials and meta-regression. Rheumatology 49:281–288
16. Ziakas PD, Pavlou M, Voulgarelis M (2010) Heparin treatment in antiphospholipid syndrome with recurrent pregnancy loss: a systematic review and meta-analysis. Obstet Gynecol 115:1256–1262
17. Lubbe WF, Butler WS, Palmer SJ et al (1983) Foetal survival after prednisolone suppression of maternal lupus-anticoagulant. Lancet 18:1361–1363
18. Lockshin MD, Druzin ML, Qamar T (1989) Prednisone does not prevent recurrent fetal death in women with antiphospholipid antibody. Am J Obstet Gynecol 160:439–443
19. Elder MG, de Swiet M, Robertson A et al (1988) Low dose aspirin in pregnancy. Lancet 1:410
20. Carmona F, Font J, Azulay M et al (2001) Risk factors associated with fetal losses in treated antiphospholipid syndrome pregnancies: a multivariate analysis. Am J Reprod Immunol 46:274–279

21. Silver RK, MacGregor SN, Sholl JS et al (1993) Comparative trial of prednisone plus aspirin versus aspirin alone in the treatment of anticardiolipin antibody-positive obstetric patients. Am J Obstet Gynecol 169:1411–1417
22. Lima F, Khamashta MA, Buchanan NMM et al (1996) A study of sixty pregnancies patients with the antiphospholipid syndrome. Clin Exp Rheumatol 14:131–136
23. Granger KA, Farquharson RG (1997) Obstetric outcome in antiphospholipid syndrome. Lupus 6:509–513
24. Huong DLT, Wechsler B, Bletry O et al (2001) A study of 75 pregnancies in patients with antiphospholipid syndrome. J Rheumatol 28:2025–2030
25. Munoz-Rodriguez FJ, Font J, Cervera R et al (1999) Clinical study of 100 patients with the antiphospholipid syndrome. Semin Arthritis Rheum 29:182–190
26. Pattison NS, Chamley LW, Birdsall M et al (2000) Does aspirin have a role in improving pregnancy outcome for women with the antiphospholipid syndrome? A randomized controlled trial. Am J Obstet Gynecol 183:1008–1012
27. Tulppala M, Marttunen M, Soderstrom-Anttila V et al (1997) Low-dose aspirin in prevention of miscarriage in women with unexplained or autoimmune related recurrent miscarriage: effect on prostacyclin and thromboxane A2 production. Hum Reprod 12:1567–1572
28. Rosove MH, Tabsh K, Wasserstrum N et al (1990) Heparin therapy for pregnant women with lupus anticoagulant or anticardiolipin antibodies. Obstet Gynecol 75:630–634
29. Cowchock FS, Reece EA, Baldan D et al (1992) Repeated fetal losses associated with antiphospholipid antibodies: a collaborative randomized trial comparing prednisone with low dose heparin treatment. Am J Obstet Gynecol 166:1318–1327
30. Laskin CA, Bombardier C, Hannah ME et al (1997) Prednisone and aspirin in women with autoantibodies and unexplained recurrent fetal loss. N Engl J Med 337:148–153
31. Kutteh WH (1996) Antiphospholipid antibody-associated recurrent pregnancy loss: treatment with heparin and low-dose aspirin is superior to low-dose aspirin alone. Am J Obstet Gynecol 174:1584–1589
32. Rai R, Cohen H, Dave M et al (1997) Randomised controlled trial of aspirin and aspirin plus heparin in pregnant women with recurrent miscarriage associated with phospholipid antibodies (or antiphospholipid antibodies). BMJ 314:253–257
33. Fishman P, Falach-Vaknin E, Sredni B et al (1996) Aspirin-interleukin-3 interrelationships in patients with anti-phospholipid syndrome. Am J Reprod Immunol 35:80–84
34. Girardi G, Redecha P, Salmon JE (2004) Heparin prevents antiphospholipid antibody-induced fetal loss by inhibiting complement activation. Nat Med 10:1222–1226
35. Di Simone N, Marana R, Castellani R et al (2010) Decreased expression of heparin-binding epidermal growth factor-like growth factor as a newly identified pathogenic mechanism of antiphospholipid-mediated defective placentation. Arthritis Rheum 62:1504–1512
36. D'Ippolito S, Marana R, Di Nicuolo F et al (2012) Effect of low molecular weight heparins (LMWHs) on antiphospholipid antibodies (aPL)–mediated inhibition of endometrial angiogenesis. PLoS One. doi:10.1371/journal.pone.0029660
37. de Carvalho JF, de Oliveira RM, Rodrigues CEM et al (2012) Heparin increases HLA-G levels in primary antiphospholipid syndrome. Clin Dev Immunol. doi:10.1155/2012/232390
38. Bates SM, Greer IA, Pabinger I et al (2008) Venous thromboembolism, thrombophilia, antithrombotic therapy, and pregnancy: American College of Chest Physicians Evidence-Based Clinical Practice Guidelines (8th Edition). Chest 133:844S–886S
39. Laskin CA, Spitzer KA, Clark CA et al (2009) Low molecular weight heparin and aspirin for recurrent pregnancy loss: results from the randomized, controlled HepASA trial. J Rheumatol 36:279–287
40. Stephenson MD, Ballem PJ, Tsang P et al (2004) Treatment of antiphospholipid antibody syndrome (APS) in pregnancy: a randomized pilot trial comparing low molecular weight heparin to unfractionated heparin. J Obstet Gynaecol Can 26:729–734
41. Noble LS, Kutteh WH, Lashey N et al (2005) Antiphospholipid antibodies associated with recurrent pregnancy loss: prospective, multicenter, controlled pilot study comparing treatment with low-molecular-weight heparin versus unfractionated heparin. Fertil Steril 83:684–690

42. Ensom MH, Stephenson MD (2004) Pharmacokinetics of low molecular weight heparin and unfractionated heparin in pregnancy. J Soc Gynecol Investig 11:377–383
43. Kutteh WH, Ermel LD (1996) A clinical trial for the treatment of antiphospholipid antibody-associated recurrent pregnancy loss with lower dose heparin and aspirin. Am J Reprod Immunol 35:402–407
44. Ruffatti A, Gervasi MT, Favaro M et al (2011) Adjusted prophylactic doses of nadroparin plus low dose aspirin therapy in obstetric antiphospholipid syndrome. A prospective cohort management study. Clin Exp Rheumatol 29:551–554
45. De Sancho MT, Khalid S, Christos PJ (2012) Outcomes in women receiving low-molecular weight heparin during pregnancy. Blood Coagul Fibrinolysis 23:51–755
46. Duckitt K, Harrington D (2005) Risk factors for pre-eclampsia at antenatal booking: systematic review of controlled studies. BMJ 330:565
47. Askie LM, Duley L, Henderson-Smart DJ, PARIS Collaborative Group et al (2007) Antiplatelet agents for prevention of preeclampsia: a meta-analysis of individual patient data. Lancet 369:1791–1798
48. Sinha J, Chowdhry I, Sedan S, Barland P (2002) Bone marrow necrosis and refractory HELLP syndrome in a patient with catastrophic antiphospholipid antibody syndrome. J Rheumatol 29:195–197
49. Pauzner R, Dulitzky M, Carp H et al (2003) Hepatic infarctions during pregnancy are associated with the antiphospholipid syndrome and in addition with complete or incomplete HELLP syndrome. J Thromb Haemost 1:1758–1763
50. Haram K, Trovik J, Sandset PM et al (2003) Severe syndrome of hemolysis, elevated liver enzymes and low platelets (HELLP) in the 18th week of pregnancy associated with the antiphospholipid-antibody syndrome. Acta Obstet Gynecol Scand 82:679–680
51. Roberts G, Gordon MM, Porter D et al (2003) Acute renal failure complicating HELLP syndrome, SLE and anti-phospholipid syndrome: successful outcome using plasma exchange therapy. Lupus 12:251–257
52. Ilbery M, Jones AR, Sampson MB, Samson J (1995) Lupus anticoagulant and HELLP syndrome complicated by placental abruption, hepatic, dermal and adrenal infarction. Aust N Z J Obstet Gynaecol 35:215–217
53. Alsulyman OM, Castro MA, Zuckerman E et al (1996) Preeclampsia and liver infarction in early pregnancy associated with the antiphospholipid syndrome. Obstet Gynecol 88:644–646
54. Amant F, Spitz B, Arnout J, Van Assche FA (1997) Hepatic necrosis and haemorrhage in pregnant patients with antiphospholipid antibodies. Lupus 6:552–555
55. Alijotas-Reis J (2013) Treatment of refractory obstetric antiphospholipid syndrome: the state of the art and new trends in the therapeutic management. Lupus 22:6–17
56. Ruffatti A, Calligaro A, Hoxha A et al (2010) Laboratory and clinical features of pregnant women with antiphospholipid syndrome and neonatal outcome. Arthritis Care Res 62:302–307
57. Bramham K, Hunt BJ, Germain S et al (2010) Pregnancy outcome in different clinical phenotypes of antiphospholipid syndrome. Lupus 19:58–64
58. Pauzner R, Dulitzki M, Langevitz P et al (2001) Low molecular weight heparin and warfarin in the treatment of patients with antiphospholipid syndrome during pregnancy. Thromb Haemost 86:1379–1384
59. Østensen M, Khamashta M, Lockshin M et al (2006) Anti-inflammatory and immunosuppressive drugs and reproduction. Arthritis Res Ther 8:209
60. Lockshin MD (2013) Anticoagulation in management of antiphospholipid antibody syndrome in pregnancy. Clin Lab Med 33:367–376
61. Erkan D, Patel S, Nuzzo M et al (2008) Management of the controversial aspects of the antiphospholipid syndrome pregnancies: a guide for clinicians and researchers. Rheumatology 47:23–27
62. Carreras LO, Perez GN, Vega H et al (1988) Lupus anticoagulant and recurrent fetal loss: successful treatment with gammaglobulin. Lancet 2:393–394

63. Parke A, Maier D, Wilson D et al (1989) Intravenous gamma-globulin, antiphospholipid antibodies, and pregnancy. Ann Intern Med 110:495–496
64. Scott JR, Branch DW, Kochenour NK et al (1989) Intravenous immunoglobulin treatment of pregnant patients with recurrent pregnancy loss caused by antiphospholipid antibodies and Rh immunization. Am J Obstet Gynecol 159:055–1056
65. Wapner RJ, Cowchock FS, Shapiro SS (1989) Successful treatment in two women with antiphospholipid antibodies and refractory pregnancy losses with intravenous immunoglobulin infusions. Am J Obstet Gynecol 161:1271–1272
66. Ron-el R, Vinder A, Golan A et al (1993) The use of intravenous gammaglobulin, heparin and aspirin in the maintenance of a pregnancy of freeze thawed embryo in a patient with lupus anticoagulant. Eur J Obstet Gynecol Reprod Biol 52:131–133
67. Kaaja R, Julkunen H, Ammala P et al (1993) Intravenous immunoglobulin treatment of pregnant patients with recurrent pregnancy losses associated with antiphospholipid antibodies. Acta Obstet Gynecol Scand 72:63–66
68. Spinnato JA, Clark AL, Pierangeli SS et al (1995) Intravenous immunoglobulin therapy for the antiphospholipid syndrome in pregnancy. Am J Obstet Gynecol 172:690–694
69. Valensise H, Vaquero E, De Carolis C et al (1995) Normal fetal growth in women with antiphospholipid syndrome treated with high-dose intravenous immunoglobulin (IVIG). Prenat Diagn 15:509–517
70. Clark AL, Branch DW, Silver RM et al (1999) Pregnancy complicated by the antiphospolipid syndrome: outcomes with intravenous immunoglobulin therapy. Obstet Gynecol 93:437–441
71. Marzusch K, Dietl J, Klein R et al (1996) Recurrent first trimester spontaneous abortion associated with antiphospholipid antibodies: a pilot study of treatment with intravenous immunoglobulin. Acta Obstet Gynecol Scand 75:922–926
72. Triolo G, Ferrante A, Accardo-Palumbo A et al (2004) IVIG in pregnancy. Lupus 13:731–735
73. Bramham K, Thomas M, Nelson-Piercy C et al (2011) First-trimester low-dose prednisolone in refractory antiphospholipid antibody-related pregnancy loss. Blood 117:6948–6951
74. Bontadi A, Ruffatti A, Tison T et al (2012) Plasma exchange and immunoadsorption effectively remove antiphospholipid antibodies in pregnant patients with antiphospholipid syndrome. J Clin Apher 27:200–204
75. Bortolati M, Marson P, Chiarelli S et al (2009) Case reports of the use of immunoadsorption or plasma exchange in high-risk pregnancies of women with antiphospholipid syndrome. Ther Apher Dial 13:157–160
76. Ruffatti A, Marson P, Pengo V et al (2007) Plasma exchange in the management of high risk pregnant patients with primary antiphospholipid syndrome. A report of 9 cases and a review of the literature. Autoimmun Rev 6:196–202
77. Cowchock S, Reece EA (1997) Do low-risk pregnant women with antiphospholipid antibodies need to be treated? Organizing group of the antiphospholipid antibody treatment trial. Am J Obstet Gynecol 176:1099–1100
78. Del Ross T, Ruffatti A, Visentin MS et al (2013) Treatment of 139 pregnancies in antiphospholipid positive women not fulfilling criteria for antiphospholipid syndrome: a retrospective study. J Rheumatol 40:425–429
79. Soh MC, Pasupathy D, Gray G et al (2013) Persistent antiphospholipid antibodies do not contribute to adverse pregnancy outcomes. Rheumatology 52:1642–1647
80. Mekinian A, Loire-Berson P, Nicaise-Roland P et al (2012) Outcomes and treatment of obstetrical antiphospholipid syndrome in women with low antiphospholipid antibody levels. J Reprod Immunol 94:222–226
81. Gardiner C, Hills J, Machin SJ et al (2013) Diagnosis of antiphospholipid syndrome in routine clinical practice. Lupus 22:18–25
82. Gris JC, Bouvier S, Molinari N et al (2012) Comparative incidence of a first thrombotic events in purely obstetric antiphospholipid syndrome with pregnancy loss: the NOH-AOS observational study. Blood 119:2624–2632

83. Martinez-Zamora MA, Peralta S, Creus M et al (2012) Risk of thrombotic events after recurrent abortion in anti-phospholipid syndrome: a case-control study. Ann Rheum Dis 71:61–66
84. Horlocker T, Wedel D, Rowlingson J et al (2010) Regional anesthesia in the patient receiving antithrombotic or thrombolytic therapy: American Society of Regional Anesthesia and Pain Medicine Evidence-Based Guidelines (Third Edition). Reg Anesth Pain Med 35:64–101
85. Douketis JD, Berger P, Dunn A et al (2008) The perioperative management of antithrombotic therapy: American College of Chest Physicians Evidence-Based Clinical Practice Guidelines (8th Edition). Chest 133:299S–339S

Antiphospholipid Antibody Carriers 17

Francesca Dall'Ara, Cecilia Nalli, and Laura Andreoli

Antiphospholipid antibodies (aPL) are a group of heterogeneous antibodies, detected by different assays (lupus anticoagulant, LA; anticardiolipin antibodies, aCL; and anti-β2-glycoprotein I antibodies, anti-β2GPI) [1]. These autoantibodies are directly involved in pathogenesis of severe clinical manifestations such as thrombosis (either venous or arterial) and pregnancy morbidity (not only pregnancy loss but also life-threatening conditions like preeclampsia) [2]. These manifestations are the hallmark of the antiphospholipid syndrome (APS) [3].

However, aPL have been increasingly detected in subjects who do not display the classical features of APS [4]. In fact, aPL may be found in patients with "non-criteria" manifestations (thrombocytopenia, hemolytic anemia, livedo reticularis) or women undergoing investigations for infertility. The presence of aPL can be discovered before a surgical procedure because of a prolonged thromboplastin time. Are these subjects at risk for thrombosis and pregnancy adverse outcomes? The answer is for sure "yes," since we know that aPL are pathogenic antibodies. However, observational studies did not report a high incidence of events in aPL carriers, ranging from 0 to 3.8 % annually [5]. This apparent discrepancy can be explained by the fact that the relationship between aPL and thrombosis is not "all or nothing."

17.1 aPL as Risk Factors

Circulating aPL should be better considered as thrombotic risk factors, with several other variables modulating the final clinical expression [6, 7]. Among these factors, the most important are the aPL profile, the coexistence of other thrombotic risk

F. Dall'Ara, MD • C. Nalli, MD • L. Andreoli, MD (✉)
Department of Clinical and Experimental Sciences, Rheumatology and Clinical Immunology, Spedali Civili of Brescia, University of Brescia, Piazzale Spedali Civili, 1, Brescia 25123, Italy
e-mail: francesca.dallara@gmail.com; cecilianalli@libero.it; laura.andreoli@unibs.it

© Springer International Publishing Switzerland 2015
P.L. Meroni (ed.), *Antiphospholipid Antibody Syndrome: From Bench to Bedside*, Rare Diseases of the Immune System, DOI 10.1007/978-3-319-11044-8_17

factors, and the presence of an underlying autoimmune disease, mainly systemic lupus erythematosus (SLE).

In terms of aPL profile, the patients may have single, double, or triple aPL; single or multiple isotypes (IgG, IgM, and IgA, although the last one is not included in the criteria); and low vs. medium to high titers of antibodies. Taken as a whole, this information means that clinicians deal every day with a wide variety of "aPL profiles" and not all antibody profiles confer the same degree of risk. According to special task forces at the 13th International Congress on Antiphospholipid Antibodies [8, 9], a high-risk profile can be defined as LA positivity, or "triple positivity" (LA + aCL + anti-β2GPI) or the isolated but persistent positivity for aCL at medium-high titers. A multicenter prospective Italian study [10] observed that the occurrence of a first thrombotic event in carriers of high-risk aPL profile is considerable and it is more frequent among male patient and in the presence of additional risk factor for venous thrombosis.

Recently, a meta-analysis [11] concluded that LA and aCL were the tests significantly associated with an increased risk of thrombosis, especially arterial thrombosis in patients without SLE. A possible limitation of this work is that the relationship with clinical manifestations was searched for single tests (either aCL or LA or anti-β2GPI) and no analysis of the aPL profile was performed. It should be actually recognized that the concept of "high-risk profile" is rather new, so many of the studies included in the meta-analysis did not apply such a definition. In any case, the international consensus of experts felt that patients with isolated aCL or anti-b2GPI at low to medium titer could be considered at low risk for future thrombosis [8].

17.2 Risk Assessment for Thrombosis in aPL-Positive Subjects

aPL alone are not sufficient to generate thrombosis. According to the "two-hit hypothesis," aPL represent only the "first hit," decreasing the thrombophilic threshold by inducing a prothrombotic and proinflammatory phenotype in endothelial cells, but a "second hit" [12] may be required as a triggering event. In fact, retrospective, cross-sectional, and prospective cohort studies demonstrated that at least half of APS patients with vascular events showed other non-aPL, reversible thrombosis risk factors at the time of the event [5]. In the general population, the thrombosis risk rises with increasing number of risk factors and age, therefore also in aPL carriers all these variables may be responsible for triggering acute events. For this reason management of aPL carriers should take into account any possible second hit, namely [13]:

1. Older age
2. Traditional cardiovascular risk factors (e.g., hypertension, diabetes mellitus, proatherogenic lipid profile, obesity, early menopause)

3. Acquired thrombosis initiators (e.g., smoking, oral contraceptives, pregnancy, immobilization, surgical procedures)
4. Genetic hypercoagulable states (e.g., protein C and protein S deficiency, factor V Leiden mutation, prothrombin 20210 gene mutation)

In addition to those "classic" risk factors, it is also important to consider the presence of an underlying systemic autoimmune disease that may also increase the risk of thrombosis. A higher incidence of vascular events, which is not completely explained by traditional vascular risk factors, is observed in patients with SLE. The inflammatory phenotypes of systemic autoimmune diseases are able to induce perturbation of the endothelium and to initiate the action of aPL, regardless of the underlying disease. Because aPL are risk factors, their assessment should become part of the routine workup of patients with a diagnosis of systemic autoimmune disease [7].

A common risk factor is cigarette smoking. A recent study [14] explored the association between smoking, aPL, and vascular events. Only aPL, among a large set of commonly occurring autoantibodies in SLE, were positively associated with a history of smoking. Among ever regular smokers who were aPL positive, a higher frequency of former venous events was observed. Smoking was shown to double the risk of stroke in LA-positive women younger than 50 years in the RATIO study (risk of arterial thrombosis in relation to oral contraceptives) [15]. Interestingly, this case-control study also found that the use of oral contraceptive multiplied sevenfold the risk of stroke.

Also genetic factors seem to play a role in risk stratification. Lundstrom [16] and coworkers described that HLA-DRB*04/*13 alleles are associated with vascular events and aPL-positive immune phenotype in SLE and demonstrated that a subset of SLE patients is genetically disposed to vascular vulnerability. Another recent work [17] investigated the role of genetic factors in arterial thrombosis in APS. No association was found between platelet glycoprotein polymorphisms and arterial thrombosis, but it was confirmed anyway that APS patients with aCL IgG antibodies, livedo reticularis, and suffering from hypertension and hypercholesterolemia are at the increased risk of arterial thrombosis.

17.3 Primary Thromboprophylaxis in aPL Carriers

Issues regarding the role of prophylaxis for patients with aPL in the absence of clinical events have long been debated [18]. Keeping in mind all previous considerations, the first approach to patients with aPL antibodies should be risk stratification. As general measures, modifiable risk factors (hypertension, diabetes mellitus, proatherogenic lipid profile, obesity, smoking) should be corrected, estrogen-containing oral contraceptives avoided, and there is a strong suggestion to thromboprophylaxis with low molecular weight heparin (LMWH) in acute high-risk situations such as surgical procedures, long periods of immobilizations, puerperium, and in less frequent conditions such as ovarian stimulation [19].

Retrospective and prospective observational studies and controlled trials of aspirin for the prevention of thrombotic events in people with aPL without history of arterial or venous thrombosis have yielded discordant results [20–22]. Up to now only one randomized, double-blind, placebo-controlled trial [22] (APLASA trial) is available in aPL-positive subjects. In this study, persistently aPL-positive patients were enrolled and they were given placebo or 81 mg/day aspirin, and a low annual incidence of acute thrombosis was observed. The APLASA trial concluded that asymptomatic individuals who are persistently positive for aPL do not benefit from low-dose aspirin since thrombotic events in this population are unlikely in the absence of additional risk factors for thrombosis. Recently, a meta-analysis of observational studies showed that the risk of first thrombotic event is significantly decreased by low-dose aspirin among asymptomatic aPL individuals with or without SLE [23]. However, no significant risk reduction was retained when considering only prospective studies or those with the best methodological quality. Furthermore, the estimated incidence of thrombosis in unselected cases (about 1 % patient-years) is equivalent to that of major bleeding associated with the use of aspirin [24]. So the dilemma is to correctly select those aPL carriers for whom the expected benefit of low-dose aspirin outweighs the risk.

The international consensus [8] on primary prevention in asymptomatic APL carriers proposed strict control of cardiovascular risk and prophylaxis with LMWH only in high-risk situations (e.g., surgery, immobilization, pregnancy). Aspirin may be useful for some subsets of APL patients at particularly high risk of arterial thrombosis, such as those with SLE or special antibody patterns such as triple positivity or isolated, persistently positive aCL at medium to high levels [24].

Also the use of warfarin has been proposed in primary thromboprophylaxis [25]. The ALIWAPAS trial compared the efficacy low-dose aspirin (LDA) with LDA in association with low-intensity warfarin. This study faced different problems, but probably the major one was the low recruitment rate because many patients refused to participate. The most likely reason for that could be that aPL carriers did not feel motivated to comply with a drug regimen that carries the risk of bleeding and requires frequent blood sampling and lifestyle modifications. Therefore the lesson to be learned is that a drug used in primary prophylaxis should be acceptable to people who carry a risk factor, not a disease [26].

Aside from drugs acting on platelets and on the coagulation system, there is evidence that immunomodulatory agents may be beneficial in primary prophylaxis of aPL carriers.

Many studies have investigated whether hydroxychloroquine (HCQ) could be useful in the prevention of thromboembolic events in patients with aPL and SLE. In fact it is well known that HCQ has several different function: may benefit patients who have aPL and high risk of vascular events through antiplatelet effects by reducing homocysteine levels, lupus disease activity titers, hyperlipidemia [27], and aPL titers [18, 28]. HCQ was also associated with lower odds of having persistently positive aPL, adjusted for age, ethnicity, and gender [28]. Several studies on SLE patients have shown a protective effect of the drug against thrombosis: prospective cohort [29, 30] and cross-sectional [31] studies suggested that HCQ decreases the risk of first thrombosis in SLE patients. In a prospective cohort study conducted by

Tektonidou et al. [32], it was shown that HCQ might reduce the thrombosis risk in both aPL-positive (hazard ratio, 0.99; 95 % CI, 0.98–1.00) and aPL-negative (hazard ratio, 0.98; 95 % CI, 0.95–0.98) patients. In another recent, case-control study, Jung et al. [33] also demonstrated that HCQ is protective against thrombosis in SLE patients (OR, 0.32; 95 % CI, 0.14–0.74). However, this potentially protective effect of HCQ was not confirmed by two other prospective cohort studies in lupus patients [34, 35]. Anyway in patients with systemic autoimmune diseases (particularly SLE), HCQ is commonly used for disease control and should be considered independently of the patients' aPL status. However, further controlled studies are needed to determine the effectiveness of HCQ for primary prophylaxis in aPL-positive patient [5].

Also statins may be useful in aPL carriers for different reasons. In the first place, statins are recommended for patients with a proatherogenic lipid profile. Secondly, they might be beneficial because of their anti-inflammatory effects and their ability to interfere with aPL-induced endothelial activation. They also have multiple effects on monocytes and lymphocytes, contributing to thrombosis prevention in APS patients [36]. In the third place statins seem to reduce the occurrence of the first major cardiovascular event and symptomatic thromboembolism also in the general population [37]. So far, two prospective studies have shown the efficacy of fluvastatin in reducing proinflammatory and prothrombotic biomarkers in persistently aPL-positive patients [38, 39].

Vitamin D deficiency was described to be common among APS patients, and it seems to be associated with a history of thrombotic events [40]. Given that vitamin D can inhibit anti-β2GPI-mediated tissue factor (TF) expression in vitro, its deficiency might be associated with decreased inhibition of TF expression and increased coagulation in APS [41]. So vitamin D supplementation could be considered as a safe and cheap complement to standard therapy in APS patients (Table 17.1).

17.4 aPL Carriers and Pregnancy Morbidity

Besides thrombosis, aPL are known risk factors for a wide range of obstetric morbidity, such as recurrent pregnancy losses, late fetal losses, preeclampsia, placental abruption, and intrauterine growth restriction. The strength of

Table 17.1 Proposed strategies of primary thrombosis prophylaxis for patients with clinically significant antiphospholipid antibody (aPL) profile

Management of aPL carriers:
Identify and reverse traditional cardio vascular risk factors
Identify concomitant systemic autoimmune diseases
Consider drugs acting on platelet and coagulation system:
ASA [20–22]
LMWH [8, 19]
Warfarin [25]
Consider drugs with immunomodulatory properties:
HCQ [27, 28]
STATINS [36–39]
Vitamin D [40, 41]

association between aPL and single manifestations may vary from study to study, mainly for "methodological" problems: most of the data are derived from small case-control studies, often results are not conclusive, and there are no large controlled-randomized trials [42]. In any case, the management of aPL carriers should include prophylaxis, not only for pregnancy outcome itself but also for maternal protection, being pregnancy and puerperium as high-risk periods for the occurrence of thrombosis.

17.5 Role of aPL in Pregnancy Morbidity: Pathogenesis

Pregnancy morbidity is not uncommon in the general population and can be due to multiple causes (anatomical defects, chromosomal aberrations, endocrine factors, subclinical infections, and, finally, immunological disturbances), but more than 50 % of the cases remain idiopathic after conventional investigations [43].

Antiphospholipid antibodies were shown to be pathogenic in several models of pregnancy wastage, both in vitro and in vivo [reviewed in [44, 45]. In particular, aPL specifically target the placenta by binding β2GPI, which is constitutively expressed on the trophoblast cell surface. This interaction may alter first-trimester human trophoblast modulating several cell biological pathways and, finally, causing unfavorable outcome [46, 47].

Suggested pathogenic mechanisms mediated by aPL are [2]:

- Placental thrombosis and infarction.
- Acute inflammation and complement activation: the complement system has been identified to be critical for the pathogenic effects of aPL, both for excessive activation or inadequate regulation [48];
- Defective placentation due to the evidence that placenta is a major target for aPL, in particular b2GPI-dependent antibodies, which bind to human trophoblast [49]. Additional manifestations were placental tissue thrombosis, syncitium-throphoblast differentiation inhibition, decidual cell inflammatory phenotype induction, complement activation, and embryo and/or placental apoptosis.
- aPL, especially anti-β2GPI, are able to disrupt the anticoagulant annexin A5 shield on trophoblast and endothelial cell monolayers [49].

A peculiar pathogenic model for aPL-induced pregnancy morbidity is preeclampsia. Preeclampsia is a vasospastic hypertensive disorders marked by abnormal maternal arteriolar reactivity to vasoactive agents such as prostacyclin, thromboxane A2, nitric oxide, and endothelins. Moreover, defective regulation of the complement system, allowing for excessive complement activation which leads to abnormal placental development and abnormal trophoblast invasion, placental damage, generalized endothelial activation, and release of antiangiogenic factors toxic to glomerular endothelium and liver sinusoids, seems to be involved in this complex model [50].

17.6 Stratification of Obstetric Risk

Association between aPL single test and pregnancy morbidity is not well defined, mainly because of lacking in randomized controlled trials and heterogeneity of design studies. Most studies are underpowered with high heterogeneity regarding association with aPL and pregnancy morbidity: there are only few studies which meet Sapporo/Sydney criteria and support association between clinical events and laboratory criteria [51, 52].

As previously discussed for the risk of thrombosis, also on the obstetric side, it is important to identify patients at high risk taking into account many variables. First of all, general obstetric risk should be assessed, taking into consideration age, concomitant autoimmune disease, previous thrombosis, family history (autoimmunity, thrombosis, abortions), hypertension, obesity, acquired thrombophilia, and so forth.

It is currently under discussion whether different aPL profiles confer the same degree of obstetric risk, and it is not easy to stratify patients into "risk classes." Routine screening for aPL antibodies is not recommended in healthy pregnant women, because they occur infrequently, at low levels, and are rarely associated with adverse pregnancy outcome. An original report at the beginning of the 1990s found that greater than 50 % of such women will go on to have uncomplicated pregnancies without any additional treatment [53].

At the moment, it is recommended to test all three validated antibodies (aCL, anti-β2GPI, LA) included in the revised Sydney criteria. There are few studies evaluating a possible role of nonclassical aPL (anti-phosphatidylcholine, anti-phosphatidylethanolamine, anti-phosphatidylinositol, anti-phosphatidylserine, and anti-sphingomyelin) in obstetric complications. They seem not to be an independent risk factor in the prediction of miscarriage in women with recurrent pregnancy loss and to have no clinical significance in obstetric complications [54].

Available meta-analysis studies evaluating the association between different aPL tests and pregnancy morbidity showed divergent results. Opatrny et al. concluded that high-risk patients are those carrying LA and IgG aCL antibodies (especially at high titers) [55]. Abou-Nassar and coworkers concluded that the association between each single aPL test and placenta-mediated complications was inconsistent and debatable [52]. However, it should be considered that most of the studies included in the meta-analysis did not test for a complete aPL profile but rather for one or two aPL tests.

More recently, some studies took into consideration a complete aPL profile and its relationships with pregnancy outcome.

The PROMISSE study (Predictors of Pregnancy Outcome: BioMarkers In Antiphospholipid Syndrome and Systemic Lupus Erythematosus), a large, multicenter observational study on pregnancies of patients with APS and/or SLE, described the pregnancy outcome of 144 aPL-positive patients. Poor pregnancy outcome was observed mainly in LAC-positive women and in women with moderate- to high-titer IgG aCL; other aPL did not independently predict adverse pregnancy outcome [56].

Other studies found out that high-risk patients are those with aPL triple positivity (aCL, anti-β2GPI, LA) [51]. A multicenter European study showed that independent risk factors for pregnancy failure despite treatment were the presence of SLE or other autoimmune diseases, history of both thrombosis and pregnancy morbidity, and triple aPL positivity [57]. On the other hand, other authors observed unfavorable pregnancy outcome also in patients with a "low-risk" aPL profile (e.g., IgM isotype or medium to low aPL titers) [58, 59].

In our opinion, those risk factors identified in pregnancy failures despite treatment could be also considered as "red flags" to be applied in for primary prophylaxis. In other words, pregnant aPL carriers with either triple aPL positivity and/or a concomitant autoimmune disease should be considered at higher risk and provided with a more generous prophylaxis.

17.7 aPL and Infertility

The main scenario in which aPL can be found incidentally is during workup for infertility. The role of aPL in infertility is controversial. aPL may interfere with several steps from implantation, placentation, to early embryonic development. At present, there is no evidence to support routine screening for aPL in patients with primary infertility, and no difference in the prevalence of aPL in women with unexplained infertility compared to fertile controls were found [51]. There is also no clear association between aPL positivity and implantation failure, clinical pregnancy, or live birth rates in women undergoing assisted reproduction.

The major point about assisted reproduction techniques is that ovarian stimulation protocols can be considered as high-risk situations for thrombosis because of artificially elevated estrogen levels [51]. One retrospective cohort study of ten APS patients who underwent 47 cycles of ovulation induction showed that no patients experienced thrombosis during treatment; all patients were treated with prophylactic LDA with or without heparin [60]. As a general measure, aPL-positive women, especially if high-risk profile, must be considered as a risk population, and so prophylactic treatment with LDA or LMWH should be considered during ovarian stimulation.

17.8 aPL Carriers and Pregnancy: Treatment

A key drug for primary obstetric prophylaxis is LDA. It is also indicated in women without aPL for the prevention of preeclampsia [61]. In clinical practice, many physicians are used to pregnant aPL carriers with LDA, in particular if the patients have already experienced one or two fetal losses or if maternal risk factors coexist (age, arterial hypertension, obesity, etc.). A large retrospective observational study showed that pregnancy outcome can be favorable without LDA in those patients with a low-risk profile [62]. According to another large cohort of pregnant aPL carriers, combination treatment of LDA and other drugs seems to be not necessary

Table 17.2 Proposed strategies of pregnancy management in women with clinically significant antiphospholipid antibody (aPL) profile and no previous obstetric events

Management of aPL-positive women during pregnancy:
High-risk profile vs. low-risk profile (what is the definition? need for a consensus definition)
Proposed treatments:
LDA (prevention of preeclampsia, possibly not necessary if low-risk aPL profile)
LMWH (maternal protection, e.g., during puerperium and ovarian stimulation, especially in high-risk profile women)
Combination of LDA and LMWH (selected high-risk cases)
HCQ (protective role suggested in experimental models)

in asymptomatic pregnant aPL carriers, even in the presence of high antibody titers [63]. Nevertheless, the experts recommend the use of LMWH in addition to LDA in selected cases (older maternal age, high-risk aPL profile, assisted reproduction techniques) [64].

In our opinion, pregnant women with a high-risk aPL profile should be granted a generous prophylaxis for both maternal and fetal protection, while patients with a low-risk profile could be candidate to a less aggressive approach. However, the definitions of "high" and "low" risk from the obstetric point of view still need to be validated in properly designed studies.

Another point of concern is the puerperium. It is considered a high-risk period for thrombosis for all women. Usually APS patients are posed in primary prophylaxis with LMWH for a few weeks after delivery (generally 4–6 weeks). Regarding aPL carriers, experts believe that is important to protect these women with a similar management [64].

Recently, a role for HCQ was proposed. Recent studies have reported that HCQ reduces the binding of aPL-β2GPI complexes in trophoblast surface [65]. In a recent study by Albert and collaborators [66], authors studied a human first-trimester trophoblast cell line exposed to a β2GPI in presence or not of HCQ. HCQ was shown to partially antagonize aPL-induced inhibition of trophoblast migration, confirming the immunomodulatory properties of HCQ and suggesting beneficial effects on the placenta in patients with aPL positivity. At least from the experimental point of view, there may be a rationale for testing HCQ in clinical studies as a preventive treatment in aPL carrier's pregnancies (Table 17.2).

References

1. Pierangeli SS, de Groot PG, Dlott J et al (2011) 'Criteria' aPL tests: report of a task force and preconference workshop at the 13th International Congress on Antiphospholipid Antibodies, Galveston, Texas, April 2010. Lupus 20:182–190
2. Meroni PL, Borghi MO, Raschi E et al (2011) Pathogenesis of antiphospholipid syndrome: understanding the antibodies. Nat Rev Rheumatol 6:330–339
3. Miyakis S, Lockshin MD, Atsumi T et al (2006) International consensus statement on an update of the classification criteria for definite antiphospholipid syndrome (APS). J Thromb Haemost 4:295–306

4. Taraborelli M, Andreoli L, Tincani A (2012) Much more than thrombosis and pregnancy loss: the antiphospholipid syndrome as a 'systemic disease'. Best Pract Res Clin Rheumatol 26:79–90
5. Barbhaiya M, Erkan D (2011) Primary thrombosis prophylaxis in antiphospholipid antibody-positive patients: where do we stand? Curr Rheumatol Rep 13:59–69
6. Roubey RA (2010) Risky business: the interpretation, use, and abuse of antiphospholipid antibody tests in clinical practice. Lupus 19:440–445
7. Andreoli L, Tincani A (2012) Beyond the "syndrome": antiphospholipid antibodies as risk factors. Arthritis Rheum 64:342–345
8. Ruiz-Irastorza G, Cuadrado MJ, Ruiz-Arruza I et al (2011) Evidence-based recommendations for the prevention and long-term management of thrombosis in antiphospholipid antibody-positive patients: report of a task force at the 13th International Congress on antiphospholipid antibodies. Lupus 20:206–218
9. Erkan D, Derksen R, Levy R et al (2011) Antiphospholipid syndrome clinical research task force report. The international consensus report on the definition of a high-risk aPL profile. Lupus 20:219–224
10. Pengo V, Ruffatti A, Legnani C et al (2011) Incidence of a first thromboembolic event in asymptomatic carriers of high-risk antiphospholipid antibody profile: a multicenter prospective study. Blood 118:4714–4718
11. Reynaud Q, Lega JC, Mismetti P et al (2014) Risk of venous and arterial thrombosis according to type of antiphospholipid antibodies in adults without systemic lupus erythematosus: a systematic review and meta-analysis. Autoimmun Rev 13:595–608
12. Raschi E, Chighizola CB, Grossi C et al (2014) β2-glycoprotein I, lipopolysaccharide and endothelial TLR4: three players in the two hit theory for anti-phospholipid-mediated thrombosis. J Autoimmun 27. pii:S0896-8411(14)00065-1
13. Nalli C, Andreoli L, Casu C et al (2014) Management of recurrent thrombosis in antiphospholipid syndrome. Curr Rheumatol Rep 16:405
14. Gustafsson JT, Gunnarsson I, Källberg H et al (2014) Cigarette smoking, antiphospholipid antibodies and vascular events in Systemic Lupus Erythematosus. Ann Rheum Dis [Epub ahead of print]
15. Urbanus RT, Siegerink B, Roest M et al (2009) Antiphospholipid antibodies and risk of myocardial infarction and ischaemic stroke in young women in the RATIO study: a case– control study. Lancet Neurol 8:998–1005
16. Lundström E, Gustafsson JT, Jönsen A et al (2013) HLA-DRB1*04/*13 alleles are associated with vascular disease and antiphospholipid antibodies in systemic lupus erythematosus. Ann Rheum Dis 72:1018–1025
17. Matyja-Bednarczyk A, Swadźba J, Iwaniec T et al (2014) Risk factors for arterial thrombosis in antiphospholipid syndrome. Thromb Res 133:173–176
18. Erkan D, Aguiar CL, Andrade D, Cohen H et al (2014) 14th international congress on antiphospholipid antibodies: task force report on antiphospholipid syndrome treatment trends. Autoimmun Rev 13:685–696
19. Ruffatti A, Del Ross T, Ciprian M, Antiphospholipid Syndrome Study Group of Italian Society of Rheumatology et al (2011) Risk factors for a first thrombotic event in antiphospholipid antibody carriers: a prospective multicentre follow-up study. Ann Rheum Dis 70:1083–1086
20. Hereng T, Lambert M, Hachulla E et al (2008) Influence of aspirin on the clinical outcomes of 103 anti-phospholipid antibodies-positive patients. Lupus 17:11–15
21. Girón-González JA, García del Río E, Rodríguez C et al (2004) Antiphospholipid syndrome and asymptomatic carriers of antiphospholipid antibody: prospective analysis of 404 individuals. J Rheumatol 31:1560–1567
22. Erkan D, Harrison MJ, Levy R et al (2007) Aspirin for primary thrombosis prevention in the antiphospholipid syndrome: a randomized, double-blind, placebo-controlled trial in asymptomatic antiphospholipid antibody-positive individuals. Arthritis Rheum 56:2382–2391
23. Arnaud L, Mathian A, Ruffatti A et al (2014) Efficacy of aspirin for the primary prevention of thrombosis in patients with antiphospholipid antibodies: an international and collaborative meta-analysis. Autoimmun Rev 13:281–291
24. Ceccarelli F, Chighizola C, Finazzi G et al (2012) Thromboprophylaxis in carriers of antiphospholipid antibodies (APL) without previous thrombosis: "Pros" and "Cons". Autoimmun Rev 11:568–571

25. Cuadrado MJ, Bertolaccini ML, Seed PT et al (2014) Low-dose aspirin vs low-dose aspirin plus low-intensity warfarin in thromboprophylaxis: a prospective, multicentre, randomized, open, controlled trial in patients positive for antiphospholipid antibodies (ALIWAPAS). Rheumatology (Oxford) 53:275–284
26. Tincani A, Andreoli L, Shoenfeld Y (2014) Anti-phospholipid antibodies. To anticoagulate or not to anticoagulate? Rheumatology (Oxford) 53:201–202
27. Petri M (2000) Detection of coronary artery disease and the role of traditional risk factors in the Hopkins Lupus Cohort. Lupus 9:170–175
28. Broder A, Putterman C (2013) Hydroxychloroquine use is associated with lower odds of persistently positive antiphospholipid antibodies and/or lupus anticoagulant in systemic lupus erythematosus. J Rheumatol 40:30–33
29. Ruiz-Irastorza G, Egurbide MV, Pijoan JI et al (2006) Effect of antimalarials on thrombosis and survival in patients with systemic lupus erythematosus. Lupus 15:577–583
30. Kaiser R, Cleveland CM, Criswell LA (2009) Risk and protective factors for thrombosis in systemic lupus erythematosus: results from a large, multi-ethnic cohort. Ann Rheum Dis 68:238–241
31. Erkan D, Yazici Y, Peterson MG et al (2002) A cross-sectional study of clinical thrombotic risk factors and preventive treatments in antiphospholipid syndrome. Rheumatology (Oxford) 41:924–929
32. Tektonidou MG, Laskari K, Panagiotakos DB et al (2009) Risk factors for thrombosis and primary thrombosis prevention in patients with systemic lupus erythematosus with or without antiphospholipid antibodies. Arthritis Rheum 61:29–36
33. Jung H, Bobbo R, Su J et al (2010) The protective effect of antimalarial drugs on thrombovascular events in systemic lupus erythematosus. Arthritis Rheum 62:863–868
34. Ho KT, Ahn CW, Alarcon GS et al (2005) Systemic lupus erythematosus in a multiethnic cohort (LUMINA): XXVIII. Factors predictive of thrombotic events. Rheumatology (Oxford) 44:1303–1307
35. Mok CC, Tang SS, To CH et al (2005) Incidence and risk factors of thromboembolism in systemic lupus erythematosus: a comparison of three ethnic groups. Arthritis Rheum 52:2774–2782
36. Erkan D, Pierangeli SS (2013) Could statins be a new therapeutic option for antiphospholipid syndrome patients? Expert Rev Hematol 6:115–117
37. Ridker PM, Danielson E, Fonseca FA, JUPITER Trial Study Group et al (2009) Reduction in C-reactive protein and LDL cholesterol and cardiovascular event rates after initiation of rosuvastatin: a prospective study of the JUPITER trial. Lancet 373:1175–1182
38. López-Pedrera C, Ruiz-Limón P, Aguirre MÁ et al (2011) Global effects of fluvastatin on the prothrombotic status of patients with antiphospholipid syndrome. Ann Rheum Dis 70: 675–682
39. Erkan D, Willis R, Murthy VL et al (2014) A prospective open-label pilot study of fluvastatin on proinflammatory and prothrombotic biomarkers in antiphospholipid antibody positive patients. Ann Rheum Dis 73:1176–1180
40. Piantoni S, Andreoli L, Allegri F et al (2012) Low levels of vitamin D are common in primary antiphospholipid syndrome with thrombotic disease. Reumatismo 64:307–313
41. Agmon-Levin N, Blank M, Zandman-Goddard G et al (2011) Vitamin D: an instrumental factor in the antiphospholipid syndrome by inhibition of tissue factor expression. Ann Rheum Dis 70:145–150
42. Andreoli L, Chighizola CB, Banzato A et al (2013) Estimated frequency of antiphospholipid antibodies in patients with pregnancy morbidity, stroke, myocardial infarction, and deep vein thrombosis: a critical review of the literature. Arthritis Care Res (Hoboken) 65(11): 1869–1873
43. Ford HB, Schust DJ (2009) Recurrent pregnancy loss: etiology, diagnosis, and therapy. Rev Obstet Gynecol 2(2):76–83
44. Meroni PL, Raschi E, Grossi C et al (2012) Obstetric and vascular APS: same autoantibodies but different diseases? Lupus 21(7):708–710, Review
45. Andreoli L, Fredi M, Nalli C et al (2012) Pregnancy implications for systemic lupus erythematosus and the antiphospholipid syndrome. J Autoimmun 38(2-3):J197–J208, Review
46. Carroll TY, Mulla MJ, Han CS et al (2011) Modulation of trophoblast angiogenic factor secretion by antiphospholipid antibodies is not reversed by heparin. Am J Reprod Immunol 66(4):286–296

47. Mulla MJ, Myrtolli K, Brosens JJ et al (2010) Antiphospholipid antibodies limit trophoblast migration by reducing IL-6 production and STAT3 activity. Am J Reprod Immunol 63(5): 339–348
48. Lynch AM, Salmon JE (2010) Dysregulated complement activation as a common pathway of injury in preeclampsia and other pregnancy complications. Placenta 31(7):561–567
49. Rand JH, Wu XX, Quinn AS et al (2010) The annexin A5-mediated pathogenic mechanism in the antiphospholipid syndrome: role in pregnancy losses and thrombosis. Lupus 19(4):460–469, Review
50. Clark EA, Silver RM, Branch DW (2007) Do antiphospholipid antibodies cause preeclampsia and HELLP syndrome? Curr Rheumatol Rep 9(3):219–225, Review
51. de Jesus GR, Agmon-Levin N, Andrade CA et al (2014) 14th International Congress on antiphospholipid antibodies task force report on obstetric antiphospholipid syndrome. Autoimmun Rev 13(8):795–813, Review
52. Abou-Nassar K, Carrier M, Ramsay T et al (2011) The association between antiphospholipid antibodies and placenta mediated complications: a systematic review and meta-analysis. Thromb Res 128(1):77–85, Review
53. Harris EN, Spinnato JA (1991) Should anticardiolipin tests be performed in otherwise healthy pregnant women? Am J Obstet Gynecol 165(5 Pt 1):1272–1277
54. Obayashi S, Ozaki Y, Sugi T et al (2010) Antiphosphatidylethanolamine antibodies might not be an independent risk factor for further miscarriage in patients suffering recurrent pregnancy loss. J Reprod Immunol 85(2):186–192
55. Opatrny L, David M, Kahn SR et al (2006) Association between antiphospholipid antibodies and recurrent fetal loss in women without autoimmune disease: a metaanalysis. J Rheumatol 33(11):2214–2221
56. Lockshin MD, Kim M, Laskin CA et al (2012) Prediction of adverse pregnancy outcome by the presence of lupus anticoagulant, but not anticardiolipin antibody, in patients with antiphospholipid antibodies. Arthritis Rheum 64(7):2311–2318
57. Ruffatti A, Tonello M, Visentin MS et al (2011) Risk factors for pregnancy failure in patients with anti-phospholipid syndrome treated with conventional therapies: a multicentre, case-control study. Rheumatology (Oxford) 50(9):1684–1689
58. Mekinian A, Loire-Berson P, Nicaise-Roland P et al (2012) Outcomes and treatment of obstetrical antiphospholipid syndrome in women with low antiphospholipid antibody levels. J Reprod Immunol 94(2):222–226
59. Gardiner C, Hills J, Machin SJ et al (2013) Diagnosis of antiphospholipid syndrome in routine clinical practice. Lupus 22(1):18–25
60. Guballa N, Sammaritano L, Schwartzman S et al (2000) Ovulation induction and in vitro fertilization in systemic lupus erythematosus and antiphospholipid syndrome. Arthritis Rheum 43(3):550–556
61. Roberge S, Giguère Y, Villa P et al (2014) Early administration of low-dose aspirin for the prevention of severe and mild preeclampsia: a systematic review and meta-analysis. Am J Perinatol 31(6):e3
62. Del Ross T, Ruffatti A, Visentin MS et al (2013) Treatment of 139 pregnancies in antiphospholipid-positive women not fulfilling criteria for antiphospholipid syndrome: a retrospective study. J Rheumatol 40(4):425–429
63. Soh MC, Pasupathy D, Gray G et al (2013) Persistent antiphospholipid antibodies do not contribute to adverse pregnancy outcomes. Rheumatology (Oxford) 52(9):1642–1647
64. Erkan D, Patel S, Nuzzo M et al (2008) Management of the controversial aspects of the antiphospholipid syndrome pregnancies: a guide for clinicians and researchers. Rheumatology (Oxford) 47(Suppl 3):iii23–iii27
65. Wu XX, Guller S, Rand JH (2011) Hydroxychloroquine reduces binding of antiphospholipid antibodies to syncytiotrophoblasts and restores annexin A5 expression. Am J Obstet Gynecol 205(6):576.e7–14
66. Albert CR, Schlesinger WJ, Viall CA et al (2014) Effect of hydroxychloroquine on antiphospholipid antibody-induced changes in first trimester trophoblast function. Am J Reprod Immunol 71:154–164

New Treatments

18

Cecilia Beatrice Chighizola and Tania Ubiali

18.1 Introduction

Antiphospholipid syndrome (APS) is an autoimmune disorder characterized by vascular thrombosis and/or pregnancy morbidity in the persistent presence of circulating antiphospholipid antibodies (aPL). Clinical management of APS patients aims not only at avoiding thrombotic and/or obstetric recurrences but also at preventing aPL-related complications as nephropathy, central nervous system involvement, and atherothrombosis. The cornerstone of APS treatment is still provided by drugs that counteract the aPL-mediated prothrombotic effects by preventing coagulation, namely, antiplatelet and anticoagulant agents. There is consensus that patients with venous events should receive long-term anticoagulation with vitamin K antagonists (VKA), while subjects who develop a stroke and present a low-risk aPL profile without any associated autoimmune condition may be prescribed with low-dose aspirin (LDASA); stroke patients at higher thrombotic risk and individuals with a history of noncerebral arterial thrombosis should receive long-term anticoagulation. A regimen combining preconceptional LDASA and low molecular weight heparin (LMWH) provides the first-line treatment for obstetric APS [1, 2].

C.B. Chighizola (✉)
Department of Clinical Sciences and Community Health, University of Milan,
Via Festa del Perdono 7, Milan 20122, Italy

Immunology Research Laboratory, IRCCS Istituto Auxologico Italiano,
Via Zucchi 18, Cusano Milanino, Milan 20095, Italy
e-mail: cecilia.chighizola@unimi.it

T. Ubiali
Department of Clinical Sciences and Community Health, University of Milan,
Via Festa del Perdono 7, Milan 20122, Italy

Division of Rheumatology, Istituto Ortopedico Gaetano Pini,
Piazza Cardinal Ferrari 1, Milan 20122, Italy

© Springer International Publishing Switzerland 2015
P.L. Meroni (ed.), *Antiphospholipid Antibody Syndrome: From Bench to Bedside*,
Rare Diseases of the Immune System, DOI 10.1007/978-3-319-11044-8_18

However, available treatments present several pitfalls. VKA, as well as LMWH, exert a strong impact on the quality of life of patients. The first agents necessitate frequent INR monitoring, as VKA interact with infections, exercise, smoking, alcohol, foods, and drugs; the latter requires a daily subcutaneous administration. In addition, despite adequate treatment, a significant rate of APS patients develops recurrences: the cumulative incidence of thromboembolic events at 10 years was 44 % in a cohort of triple positive APS patients. Remarkably, rethromboses provide the most common cause of death in APS [3]. Similarly, approximately 30 % of pregnant APS women receiving standard care have a poor obstetric outcome, with any alternative strategy being effective in this setting. Anticoagulation also carries a significant bleeding risk: a systematic review reported a major bleeding rate in APS patients on VKA between 0.57 and 10 % per year [4].

It clearly emerges that novel pharmacological tools are strongly warranted in APS to overcome the limitations of available treatments. A potential strategy consists in considering drugs implementing the anticoagulant and antiplatelet effect of standard treatment: new oral and nonoral anticoagulants, hydroxychloroquine (HCQ), and statins. Alternatively, the therapeutic approach could be completely modified using molecules modulating the interaction of aPL with their molecular targets and counteracting their downstream cellular effects. Potential pharmacological strategies include modulation of B cell and complement activation, receptor antagonism, and inhibition of aPL-induced intracellular and extracellular mediators such as NFκB, p38MAK, tissue factor (TF), interleukin (IL)-6, and tumor necrosis factor (TNF)-α [5]. Surely, a deeper unraveling of APS pathogenic mechanisms may allow identifying additional alternative therapeutic targets (Fig. 18.1).

18.2 aPL-Mediated Pathogenic Mechanisms

aPL are a heterogeneous family of autoantibodies reacting against proteins with affinity for negatively charged phospholipids (PL). In particular, beta-2 glycoprotein I (β2GPI) provides, together with prothrombin, the most important epitope targeted by aPL. Three configurations of β2GPI have been described: circulating plasma β2GPI exists in a circular form; upon binding to suitable anionic surfaces as cardiolipin (CL) and other PL or to LPS, the molecule opens into a J-shaped fishhook configuration; recently an intermediate S shape of β2GPI has been observed. β2GPI consists of 5 domains (D): DI-IV comprise 60 amino acids and contain two disulfide bridges each, while DV is aberrant, as it includes 82 amino acids due to a 6-residue insertion and a 19-residue C-terminal extension cross-linked by an additional disulfide bond. DI has been identified as the most relevant antigenic target involved in β2GPI/anti-β2GPI antibody binding. This epitope is a cryptic and conformation-dependent structure: in the circular conformation of β2GPI, DI interacts with DV and the critical epitope is thus hidden. When β2GPI adopts the S shape, the epitope is covered by DIII–IV carbohydrate chains, thus preventing antibodies from binding β2GPI. Upon opening to a J configuration, the critical epitope is exposed, becoming available for antibody binding. Several factors might lead to

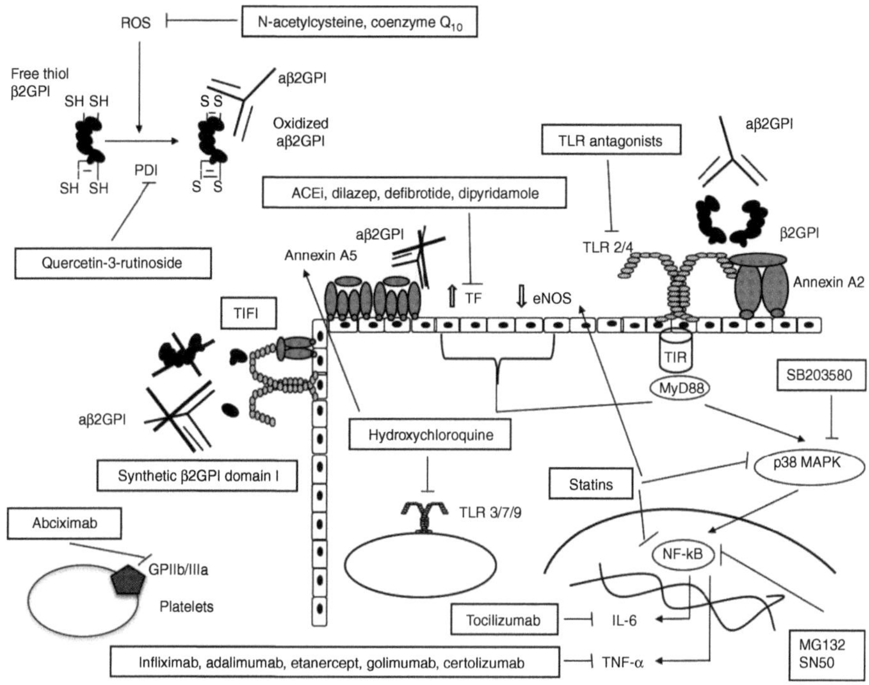

Fig. 18.1 Mechanisms of action of potential future therapeutic tools in APS. *ROS* reactive oxygen species, *β2GPI* β2 glycoprotein I, *aβ2GPI* antibodies against β2GPI, *PDI* protein disulfide-isomerase, *ACEi* angiotensin-converting enzyme inhibitors, *TLR* toll-like receptor, *TF* tissue factor, *eNOS* endothelial nitric oxide synthase, *GP* glycoprotein

the surface exposition of the critical epitope, such as oxidative stress. Indeed, under oxidative conditions, disulfide bonds form in the molecule leading to the unmasking of the critical B-cell structure [6].

aPL exert a thrombogenic effect by interfering with both soluble components and cells involved in the coagulation cascade [5]. aPL promote aggregation and activation of platelets, neutralizing β2GPI interaction with von Willebrand factor and enhancing the expression of platelet membrane glycoprotein (GP) IIb/IIIa. Moreover, aPL induce a proinflammatory and procoagulant endothelial phenotype upregulating cellular adhesion molecules, promoting the synthesis of endothelial nitric oxide synthase (eNOS) and of proinflammatory cytokines as IL-6 and TNF-α. Lastly, aPL have been shown to significantly increase in both ECs and monocytes the expression of TF, the major initiator of the clotting cascade. Many molecules have been advocated as potential mediators of β2GPI interaction with target cells: annexin A2, toll-like receptor (TLR) 2 and 4, heparan sulfate, and ApoER2'. There is general agreement that NFκB and p38MAPK are involved in the downstream signaling pathways engaged by aPL [7].

aPL exert a thrombophilic effect also at a placental level, inducing intraplacental thrombosis and infarction, leading to an impairment of the maternal-fetal blood exchange. aPL were also shown to contribute to the prothrombotic state by activating complement and disrupting the anticoagulant annexin A5 shield on trophoblast and endothelial cell (EC) monolayers [7].

Hereby, cutting-the-edge therapeutic strategies are widely discussed, presenting the pioneer reports about the efficacy of novel pharmacological agents in APS based on the recent advances in understanding of aPL pathogenic mechanisms.

18.3 Novel Nonoral Anticoagulants

Fondaparinux and idraparinux are synthetic pentasaccharides homologous to heparin-binding site; their activity is limited on factor Xa. Both administered subcutaneously, fondaparinux is given daily, whereas idraparinux has a longer half-life, which allows a weekly administration. Given the low affinity to platelet factor 4, fondaparinux and idraparinux can be safely prescribed to patients with a history of heparin-induced thrombocytopenia. Fondaparinux has been licensed for VTE prophylaxis; idraparinux has not yet been patented: even though it was as effective as warfarin in preventing recurrence, it was associated with a significantly higher bleeding rate. Neither fondaparinux nor idraparinux has been yet evaluated in the setting of APS [8].

18.4 Novel Oral Direct Anticoagulants

Most recently, a novel class of anticoagulants has been synthesized: all administered orally, such pharmacological agents inhibit a single enzyme of the coagulation cascade, being thus called direct oral anticoagulants (DOA). Dabigatran is a potent, competitive, reversible direct thrombin inhibitor, which binds to thrombin and blocks its interaction with substrates. Direct FXa inhibitors include rivaroxaban, apixaban, and edoxaban. All these agents are highly selective, reversible, competitive, and dose dependent. They represent an advance over VKA mainly in terms of a better quality of life for patients: since they display a predictable anticoagulant effect, DOA are administered at a fixed dose. In addition, not being metabolized by the cytochrome P450 system, they do not interact with dietary constituents or alcohol and have few reported drug interactions, therefore not requiring routine monitoring of anticoagulant intensity. However, these novel DOA do not allow overcoming some other limitations affecting treatment with VKA. The main issue lies in the significant bleeding risk that any anticoagulant regimen carries and in the absence of an available pharmacological reversal agent [9].

The role of these emerging anticoagulants in APS management is still to be determined: there are three ongoing randomized controlled clinical trials evaluating rivaroxaban in the management of APS, as compared to low-intensity anticoagulation. The RAPS trial has been promoted by a UK group; it is a phase II/III study that has recruited 156 APS patients with a history of venous thromboembolism. A Spanish phase III trial has been started in Spain on 218 patients with venous or arterial events [10]. Most recently, an Italian trial considering triple positive APS patients only is going to start recruiting.

18.5 Hydroxychloroquine

HCQ is an antimalarial drug with anti-inflammatory and antithrombotic properties. In addition, HCQ has been shown to exert immunomodulatory effects: it prevents activation of TLR3, TLR7, and TLR9; inhibits antigen processing and presentation; and reduces circulating immune complexes [11, 12]. In in vitro models of thrombotic APS, HCQ has been demonstrated to inhibit GPIIb/IIIa expression on aPL-activated platelets [13], to reverse the formation of aPL-β2GPI-PL bilayer complexes [14], and to prevent the aPL-induced disruption of the annexin A5 shield [15]. Its antithrombogenic properties have been confirmed in in vivo models of APS: HCQ injection in mice induced a dose dependent decrease in thrombus size [16]. HCQ might be effective even in obstetric APS, as it was shown to reverse the binding of aPL to human placental syncytiotrophoblasts [17] and the aPL-inhibition of trophoblast IL-6 secretion [18].

Clinical data on the effectiveness of HCQ in preventing aPL-related thrombotic events have been derived from studies in SLE cohorts. Recently, a cross-sectional study on 77 APS patients and 56 asymptomatic aPL carriers from an SLE registry proved that the probability of a thrombotic event was decreased by LDASA or HCQ use [19]. In a still unpublished work, Petri and coworkers observed a decrease in arterial as well as venous thrombosis in aPL-positive lupus patients receiving HCQ [20].

In primary thrombotic APS, HCQ has been to date evaluated as an adjunctive pharmacological tool: patients receiving a combo regimen comprising HCQ plus oral anticoagulation experienced less recurrences compared to those on anticoagulants only. However, the extrapolation of data is affected by the limitations biasing this work: the study cohort was limited to 40 patients, and the follow-up lasted 36 months only [21]. HCQ is currently catalyzing much attention in APS: an ongoing study is assessing the effect of HCQ on annexin A5 resistance assay in aPL patients with or without SLE; a randomized controlled trial promoted by the international research organization APS ACTION is evaluating HCQ in the primary prevention of thrombosis in aPL asymptomatic carriers at 5 years of follow-up [22].

Even though there is limited clinical evidence of its antithrombotic effects in primary APS, treatment guidelines consider HCQ as a potential adjunctive therapy, particularly in consideration of its excellent safety profile [2].

18.6 Statins

Statins inhibit cholesterol synthesis in the mevalonate pathway by blocking the 3-hydroxy-3-methyl-glutaryl-coenzyme A (HMG-CoA) reductase. The use of statins in the treatment of APS might thus be beneficial in the prevention of thrombosis since hypertriglyceridemia and low HDL cholesterol levels provide the most frequent cardiovascular risk factor reported in APS patients [23]. However, these pharmacological compounds have also been shown to exert a wide array of additional pleiotropic antithrombotic and anti-inflammatory effects in APS. In vitro, fluvastatin, simvastatin, and rosuvastatin have been demonstrated to inhibit TF synthesis in EC [24]; fluvastatin and simvastatin were both reported to suppress anti-β2GPI antibody-induced endothelial adhesiveness and to reduce monocyte adhesion to the endothelium [25], while rosuvastatin inhibited the upregulation of VCAM induced by aPL [26]. In vivo, fluvastatin reduced the size of the thrombus induced by aPL infusion and the leukocyte adhesion to EC. In models of obstetric APS, pravastatin did not prevent aPL-mediated functional effects on human trophoblasts in vitro [27], while in vivo simvastatin and pravastatin reduced fetal death [28]. These findings have been later confirmed in ex vivo studies. A trial in 42 patients with APS treated with fluvastatin for 30 days reported a decline in several thrombogenic and inflammatory mediators in monocytes [29]. More recently, Erkan observed a significant reduction of half of the evaluated proinflammatory and procoagulant parameters (IL-1β, VEGF, TNF-α, IP10, CD40L, and TF) in a cohort of 41 aPL asymptomatic carriers after 3 months of treatment with fluvastatin [30].

As a whole, statins could have a role a potential treatment for APS, beyond their lipid-lowering activity with no intrinsic additional risk of bleeding [31].

18.7 Vitamin D

In vitro, vitamin D exerts an antithrombotic and immunomodulator function by inhibiting β2GPI-mediated TF expression [32]. Retrospective studies indicated that the prevalence of vitamin D deficiency in APS patients ranges from 10 to 50 %, while insufficiency may occur in up to 70 % of patients [32–36]. Low vitamin D levels correlate with arterial and venous thrombosis as well as with non-criteria APS manifestations [32–34]. Conversely, most studies supported no association between low vitamin D levels and obstetric APS [32–35]. Prospective studies are warranted to evaluate the therapeutic value of supplementation with vitamin D in aPL carriers.

18.8 Intravenous Immunoglobulins

In vivo and in vitro models suggest the therapeutic potential of intravenous immunoglobulins (IVIg) in APS. IVIg were shown to inhibit aPL, by partially neutralizing LA activity and preventing aCL binding to cardiolipin by Fab. IVIg exert an anti-idiotype activity, with inactivation of idiotype-bearing B-cell clones. Furthermore, IVIg have been demonstrated to increase IgG catabolism, to modulate complement activation, to block Fcγ receptor on macrophages, and to downregulate proinflammatory cytokines [37]. Treatment with IVIg resulted in an inhibition of aPL thrombogenic effects, with a reduction of circulating aCL levels [38]. There are few reports about successful treatment with IVIg in the management of aPL-related clinical manifestations, mainly hematogical (thrombocytopenia, hemolytic anemia, hypoprothrombinemia). Treatment response was observed in all cases but one [39]. Recently, IVIg were found to be effective in preventing recurrent thrombosis among five patients with refractory APS in a 5-year open study [40].

18.9 Rituximab

The pivotal role exerted by B cells in APS has been progressively deciphered: B lymphocytes contribute to APS etiopathogenesis by producing autoantibodies, inducing the formation of germinal centers and the synthesis of cytokines. Accordingly, in NZW x BXSB mice, treatment with IgG against B-cell activating factor (BAFF) receptor did not prevent the development of aCL even though it prevented aPL-related thrombotic vasculopathy, prolonging survival [41]. In the same murine models, IgG against cytotoxic T-lymphocyte antigen 4 immunoglobulin (CTLA4) affected initiation but not development of APS. These data suggest the potential efficacy of belimumab and abatacept in APS [42]. Interestingly, in belimumab-treated patients with systemic lupus erythematosus (SLE) a positive-to-negative conversion rate was reported for aCL [43]. To date, clinical experience of B-cell inhibitory agents specifically in APS patients are restricted to the use of rituximab, a chimeric monoclonal antibody targeting CD20 on the surface of B cells. Successful treatment with rituximab has been reported in anecdotal reports and in one case series from the BIOGEAS registry. In this multicenter Spanish registry, a therapeutic response was observed in 92 % of 12 cases [44]. In 2012, a review collected all the published cases, identifying 27 APS patients treated with rituximab [45]. The anti-CD20 monoclonal resulted in a decrease of aPL titers; among those receiving rituximab because of thrombotic recurrences, clinical improvement was observed in all cases. Moreover, rituximab was beneficial for a plethora of aPL-related clinical manifestations. At this regard, an open-label phase IIa descriptive pilot study (RITAPS) has been carried out in 20 patients with non-criteria APS manifestations refractory to conventional treatments [46]. Rituximab resulted to be effective in controlling some but not all non-criteria manifestations, without substantial change in aPL profile. Notably, caution should be paid to its use in APS: episodes of severe acute thrombotic exacerbations (lacunar infarctions and transverse myelitis) have been reported in two APS/SLE patients receiving rituximab [47].

Rituximab has been used in 20 cases of catastrophic APS (CAPS), in different combination with anticoagulation, high doses of steroids, plasma exchange, and IVIg. Despite the difficulties in determining the effects of rituximab, a lower mortality compared to larger series emerged [48].

18.10 Eculizumab

The complement system, in particular the mediator C5a, has been shown to play a central role in APS. C5a, a potent anaphylatoxic, proinflammatory, and chemotactic molecule, was demonstrated to induce the expression of TF on EC [49] and neutrophils [50]. In vivo, C5a was involved in deposition of fibrin in a growing thrombus induced by aPL injection [51]. C5a-induced recruitment and activation of neutrophils lead to trophoblast injury and angiogenic factor imbalance in aPL-induced fetal injury [52]. Eculizumab is a humanized monoclonal antibody which binds to the C5 protein with high affinity, thereby inhibiting its cleavage to C5a and C5b and preventing the generation of membrane attack complex [53]. In vivo, anti-C5 antibody was shown to attenuate thrombosis and to prevent aPL-mediated pregnancy loss [49]. To date, eculizumab has been administered to few CAPS patients in which all the other therapeutic strategies proved to be ineffective. A favorable response was described in two cases [54, 55] and a negative outcome in the others [22]. Eculizumab has also been investigated as a tool to manage APS patients after renal transplantation. In a first report on three consecutive kidney transplant recipients with posttransplant aPL-mediated thrombotic microangiopathy (TMA) resistant to plasmapheresis, treatment with eculizumab improved TMA [56]. In another case series of three patients treated with anticoagulation and eculizumab, no systemic thrombotic events or early graft losses were reported after a follow-up ranging from 4 months to 4 years [57].

18.11 Defibrotide

Defibrotide is a polydisperse mixture of 90 % single-stranded and 10 % double-stranded phosphodiester oligonucleotides derived from the controlled depolymerization of porcine intestinal mucosal DNA. This pharmacological compound acts by upregulating the release of prostacyclin and prostaglandin E2, reducing concentrations of leukotriene B4, inhibiting monocyte superoxide anion generation, stimulating expression of thrombomodulin in human vascular EC, and modulating platelet activity [58]. More recently, defibrotide was shown to downregulate TF expression on monocytes [59]. To date, it has been used in two patients with CAPS: in one case this treatment was successful, while the second patient died [60, 61].

18.12 Novel Molecules Blocking β2GPI/Anti-β2GPI Antibody Binding

TIFI is a 20 amino acid synthetic peptide that spans Thr101–Thr120 of ULB0-HCMVA from human cytomegalovirus, which shares similarities with the PL-binding site in β2GPI molecule, DV. TIFI is not targeted by aPL; in vitro evidence suggest that TIFI inhibits the binding of labeled β2GPI to human EC and mouse monocytes [62]. Similarly, the peptide prevented anti-β2GPI reactivity toward human trophoblast monolayers. These findings were also confirmed in animal models: the infusion of this synthetic peptide inhibited aPL-mediated thrombosis by decreasing the thrombus size produced in response to aPL and by reducing the binding of fluoresceinated β2GPI to EC. Pregnant naïve mice treated with TIFI were protected from fetal loss induced by human aPL IgG [63].

Accordingly, a *synthetic β2GPI-DI* was shown to inhibit aPL-mediated prothrombic effects both in vivo and in vitro [64].

MBB2 is a novel single-chain variable fragment (scFv)-Fc monoclonal antibody targeting DI of human, rat, and mouse β2GPI. When infused to experimental animals, MBB2 caused blood clots in rat mesenteric microcirculation after LPS priming. A non-complement-fixing variant of MBB2, *MBB2ΔCH2*, has also been developed. MBB2ΔCH2 displays the same antigen specificity of MBB2 but, lacking the CH2 domain, is unable to activate the complement cascade. MBB2ΔCH2 has been shown to prevent the aPL procoagulant effects in vivo by competing with circulating aPL for binding to β2GPI. In vivo, the CH2-deleted monoclonal antibody significantly reduced mesenteric thrombus formation and vessel occlusion [65].

Such antibody can be used in the future even in the management of obstetric APS, as MBB2ΔCH2 leaves bound β2GPI untouched. This is important because cell-bound β2GPI exerts a key role at the placental level, as supported by the defective embryo implantation and placental morphogenesis displayed by β2GPI$^{-/-}$ mice. Hence, any tool able to block the pathogenic effects of aPL leaving untouched β2GPI represents a useful approach.

It can also be postulated that *antagonists of the receptors involved in β2GPI cell binding* may exert a therapeutic potential [66]. The use of antagonists or neutralizing monoclonal antibodies acting on TLR2/4 might be speculated in APS. In addition, DV of β2GPI binds the A1 ligand-binding type A module of ApoER2'; a dimer composed of two A1 molecules joined by a flexible linker has been shown to inhibit anti-β2GPI antibody/dimerized β2GPI immune complexes from binding negatively charged PL and ApoER2' in vitro, more potently than A1 in the monomeric form [67]. More recently, proofs of the effectiveness of this dimeric molecule were obtained in vivo, in two animal models of APS. Indeed, treatment with A1-A1 efficiently reduced thrombus size in vivo in the presence of chronic autoimmune anti-β2GPI antibody in lupus-prone (NZW3BXSB)F1 male mice as well as in wild-type mice after infusion with anti-β2GPI antibodies [68].

Similarly, *blockers of the intracellular mediators involved in aPL-activated signaling pathways* may reverse the prothrombotic phenotype: NFkB and p38MAPK inhibitors have been shown to be effective in preventing aPL-mediated prothrombotic and proinflammatory effects in vitro [69]. More recently, the NFkB inhibitor DHMEQ was demonstrated to ameliorate the prothrombotic state induced by the infusion of the monoclonal antibody WB-6 in normal BALB/c mice [70].

18.13 Novel Molecules Interfering with aPL-Induced Mediators

It is can be speculated that TF inhibition may prevent thrombosis in APS [71]. Currently, there are few drugs available on the market blocking TF expression: *ACE inhibitors, dilazep, defibrotide,* and *dipyridamole.* In particular, both dilazep and dipyridamole have been shown to block the upregulation of TF specifically induced by polyclonal IgG purified from APS patients in monocytes [72, 73]. However, their role in APS management has been scarcely documented. Dual antiplatelet treatment (different combination of LDASA, ticlopidine, clopidogrel, cilostazol) has been recently proposed: a Japanese study on 82 APS patients with refractory arterial events documented no recurrences among those subjects receiving two antiplatelet agents [74].

aPL also upregulate GPIIb/IIIa, thus leading to platelet aggregation. *Abciximab* is a specific GPIIb/IIIa inhibitor routinely prescribed in stroke and acute coronary syndromes, which might be beneficial in APS [75].

Protein disulfide-isomerase is the enzyme responsible of the formation of two disulfide bridges within β2GPI molecule, a reaction leading to an oxidized and immunogenic molecule. This enzyme is inhibited by *quercetin-3-rutinoside*, whose potential pharmacological effect in APS has to be investigated [76]. In animal models, inhibitors of PDI were effective in treating thrombosis [76].

Given that oxidation leads to the unmasking of the critical B-cell epitope, it might be worth exploring the role of antioxidant compounds as *N-acetylcysteine, vitamin C,* and *coenzyme* Q_{10} in APS [66]. In an in vitro study, the inhibition of intracellular reactive oxygen species in monocytes prevented the upregulation of TF induced by aPL [77]. Similarly, TNF-α and IL-6 are proinflammatory mediators induced by aPL: it is therefore reasonable to hypothesize that the blockade of these cytokines with biologic agents may be clinically beneficial. Interestingly, in a mice model *anti-TNF-α agents* proved to be protective against aPL-induced pregnancy loss [69].

Conclusions

Much research attention is currently focused at identifying novel pharmacological tools in APS: some of these compounds have already been used in clinical practice, although in many cases experience is yet limited to anecdotal reports. Some others are currently under evaluation in randomized clinical trial in order to test their efficacy in the setting of APS.

However, the impact of a tight control of traditional vascular risk factors on clinical outcome of APS patients has not been ascertained yet. At this regard, the pleiotropic effects of agents such as statins and HCQ should be further assessed: the addition of these drugs to standard anticoagulation may lead to a better disease control. Moreover, the identification of novel diagnostic tools, such as antibodies against domain I of β2GPI or against phosphatidylserine/prothrombin, may allow a more precise stratification of thrombotic risk, leading to a tailored treatment strategy.

Forthcoming years will be essential to understand whether the above cited agents might eventually revolutionize APS management.

References

1. Lim W, Crowther MA, Eikelboom JW (2006) Management of antiphospholipid antibody syndrome. JAMA 295:1050–1057

2. Ruiz-Irastorza G, Cuadrado MJ, Ruiz-Arruza I et al (2011) Evidence-based recommendations for the prevention and long-term management of thrombosis in antiphospholipid antibody-positive patients: report of a task force at the 13th International Congress on Antiphospholipid Antibodies. Lupus 20:206–218
3. Cervera R, Serrano R, Pons-Estel GJ et al; On behalf of the Euro-Phospholipid Project Group (European Forum on Antiphospholipid Antibodies) (2014) Morbidity and mortality in the antiphospholipid syndrome during a 10-year period: a multicentre prospective study of 1000 patients. Ann Rheum Dis. doi:10.1136/annrheumdis-2013-204838
4. Les I, Ruiz-Irastorza G, Khamashta MA (2012) Intensity and duration of anticoagulation therapy in antiphospholipid syndrome. Semin Thromb Hemost 38:339–347
5. Meroni PL, Chighizola C (2012) Pathophysiology of the antiphospholipid syndrome (APS). Rev Med Interne 33:A2–A4
6. Chighizola CB, Gerosa M, Meroni PL (2014) New tests to detect antiphospholipid antibodies: anti-domain I beta-2-glycoprotein-I antibodies. Curr Rheumatol Rep 16:402
7. Meroni PL, Borghi MO, Raschi E et al (2011) Pathogenesis of antiphospholipid syndrome: understanding the antibodies. Nat Rev Rheumatol 7:330–339
8. Alijotas-Reig J (2013) Treatment of refractory obstetric antiphospholipid syndrome: the state of the art and new trends in the therapeutic management. Lupus 22:6–17
9. Chighizola C, Moia M, Meroni PL (2014) New oral anticoagulants in thrombotic antiphospholipid syndrome. Lupus 23:1279–82
10. Giles I, Khamashta M, D'Cruz D et al (2012) A new dawn of anticoagulation for patients with antiphospholipid syndrome? Lupus 21:1263–1265
11. Petri M (2011) Use of hydroxychloroquine to prevent thrombosis in systemic lupus erythematosus and in antiphospholipid antibody-positive patients. Curr Rheumatol Rep 13:77–80
12. Kuznik A, Bencina M, Svajger U et al (2011) Mechanism of endosomal TLR inhibition by antimalarial drugs and imidazoquinolines. J Immunol 186:4794–4804
13. Espinola RG, Pierangeli SS, Gharavi AE et al (2002) Hydroxychloroquine reverses platelet activation induced by human IgG antiphospholipid antibodies. Thromb Haemost 87:518–522
14. Rand J, Wu X, Quinn A et al (2008) Hydroxychloroquine directly reduces the binding of antiphospholipid antibody-beta2-glycoprotein I complexes to phospholipid bilayers. Blood 112:1687–1695
15. Rand JH, Wu XX, Quinn AS et al (2010) Hydroxychloroquine protects the annexin A5 anticoagulant shield from disruption by antiphospholipid antibodies: evidence for a novel effect for an old antimalarial drug. Blood 115:2292–2299
16. Edwards MH, Pierangeli S, Liu X et al (1997) Hydroxychloroquine reverses thrombogenic properties of antiphospholipid antibodies in mice. Circulation 96:4380–4384
17. Wu XX, Guller S, Rand JH (2011) Hydroxychloroquine reduces binding of antiphospholipid antibodies to syncytiotrophoblasts and restores annexin A5 expression. Am J Obstet Gynecol 205:e7–e14
18. Albert CR, Schlesinger WJ, Viall CA et al (2014) Effect of hydroxychloroquine on antiphospholipid antibody-induced changes in first trimester trophoblast function. Am J Reprod Immunol 71:154–164
19. Erkan D, Yazici Y, Peterson MG et al (2002) A cross-sectional study of clinical thrombotic risk factors and preventive treatments in antiphospholipid syndrome. Rheumatology (Oxford) 41:924–929
20. Law G, Magder LS, Fang H et al (2012) Hydroxychloroquine reduces thrombosis in systemic lupus erythematosus, particularly in antiphospholipid positive patients [abstract]. Arthritis Rheum 64:2569
21. Schmidt-Tanguy A, Voswinkel J, Henrion D et al (2013) Antithrombotic effects of hydroxychloroquine in primary antiphospholipid syndrome patients. J Thromb Haemost 11:1927–1929
22. Erkan D, Aguiar CL, Andrade D et al (2014) 14th international congress on antiphospholipid antibodies task force report on antiphospholipid syndrome treatment trends. Autoimmun Rev 13:685–696

23. Medina G, Gutiérrez-Moreno AL, Vera-Lastra O et al (2011) Prevalence of metabolic syndrome in primary antiphospholipid syndrome patients. Autoimmun Rev 10:214–217
24. Ferrara D, Swerlick R, Casper K et al (2004) Fluvastatin inhibits up-regulation of tissue factor expression by antiphospholipid antibodies on endothelial cells. J Thromb Haemost 2:1558–1563
25. Meroni PL, Raschi E, Testoni C et al (2001) Statins prevent endothelial cell activation induced by antiphospholipid (anti-beta2-glycoprotein I) antibodies: effect on the proadhesive and proinflammatory phenotype. Arthritis Rheum 44:2870–2878
26. Martínez-Martínez LA, Amigo MC, Orozco A et al (2006) Effect of rosuvastatin on vascular cell adhesion molecule 1 (vcam-1) expression by human endothelial cells exposed to antiphospholipid syndrome serum. J Clin Rheumatol 12:S80
27. Odiari EA, Mulla MJ, Sfakianaki AK et al (2012) Pravastatin does not prevent antiphospholipid antibody-mediated changes in human first trimester trophoblast function. Hum Reprod 27:2933–2940
28. Redecha P (2008) Neutrophil activation by the tissue factor/Factor VIIa/PAR2 axis mediates fetal death in a mouse model of antiphospholipid syndrome. J Clin Invest 118:3453–3461
29. Lòpez-Pedrera C, Ruiz-Limòn P, Aguirre MÀ et al (2011) Global effects of fluvastatin on the prothrombotic status of patients with antiphospholipid syndrome. Ann Rheum Dis 70:675–682
30. Erkan D, Willis R, Vega JA et al (2012) An open-label prospective pilot mechanistic study of fluvastatin in persistently antiphospholipid antibody-positive patients. Arthritis Rheum 64:S1034
31. Ruiz-Irastorza G, Crowther M, Branch W et al (2010) Antiphospholipid syndrome. Lancet 376:1498–1509
32. Agmon-Levin N, Blank M, Zandman-Goddard G et al (2011) Vitamin D: an instrumental factor in the anti-phospholipid syndrome by inhibition of tissue factor expression. Ann Rheum Dis 70:145–150
33. Andreoli L, Piantoni S, Dall'Ara F et al (2012) Vitamin D and antiphospholipid syndrome. Lupus 21:736–740
34. Piantoni S, Andreoli L, Allegri F et al (2012) Low levels of vitamin D are common in primary antiphospholipid syndrome with thrombotic disease. Reumatismo 64:307–313
35. Klack K, Carvalho JF (2010) High frequency of vitamin D insufficiency in primary antiphospholipid syndrome. Joint Bone Spine 77:489–490
36. Paupitz JA, Freire de Carvalho J, Caparbo VF et al (2010) Primary antiphospholipid syndrome in premenopausal women: low vitamin D, high fat mass and maintained bone mineral mass. Lupus 19:1302–1306
37. Konova E (2005) Intravenous Immunoglobulin therapy in anti-phospholipid syndrome. Clin Rev Allergy Immunol 29:229–236
38. Pierangeli SS, Espinola R, Liu X et al (2001) Identification of an Fc gamma receptor-independent mechanism by which intravenous immunoglobulin ameliorates antiphospholipid antibody-induced thrombogenic phenotype. Arthritis Rheum 44:876–883
39. Sherer Y, Levy Y, Shoenfeld Y (2000) Intravenous immunoglobulin therapy of antiphospholipid syndrome. Rheumatology (Oxford) 39:421–426
40. Sciascia S, Giachino O, Roccatello D (2012) Prevention of thrombosis in antiphospholipid syndrome patients refractory to conventional therapy using intravenous immunoglobulin. Clin Exp Rheumatol 30:409–413
41. Kahn P, Ramanujam M, Bethunaickan R et al (2008) Prevention of murine antiphospholipid syndrome by BAFF blockade. Arthritis Rheum 58:2824–2834
42. Akkermann A, Huang W, Wang X et al (2004) CTLA4Ig prevents initiation but not evolution of anti-phospholipid syndrome in NZW/BXSB mice. Autoimmunity 37:445–451
43. Stohl W, Hiepe F, Latinis KM et al (2012) Belimumab reduces autoantibodies, normalizes low complement levels, and reduces select B cell population in patients with systemic lupus erythematosus. Arthritis Rheum 64:2328–2337

44. Ramos-Casals M, Brito-Zeròn P, Muñoz S et al (2008) A systematic review of the off-label use of biological therapies in systemic autoimmune diseases. Medicine (Baltimore) 87: 345–364
45. Khattri S, Zandman Goddard G, Peeva E (2012) B-cell directed therapies in antiphospholipid antibody syndrome – new directions based on murine and human data. Autoimmun Rev 11:717–722
46. Erkan D, Vega J, Ramòn G et al (2013) A pilot open-label phase II trial of rituximab for non criteria manifestations of antiphospholipid syndrome. Arthritis Rheum 65:464–471
47. Suzuki K, Nagasawa H, Kameda H et al (2009) Severe acute thrombotic exacerbation in two cases with anti-phospholipid syndrome after retreatment with rituximab in phase I/II clinical trial for refractory systemic lupus erythematosus. Rheumatology (Oxford) 48:198–199
48. Berman H, Rodrìguez-Pintò I, Cervera R et al (2013) Rituximab use in the catastrophic antiphospholipid syndrome: descriptive analysis of the CAPS registry. Autoimmun Rev 1:1085–1090
49. Ikeda K, Nagasawa K, Horiuchi T et al (1997) C5a induces tissue factor activity on endothelial cells. Thromb Haemost 77:394–398
50. Ritis K, Doumas M, Mastellos D et al (2006) A novel C5a receptor-tissue factor cross-talk in neutrophils links innate immunity to coagulation pathways. J Immunol 177:4794–4802
51. Fischetti F, Durigutto P, Pellis V et al (2005) Thrombus formation induced by antibodies to beta2-glycoprotein I is complement dependent and requires a priming factor. Blood 106:2340–2346
52. Lubbe WF, Butler WS, Palmer SJ et al (1983) Fetal survival after prednisolone suppression of maternal lupus-anticoagulant. Lancet 18:1361–1363
53. Schmidtko J, Peine S, El-Housseini Y et al (2013) Treatment of atypical hemolytic uremic syndrome and thrombotic microangiopathies: a focus on eculizumab. Am J Kidney Dis 61:289–299
54. Lonze BE, Singer AL, Montgomery RA (2010) Eculizumab and renal transplantation in a patient with CAPS. N Engl J Med 362:1744–1745
55. Shapira I, Andrade D, Allen SL et al (2012) Brief report: induction of sustained remission in recurrent catastrophic antiphospholipid syndrome via inhibition of terminal complement with eculizumab. Arthritis Rheum 64:2719–2723
56. Canaud G, Kamar N, Anglicheau D et al (2013) Eculizumab improves posttransplant thrombotic microangiopathy due to antiphospholipid syndrome recurrence but fails to prevent chronic vascular changes. Am J Transplant 13:2179–2185
57. Lonze BE, Zachary AA, Magro CM et al (2014) Eculizumab prevents recurrent antiphospholipid antibody syndrome and enables successful renal transplantation. Am J Transplant 14:459–465
58. Morabito F, Gentile M, Gay F et al (2009) Insights into defibrotide: an updated review. Expert Opin Biol Ther 9:763–767
59. Falanga A, Vignoli A, Marchetti M et al (2003) Defibrotide reduces procoagulant activity and increases fibrinolytic properties of endothelial cells. Leukemia 17:1636–1642
60. Asherson RA, Cervera R, Piette JC et al (2001) Catastrophic antiphospholipid syndrome: clues to the pathogenesis from a series of 80 patients. Medicine (Baltimore) 80:355–376
61. Burcoglu-O'Ral A, Erkan D, Asherson R (2002) Treatment of catastrophic antiphospholipid syndrome with defibrotide, a proposed vascular endothelial cell modulator. J Rheumatol 29:2006–2011
62. Ostertag MV, Liu X, Henderson V et al (2006) A peptide that mimics the Vth region of β2-glycoprotein I reverses antiphospholipid-mediated thrombosis in mice. Lupus 15:358–365
63. de la Torre YM, Pregnolato F, D'Amelio F et al (2012) Anti-phospholipid induced murine fetal loss: novel protective effects of a peptide targeting the beta-2 glycoprotein I phospholipid-binding site. Implication for human fetal loss. J Autoimmun 38:209–215
64. Ioannou Y, Romay-Penabad Z, Pericleous C et al (2009) In vivo inhibition of antiphospholipid antibody-induced pathogenicity utilizing the antigenic target peptide domain I of beta2-glycoprotein I: proof of concept. J Thromb Haemost 7:833–842

65. Agostinis C, Durigutto P, Sblattero D et al (2014) A non complement-fixing antibody to b2 glycoprotein I as a novel therapy to control abortions and thrombosis in antiphospholipid syndrome. Blood. doi:10.1182/blood-2013-11-537704
66. Giannakopoulos B, Krilis SA (2013) The pathogenesis of the anti-phospholipid syndrome. N Engl J Med 368:1033–1044
67. Kolyada A, Chang-Jin L, De Biasio A et al (2010) A novel dimeric inhibitor targeting Beta2GPI in Beta2GPI/antibody complexes implicated in antiphospholipid syndrome. PLoS One 5:e15345
68. Kolyada A, Porter A, Beglova N (2014) Inhibition of thrombotic properties of persistent autoimmune anti-b2GPI antibodies in the mouse model of antiphospholipid syndrome. Blood 123:1090–1097
69. Comarmond C, Cacoub P (2013) Antiphospholipid syndrome: from pathogenesis to novel immunomodulatory therapies. Autoimmun Rev 12:752–757
70. Nishimura M, Nii T, Trimova G et al (2013) The NF-κB specific inhibitor DHMEQ prevents thrombus formation in a mouse model of antiphospholipid syndrome. J Nephropathol 2:114–121
71. Pierangeli SS, Erkan D (2010) Antiphospholipid syndrome treatment beyond anticoagulation: are we there yet? Lupus 19:475–485
72. Zhou H, Wolberg AS, Roubey RA (2004) Characterization of monocyte tissue factor activity induced by IgG antiphospholipid antibodies and inhibition by dilazep. Blood 104:2353–2358
73. Zhou H (2004) Dilazep and dipyridamole inhibit tissue factor expression on monocytes induced by IgG from patients with antiphospholipid syndrome. Acta Pharmacol Sin 25:1366–1371
74. Fujieda Y, Amengual O, Watanabe T et al (2012) Dual antiplatelet therapy as prophylaxis of recurrent arterial thrombosis in patients with antiphospholipid syndrome. Arthritis Rheum 64:S1036
75. Scoble T, Wijetilleka S, Khamashta MA et al (2011) Management of refractory antiphospholipid syndrome. Autoimmun Rev 10:669–673
76. Jasuja R, Passam FH, Kennedy DR et al (2012) Protein disulphide isomerase inhibitors constitute a new class of antithrombotic agent. J Clin Invest 122:2104–2113
77. Perez-Sanchez C, Ruiz-Limon P, Aguirre MA et al (2012) Mitochondrial dysfunction in antiphospholipid syndrome: implications in the pathogenesis of the disease and effects of coenzyme Q10 treatment. Blood 119:5859–5870

Secondary Antiphospholipid Syndrome 19

Anisur Rahman and Maria Gabriella Raimondo

19.1 What Is Secondary APS (SAPS)?

The antiphospholipid syndrome (APS) is a prothrombotic disorder characterized by the occurrence of recurrent venous and arterial thromboses and/or pregnancy morbidity in association with the presence of antiphospholipid antibodies (aPL). aPL are autoantibodies that target negatively charged phospholipids and/or their complexes with plasma proteins like β2-glycoprotein I. The aPL are formally detected by functional coagulation assay (lupus anticoagulant, LAC) and/or by solid-phase binding assays: anticardiolipin (aCL) or anti-β2 glycoprotein I (anti-β2GPI) enzyme-linked immunosorbent assays (ELISAs) [1].

Preliminary classification criteria for APS were developed in 1999 after an expert workshop in Sapporo, Japan, and then updated after another international meeting in Sydney, Australia, in 2006 (Table 19.1) [2, 3]. Like the preliminary classification, the revised one was divided into clinical and laboratory criteria with the recommendation to stratify APS patients according to the presence or absence of inherited and acquired risk factors for arterial or venous thrombosis. These risk factors include age (>55 in men and >65 in women), the presence of any of the established risk factors for cardiovascular diseases, inherited thrombophilias, oral contraceptives,

A. Rahman (✉)
Division of Medicine, Centre for Rheumatology Research, University College London,
5 University Street, London WC1E 6JF, UK
e-mail: anisur.rahman@ucl.ac.uk

M.G. Raimondo (✉)
Department of Rheumatology, Department of Internal Medicine,
Università degli Studi di Milano, Istituto Ortopedico Gaetano Pini,
Piazza Cardinale Andrea Ferrari 1, Milan 20122, Italy
e-mail: maria.raimondo@unimi.it; mg.raimondo@gmail.com

© Springer International Publishing Switzerland 2015
P.L. Meroni (ed.), *Antiphospholipid Antibody Syndrome: From Bench to Bedside*,
Rare Diseases of the Immune System, DOI 10.1007/978-3-319-11044-8_19

Table 19.1 Classification criteria for APS

Clinical criteria
One or more episodes of arterial, venous, or small vessel thrombosis by validated criteria with no vessel wall inflammation
One or more unexplained fetal deaths later than 10 weeks' gestation (morphologically normal fetus)
One or more premature births of morphologically normal neonate before 34 weeks' gestation due to eclampsia or preeclampsia or recognized features of placental failure
Three or more unexplained consecutive spontaneous abortions before 10 weeks' gestation, excluding hormonal or chromosomal causes
Laboratory criteria
Lupus anticoagulant in plasma on two or more occasions at least 12 weeks apart
IgG and/or IgM anticardiolipin antibodies in serum or plasma at medium or high titer on two or more occasions at least 12 weeks apart measured by a standardized ELISA
IgG and/or IgM anti-beta2glycoprotein I antibodies in serum or plasma at titer >99th percentile of healthy population on two or more occasions at least 12 weeks apart measured by a standardized ELISA

APS is present if at least one of the clinical criteria and one of the laboratory criteria are met [2]

nephrotic syndrome, malignancy, immobilization, and surgery. Moreover, a new correct definition of placental insufficiency was provided, and correct interpretation of preeclampsia and eclampsia was highlighted. Within the laboratory criteria IgM and IgG anti β2 GPI were added with a specific indication concerning the positive threshold for each.

According to these recommendations, APS is defined by the presence of at least one clinical and one laboratory criterion (Table 19.1) [2, 3].

Patients with primary APS (PAPS) have no other autoimmune conditions, whereas secondary APS (SAPS) is diagnosed where the criteria for APS are fulfilled in the presence of another condition – most commonly systemic lupus erythematosus (SLE) [4]. The use of this term, however, does not imply that SLE causes APS to develop, and there are some cases where APS precedes SLE chronologically. Large cohort studies have found no differences in clinical features or consequences between PAPS and SAPS. Thus some experts suggested that the term SAPS should be abandoned in favor of terms such as SLE-associated APS, to document the coexistence of APS with other diseases [2].

The catastrophic APS (CAPS), a dramatic variant of APS, is characterized by acute widespread coagulopathy affecting small vessels leading to rapid multi-organ failure with high mortality rate [5].

The aPL can appear in different scenarios: asymptomatic carriers of aPL, "classical" APS with recurrent venous and/or arterial thrombosis with or without pregnancy morbidity, pure obstetric APS causing recurrent pregnancy loss with no thrombosis, aPL positivity with nonthrombotic manifestations (i.e., thrombocytopenia, hemolytic anemia, or livedo reticularis), or CAPS [6].

aPL have been reported in patients with:

- Autoimmune rheumatic diseases
- Infections
- Malignancies
- In association with certain drugs

But these aPL only seem to cause true APS in association with autoimmune rheumatic diseases and, rarely, with some infections. In this chapter, we will briefly discuss aPL found in infections and malignancies and in association with drugs and then concentrate on aPL and APS found in autoimmune rheumatic diseases, especially SLE.

19.2 Epidemiology of aPL and APS

Some evidence indicates that the incidence of the APS is around 5 new cases per 100,000 persons per year and the prevalence around 40–50 cases per 100,000 persons [6]. However, it is important to be aware that aPL can also occur in healthy people, in contrast to other autoantibodies, such as anti-dsDNA and anti-Sm, that are almost specific for patients with SLE [7].

Several studies evaluated the presence of aPL among healthy young people showing a prevalence range between 1 and 5 % for both aCL and LAC antibodies. Prevalence of anti-β2GPI and aCL (both IgM and IgG) antibodies in a large cohort of 510 healthy pregnant women studied prospectively at 15–18 weeks' gestation was found to be 3.9 and 1.6 %, respectively. However, in most cases the antibodies were present at low titers, and only a minority of these individuals developed APS [8]. Prevalence of aPL antibodies (by all three standard assays) increases with age and, in particular, in elderly people with chronic diseases. However, in most cases these subjects do not develop APS clinical manifestations [9].

Recently, the APS ACTION group (AntiPhospholipid Syndrome Alliance For Clinical Trials and InternatiOnal Networking) published a literature review concerning the prevalence of aPL in the general population with pregnancy morbidity, stroke, myocardial infarction (MI), and deep vein thrombosis (DVT). Although 120 papers were included in the review, the authors noted a number of limitations in the evidence; the majority of studies were published several years ago, all three criteria aPL tests were performed in only 11 % of the papers, most studies used a low-titer aCL ELISA cutoff, the method of reporting the cutoff for anti-β2GPI ELISA was quite heterogeneous, confirmation tests for positive aPL were performed in only one-fifth of the papers, and the study design was retrospective in nearly half of the papers. The authors concluded the literature review by estimating that aPL are positive in approximately 13 % of patients with stroke, 11 % with MI, 9.5 % with DVT, and 6 % of patients with pregnancy morbidity [10].

Table 19.2 Frequency of aCL in infectious diseases [16, 17]

Organism/infection	aCL frequency (%)
Leprosy	21–67
Mycobacterium tuberculosis	27–53
Syphilis	8–67
Leptospirosis	23–50
Mycoplasma	20–53
Streptococcus	80
Staphylococcus aureus	43
Escherichia coli	67
Malaria	12–30
Kala-azar	6
Rickettsia	42–84

The reported prevalence of aPL antibodies in children without any underlying disorder ranges from 3 to 28 % for aCL and from 3 to 7 % for anti-β2GPI. These figures are generally higher than those reported for adults. The reason for this is not yet understood but may be related to the frequent occurrence of infectious processes during childhood [11].

19.3 APS and Infection

19.3.1 aPL in Infectious Diseases

Wasserman described a complement fixation test for the serological diagnosis of syphilis (Wasserman test). This test can be falsely positive in the presence of aPL. This link between aPL and a false-positive test for syphilis was the first recognized association between APS and infectious diseases [12].

Since the association of aPL and syphilis was first described, many other viral, bacterial, and parasitic infections have been shown to induce the production of aPL. It is important, however, to emphasize that no particular infection or organism shows a high rate of association with aPL. Although molecular mimicry between infectious organisms and β2GPI has been suggested to play a possible key role in the pathogenesis of APS [13], this has not been ascribed convincingly to particular organisms. Although aPL have been reported in all the infections listed in Table 19.2, most patients who suffer these infections do NOT develop aPL.

Reports of aPL in infections have concentrated especially on viral illnesses. The prevalence of aPL in hepatitis C virus (HCV) infection has been reported to range from 3.3 to 46 % [8]. Sène and colleagues in a literature review published in 2008 estimated aCL prevalence of 18.6 % in HCV-infected patients compared with 1.78 % in control groups, while the anti-β2GPI prevalence was 1.65 % in the infected patients compared with 0.75 % in the controls [12]. In analogy, patients with hepatitis B virus (HBV) were found to be positive for aCL with a range between 18 and 42 %, while the figure for anti-β2GPI was lower (2–7.5 %) and no association has been demonstrated with APS-related phenomena [12, 14]. The reported prevalence of aCL and anti-β2GPI in patients with human immunodeficiency virus (HIV) ranges between 7–75 % and 3–20 %, respectively, but these antibodies are not significantly associated with thrombotic events or other APS manifestations [15].

aPL have been detected in patients with serology suggestive of other viral infections, including cytomegalovirus (CMV), Epstein-Barr virus (EBV), varicella-zoster virus (VZV), human T-cell lymphotropic virus type 1 (HTLV-1), adenoviruses, and parvovirus B19 with only anecdotal correlation with APS manifestations [16, 17]. In another study, a high prevalence of IgG aCL was found in patients with CMV infections after bone marrow transplantation, and a transient and high titer of aCL was found in pregnant women with primary parvovirus B19 infection [8, 12].

aCL have been also observed in various bacterial, mycobacterial, and parasitic infections without any association with thrombotic events (Table 19.2), whereas high levels of anti-β2GPI were observed in patients with leprosy and syphilis (3–89 % and 4–10 %, respectively) [16].

19.3.2 APS in Infectious Diseases

An important distinction in antigen-binding properties between infection-associated and APS-associated aPL has been recognized. Anti-CL antibodies detected in APS are thrombogenic and require the presence of serum cofactors, chiefly β2GPI, to bind CL. They are thus classified as "β2GPI dependent." In contrast, aCL from patients with infections bind CL in the absence of serum cofactors and are described as "β2GPI independent" [18]. Moreover, aCL found in infections are more likely to be of IgM rather than IgG isotype [8]. The aPL occurring in infections may be transient and disappear within 2 or 3 months [19]. These largely IgM, often transient, β2GPI-independent aPL are rarely associated with clinical features of APS, and thus it is unusual for a positive aPL test in a patient suffering from infection to alter clinical management. However, it has been reported that certain infections, such as leprosy and parvovirus B19, are sometimes associated with anti-β2GPI or β2GPI-dependent aCL that are more likely to cause thrombotic events [16].

Rare cases of thrombosis with aPL occurring with HCV have been described: one venous thrombosis in a thalassemic patient with lupus anticoagulant and one lacunar cerebral infarction with high level of aCL [12].

Several isolated cases of thrombosis in patients with HIV were associated with the presence of aPL, including digital ischemia, deep vein thrombosis, arterial pulmonary embolism, portal vein thrombosis, cutaneous necrosis, testicular thrombosis, stroke, and bone avascular necrosis [8].

Ramos-Casals et al. reported a literature review of clinical features related to APS in patients with chronic viral infections, including HCV and HIV. They selected 82 patients (45 had chronic HCV infection, 32 had HIV infection, and 5 had HCV-HIV coinfection) and found that the main APS-related features in HCV-infected patients were intra-abdominal thrombosis and myocardial infarction, whereas, in HIV-infected patients, the main features were avascular bone and cutaneous necrosis.

This evidence suggests that these viruses might act in some patients as chronic triggering agents inducing atypical presentation of APS [20].

Cervera et al. described the clinical and serological characteristics of 100 patients with APS related to infections (68 had primary APS, 27 had SLE, 2 had LLD, 2 had inflammatory bowel diseases, and 1 had RA). The main clinical manifestations of APS included pulmonary involvement (39 %), skin involvement (36 %), and renal involvement (35 %). The main associated infections and agents included skin infection (18 %), HIV (17 %), pneumonia (14 %), hepatitis C (13 %), and urinary tract infection (10 %) [21]. Of particular note, APS presented as a catastrophic syndrome in 40 % of these infection-related cases, whereas CAPS constitutes fewer than 2 % of all APS cases. CAPS is an exception to the rule that infection and APS are rarely linked. CAPS develops after a specific precipitating event in 60 % of cases, and 25 % of these events are infections [22].

19.4 APS and Malignancy

Isolated case reports and some retrospective studies showed the association of aCL with vascular events in patients with a variety of malignant conditions, including solid tumors and lymphoproliferative malignancies, compared with the general population. Since malignancy is also a hypercoagulable state, it is controversial whether the aPL have a pathogenic role in the thrombosis or are just an epiphenomenon in cancer patients [23]. From the literature, the incidence of aPL positivity in cancer varies with few reports on the persistence of aPL positivity.

Yoon et al. observed an incidence of aPL antibodies in up to 60 % of cancer patients in a small cohort of 33 Asian subjects, although the most prevalent antibody was anti-β2GPI IgA [24]. Additionally, Miesbach et al. performed a retrospective study in which a history of malignancy was found in 58 of 425 aPL-positive patients [25]. Armas et al. found a significantly higher aCL IgG levels in cancer patients compared with general population, although no differences in the incidence of thrombotic events were observed between aCL-positive and aCL-negative patients with cancer [26]. In contrast, another study demonstrated a higher prevalence of aCL IgM in patients with malignancies but without thrombosis compared with healthy controls [27]. Additionally, a prospective study evaluated the occurrence of malignancy in patients with aPL antibodies and found that 19 % developed cancer. None of these patients with malignancy and aPL antibodies were noted to develop any thromboembolism [28].

In another study the prevalence of aCL was compared between cancer patients with positive or negative history for acute thrombosis and healthy controls. No differences in mean value of aCL IgG were found, whereas a higher prevalence of aCL IgM was observed in patients with thrombotic events than without [29].

Pusterla and colleagues demonstrated an increased rate of thrombosis among patients with lymphoma and aPL compared with aPL-negative patients. In contrast, Genvresse reported a prevalence of 26.6 % of aPL in patients with non-Hodgkin lymphoma, but none of these patients presented clinical manifestations suggestive for APS [30].

Table 19.3 Studies on aPL and malignancies

Study	No. of cancer patients/healthy controls	No. of cancer patients with aPL	aPL antibodies	No. of patients with aPL, malignancy, and thrombosis
Zuckerman et al.	216/88	47	aCL IgG, IgM	13
Ozguroglu et al.	61/20	NA	aCL IgG, IgM	NA
Yook et al.	33/0	20	aCL IgG, IgM	NA
			anti-β2GPI IgG, IgM, IgA	
Miesbach et al.	58/0	58	LAC	24
			aCL IgG, IgM	
Pusterla et al.	100/100	27	LAC	6
			aCL IgG, IgM	
Bazzan et al.	137/137	33	aCL IgG, IgM	1
			anti-β2GPI IgG, IgM	
Font et al.	258/142	23	LAC	21
			aCL IgG, IgM	
			anti-β2GPI IgG, IgM	
Genvresse et al.	90/0	24	aCL IgG, IgM	0
			anti-β2GPI IgG, IgM	

NA: not available literature reviewed in [35]

Zuckerman et al. found a higher prevalence of aCL in a study of 216 patients with solid and nonsolid tumors compared with 88 healthy controls (22 % vs. 3 %), and, moreover, only those patients with high level of aCL had a higher rate of thromboembolic events [31]. Bazzan et al. found a higher prevalence of low titers of aPL in a series of 137 cancer patients compared with healthy controls. No significant difference was found between rates of thromboembolic events between aPL-positive and aPL-negative patients [32]. Font et al. found a low prevalence and transience of aPL positivity in patients with solid malignancies who developed venous thromboembolism [23]. In contrast, De Meis and colleagues found a strong correlation between thrombosis and LAC positivity in a cohort of patients with lung adenocarcinoma [33].

In conclusion, conflicting data are available regarding the role of aPL in patients with cancer. The reported aPL prevalences varied widely between studies, probably related to different clinical characteristics of the study populations and different ELISA techniques for aPL detection. However, there is no clear evidence that the aPL are necessarily associated with an increased thrombophilic risk. Conversely, presence of aPL may be a risk for hematological malignancies [34] (Table 19.3).

19.5 APS and Drugs

Several drugs may induce generation of aPL with a low prevalence and no clear association with APS clinical manifestations. Some reports include phenothiazines (chlorpromazine), phenytoin, hydralazine, procainamide, quinidine, quinine, Dilantin, ethosuximide, interferon-alfa, amoxicillin, chlorothiazide, oral contraceptives, and propranolol [4].

Biologic medications and in particular tumor necrosis factor-alpha (TNF-α) inhibitors (adalimumab, etanercept, infliximab) induce the production of autoantibodies including aCL. One possible explanation for the induction of aPL positivity in patients treated with anti-TNF-α is that downregulation of TNF-α leads to upregulation of interleukin-10 (IL-10), which in turn activates autoreactive B cells and thus induces autoantibody production [36]. Ferraccioli et al. observed the induction of aCL in 5 of 8 RA patients treated with etanercept and followed for 85 weeks. The authors showed that the appearance of these autoantibodies correlated with infections including urinary or upper respiratory tract infections and that antibiotic treatment restored normal aCL antibody levels [37]. Another study evaluated 39 RA patients treated with infliximab and followed over 78 weeks. Among these a significant increase level of aCL was observed, starting at 30 weeks for IgM antibodies but not till the final time point (78 weeks) for IgG antibodies. However, the levels were low and none of the patients exhibited any clinical features related to APS [38]. Two case reports provide evidence of APS related to anti-TNF-α treatment. Hemmati et al. described a 67-year-old woman who developed APS and vasculitis associated with de novo positive aCL antibody following the third dose of adalimumab therapy for the treatment of spondyloarthropathy [39]. Vereckei and colleagues reported a case of infliximab-induced APS with manifestation as necrotizing vasculitis of toes and fingers in a patient with RA [40].

19.6 APS Associated with Autoimmune Rheumatic Diseases

In 1983 Graham Hughes identified a group of patients with SLE, who suffered from obstetric morbidity and/or recurrent thromboses and with serum IgG aCL positivity [41]. Since then, the majority of publications related to APS in the setting of another autoimmune rheumatic disease have continued to relate to SLE, as this is by far the most commonly associated condition. In this section, therefore, we will concentrate on SLE-associated APS before covering the relatively sparse literature on APS in association with other autoimmune rheumatic diseases.

19.6.1 APS Developing in Patients with Preexisting SLE

The prevalence of aPL among patients with SLE ranges from 12 to 44 % for aCL, from 15 to 34 % for LAC, and from 10 to 19 % for anti-β2GPI [34]. Interestingly, a meta-analysis of the published studies was performed by Avcin and colleagues showing a global prevalence of 44 % for aCL, 40 % for anti-beta2GPI, and 22 % for LAC among the SLE pediatric population [42]. It is possible that the real frequency of aPL in patients with SLE is underestimated, especially if patients develop these antibodies intermittently or if levels are altered by treatment [43].

APS may develop in 30–70 % of aPL-positive patients with SLE within 20 years of follow-up [8]. Alarcon-Segovia et al. showed that up to 30 % of patients with SLE and positive aCL have no clinical manifestation of APS during an average follow-up of 7 years. Conversely, in the Hopkins lupus cohort the risk of developing thrombosis in SLE patients with LAC positivity was about 50 % at 20 years of follow-up [43, 44].

19.6.2 SLE Developing in Patients with Preexisting APS

Progression from primary APS to a full-blown SLE is rare event. To date, there are several reported cases of patients whose PAPS evolved to SLE or LLD. Moreover, some large studies have addressed this issue in detail.

In a retrospective study, Gomez-Puerta et al. followed up for about 9 years 128 patients with PAPS of whom 11 (8 %) patients developed SLE, 6 (5 %) developed lupus-like disease, and 1 (1 %) developed myasthenia gravis. The remaining 110 patients (86 %) continued to have primary APS. In this study a positive Coombs test was a clinically significant predictor of progression to SLE [45].

Recently, Freire PV et al. retrospectively analyzed a cohort of 80 patients with primary APS. Among these 14 (17.5 %) patients who were significantly younger at the time of diagnosis, with a longer disease duration, progressed within 5.2+/-4 years to SLE-related APS. All these patients were ANA positive before the diagnosis of SLE, compared to 51 % of the 66 patients who did not develop SLE [46].

A retrospective study performed by Tarr and colleagues evaluated a large cohort of lupus patients. The authors observed that in 26 cases (7.2 %) lupus started in the form of PAPS [47].

In a 5-year prospective follow-up of 531 patients with PAPS included in the 1000 APS subjects of the Europhospholipid study [48], only 6 patients developed SLE.

Interestingly, the percentage of progression to SLE or lupus-like disease in pediatric patients with PAPS is almost double compared with that found in the adult PAPS patients [49].

19.6.3 Genetic Comparisons Between Patients with PAPS and SLE-Associated APS

Like other autoimmune diseases, the etiology of APS is linked to genetic predisposition as demonstrated by animal models and by familial occurrence of this syndrome. The genes of the major histocompatibility complex (HLA system) have been the most investigated, and some evidence shows the association of some HLA alleles with increased risk of developing aPL independent of the clinical context and across various ethnic groups [50].

Overall, very similar associations between HLA and aPL have been reported in primary APS and in APS secondary to SLE. An association of HLA-DR4, HLA-DR7, DRw53, and HLA-DQB1*0302 with aCL has been found in primary APS and in patients with SLE [51]. In contrast, Freitas et al. studied 123 patients (34 of whom had PAPS and 35 SAPS due to SLE, 54 SLE patients without APS, and 166 controls) to assess whether the major histocompatibility complex (MHC) profile of patients presenting with PAPS was different from that of patients with SAPS. The results indicate that the association of SAPS with HLA-DRB1*03 is due to the association with SLE and is not due to aCL and suggest that the HLA class II profile of PAPS is different from that of SAPS [52].

Several other studies investigate the HLA alleles and haplotypes in APS patients. Caliz et al. observed that the DQB1*0604/5/6/7/9-DQA1*0102-DRB1*1302 haplotype was the major association in APS and its frequency was more strikingly increased in 53 British Caucasoid patients with primary APS than in secondary APS. Moreover, it is suggested that this haplotype predisposes to anti-β2GPI positivity. The authors proposed that a molecule encoded by the DQB1*0604/5/6/7/9-DQA1*0102-DRB1*1302 haplotype may preferentially present peptides derived from β2 glycoprotein I, thus leading to the generation of autoantibodies [53]. Another study reports the association of HLA-DR5 with primary APS in Mexican patients [51].

Non HLA-genes, in particular the FcγR and PDCD1 polymorphisms, seem to support lupus susceptibility, but without any associations with APS patients [54]. In conclusion, genetic studies suggest that APS differs from SLE, although the genetic predisposition of HLA and non-HLA-genes to APS can only in part explain this differences [51].

19.6.4 Clinical Comparisons Between Patients with PAPS and SLE-Associated APS

In 1994 Vianna and colleagues published a study in which 114 patients (56 had APS plus SLE and 58 had PAPS) were compared over 10 years of follow-up. The authors found that patients with PAPS and SLE-associated APS had similar clinical and laboratory profiles, with some exceptions. Indeed, autoimmune hemolytic anemia, endocardial valve disease, neutropenia, and low C4 levels were found more frequently in patients with SLE and APS (SAPS). No patient with PAPS had either anti-DNA or anti-extractable nuclear antigen antibodies, and these patients had a significantly lower prevalence of antinuclear antibodies (41 %) compared with SAPS ones (89 %) [55].

Soltesz et al. studied a large cohort of Hungarian APS patients (218 PAPS and 288 SLE-related APS). They found more men among the primary APS (39/128) compared with the SLE-associated APS (27/288) patients. Cerebrovascular thrombosis was significantly higher in SLE patients with APS (128/288) than among the PAPS (77/128), but no differences were found among the two groups in terms of laboratory and other clinical manifestations (i.e., LAC and IgM and IgG aCL, venous thrombosis, coronary, carotid and peripheral arterial thrombosis, and fetal loss respectively) [56].

Thrombotic events occur more often in SLE patients positive for aPL compared to aPL-positive patients without lupus or with other systemic autoimmune diseases [34]. Similar results have been obtained by another study with a higher frequency of thrombosis and pregnancy loss in APS associated with SLE than in PAPS [57]. Interestingly, all SLE patients with thrombosis were reported to be positive for anti-β2GPI in comparison with controls, while aCL IgG and IgM were similar in lupus patients with or without thrombosis [8]. In contrast, aCL IgG and/or IgM were found in 18.5 % of 130 SLE patients before the diagnosis of SLE and this was predictive of a more severe clinical outcome [58]. Both the Hopkins lupus cohort study and a meta-analysis on the association between aPL and venous thromboembolism (VTE) in SLE patients found that those with LAC positivity have a sixfold greater risk for VTE compared to LAC-negative patients, whereas aCL-positive patients have a twofold greater risk for VTE than the negative ones [59, 60]. Moreover, the diagnosis of secondary APS led to a threefold increase in pregnancy loss, predominantly after 20 weeks of gestation, and was an independent risk factor for further pregnancy losses in a cohort study of 166 pregnancies in women with SLE at Hopkins lupus center. In this study, the presence of aPL (aCL and/or LAC) without the clinical criteria for secondary APS did not increase the risk for pregnancy loss in the same series [61].

Moreover, aPL were associated with an increased risk for chronic renal insufficiency in patients with lupus nephritis, and they were also found to be associated with neuropsychiatric events in SLE [54].

The Europhospholipid project is a cross-sectional study of 1,000 patients with APS from 20 centers in 13 countries. In a publication of the baseline characteristics of the cohort in 2002, Cervera et al. [48] reported that 531 patients in the study had PAPS, 362 had SLE-associated APS, and 59 had APS associated with other conditions. Only 3 % of PAPS subjects had arthritis, compared to 56 % of those with SLE-associated APS, and SLE-associated APS was also associated with a higher frequency of leukopenia, livedo reticularis, and thrombocytopenia. However, in a 5-year follow-up of the same cohort, there were no differences in clinical outcomes between the PAPS and SLE-associated APS groups [62].

Overall, therefore, the majority of the evidence suggests that clinical features and outcomes of APS are broadly similar, whether or not patients also have SLE. Naturally features due to SLE itself (e.g., arthritis) would be expected to occur more frequently in SLE-associated APS than in PAPS.

19.6.5 Management of SLE-Associated APS

There is no evidence to suggest that management of either thrombosis risk or pregnancy should be any different in SLE-associated APS than in primary APS. This point has been specified in recent Treat-to-Target guidelines for patients with SLE [63].

Both retrospective studies [64] and prospective randomized controlled trials [65, 66] included both patients with PAPS and patients with SLE-associated APS and found that clinical outcomes did not differ between those groups. For example, Khamashta et al. [64] in a seminal retrospective study including nearly 1,000 patient-years follow-up studied 62 patients with PAPS, 66 patients with SLE-associated APS, and 19 with lupus-like disease and APS. Their recommendations of long-term high-dose anticoagulation to prevent recurrent thrombosis applied equally to both groups. In RCTs 32 of the 109 patients randomized by Finazzi et al. [66] had SAPS and 16 of the 114 randomized by Crowther et al. [65] had SLE-associated APS. Both trials suggested that moderate-intensity anticoagulation would be as effective as high-intensity anticoagulation in preventing recurrent thrombosis and did not distinguish between PAPS and SAPS patients. In two systematic reviews of the management of APS by Lim et al. [67] and Ruiz-Irastorza et al. [68], recommendations were not classified in terms of PAPS and SLE-associated APS, again showing that there is no difference between the recommended management regimes for these two forms of APS.

However, as a detailed description of therapy for APS is provided in Chaps. 15 and 16 of this book, we will not repeat it here.

19.6.6 Are the Symptoms Due to SLE or APS?

In patients with SLE-associated APS, there may sometimes be confusion as to whether particular clinical manifestations are caused by thrombosis (i.e., the APS component) or autoimmune inflammation (the SLE component). It is important to distinguish the two scenarios to decide whether immunosuppression, anticoagulation, or both is the appropriate treatment. For example, renal biopsies may show classic lupus glomerulonephritis or, less commonly, microthrombi and intimal proliferation [69, 70]. However, the latter appearance is typically associated with falling creatinine clearance rather than proteinuria and active urinary sediment [71].

Neuropsychiatric symptoms such as seizures or migraine may also be features of either APS or SLE. Cerebral imaging may not help distinguish the two as both may be characterized by small white matter lesions. Elevated anti-dsDNA antibodies and low complement would suggest active SLE, whereas very high aPL levels would be more in favor of APS. Hanly et al. [72] suggested that presence of IgG or IgM aCL might be associated with increased risk of cognitive dysfunction in patients with SLE. A more recent, much larger multicenter study did not confirm that finding [73] and only described an association between LAC positivity and intracerebral thrombosis.

19.6.7 APS and Other Autoimmune Rheumatic Diseases

Although aPL antibodies have been studied most extensively in association with SLE, they have also been reported in patients with other autoimmune disorders [4]. One report described a high frequency of aPL of up to 28 % in patients with rheumatoid arthritis (RA), while lower values close to the general population prevalence were found in other autoimmune diseases [34].

A prospective study of patients with different autoimmune rheumatic diseases was performed by Merkel and colleagues in 1996. The investigators found different prevalences of either IgG or IgM aCL among each of these groups: SLE 15.76 %,

RA 15.7 %, systemic sclerosis (SSc) 6.7 %, polymyositis/dermatomyositis (PM/DM) 8.3 %, early undifferentiated connective tissue diseases (EUCTD) 9.1 %, Sjögren's syndrome (SS) 6.8 %, ANCA-related renal vasculitis 3.8 %, and blood bank controls 4 %. In this study the prevalence of aCL was significantly higher in patients with RA or SLE compared with controls, whereas the prevalence in the other diseases was comparable with that of the healthy controls [74]. Other studies investigated the prevalence of aCL in SLE, RA, and SSc with higher ranges of results (4–49 %, 12–39 %, and 0–41 %, respectively) [8]. However, the presence of aPL did not correlate with consistent clinical manifestations so the clinical importance and specificity of these antibodies has yet to be determined.

Sanna et al. in 2005 confirmed that aCL IgG and/or IgM were more frequently found in patients with SSc than in controls, whereas the prevalence of anti-β2GPI did not differ between the two groups. In the same paper, the authors also showed a slight association of anti-phosphatidylserine-prothrombin complex antibodies (anti-PS/PT) with vascular complications in patients with SSc [75].

Increased prevalence of anti-β2GPI antibodies (up to 42 %) was also detected in children suffering from atopic dermatitis with no APS clinical manifestations. Authors suggested that a repeated exposure to nutritional β2GPI as the consequence of the abnormal intestinal permeability may be responsible for the induction of autoantibodies cross-reacting with self and exogenous molecule in susceptible children [42].

References

1. Giannakopoulos B, Krilis SA (2013) The pathogenesis of the antiphospholipid syndrome. N Engl J Med 368(11):1033–1044
2. Miyakis S et al (2006) International consensus statement on an update of the classification criteria for definite antiphospholipid syndrome (APS). J Thromb Haemost 4(2):295–306
3. Wilson WA et al (1999) International consensus statement on preliminary classification criteria for definite antiphospholipid syndrome: report of an international workshop. Arthritis Rheum 42(7):1309–1311
4. Asherson RA et al (2009) History, classification, and subsets of the antiphospholipid syndrome. In: Antiphospholipid syndrome in systemic autoimmune diseases, vol 10. Elsevier Science, Amsterdam/London, pp 1–11
5. Asherson RA et al (2003) Catastrophic antiphospholipid syndrome: international consensus statement on classification criteria and treatment guidelines. Lupus 12(7):530–534
6. Gomez-Puerta JA, Cervera R (2014) Diagnosis and classification of the antiphospholipid syndrome. J Autoimmun 48–49:20–25
7. Swaak AJ et al (1979) Anti-dsDNA and complement profiles as prognostic guides in systemic lupus erythematosus. Arthritis Rheum 22(3):226–235
8. Mehrani T, Petri M (2009) Epidemiology of the antiphospholipid syndrome. In: Antiphospholipid syndrome in systemic autoimmune diseases, vol 10. Elsevier Science, Amsterdam/London, pp 13–34
9. Meroni PL et al (2004) Anti-beta 2 glycoprotein I antibodies in centenarians. Exp Gerontol 39(10):1459–1465
10. Andreoli L et al (2013) The estimated frequency of antiphospholipid antibodies in patients with pregnancy morbidity, stroke, myocardial infarction, and deep vein thrombosis: a critical review of the literature. Arthritis Care Res (Hoboken) 65(11):1869–1873

11. Cabiedes J et al (2002) Anti-cardiolipin, anti-cardiolipin plus bovine, or human beta(2)-glycoprotein-I and anti-human beta(2)glycoprotein-I antibodies in a healthy infant population. Arch Med Res 33(2):175–179
12. Sene D, Piette JC, Cacoub P (2008) Antiphospholipid antibodies, antiphospholipid syndrome and infections. Autoimmun Rev 7(4):272–277
13. Harel M et al (2005) The infectious etiology of the antiphospholipid syndrome: links between infection and autoimmunity. Immunobiology 210(10):743–747
14. Zachou K et al (2003) Anti-cardiolipin antibodies in patients with chronic viral hepatitis are independent of beta2-glycoprotein I cofactor or features of antiphospholipid syndrome. Eur J Clin Invest 33(2):161–168
15. Palomo I et al (2003) Prevalence of antiphospholipid and antiplatelet antibodies in human immunodeficiency virus (HIV)-infected Chilean patients. J Clin Lab Anal 17(6):209–215
16. Asherson RA, Cervera R (2003) Antiphospholipid antibodies and infections. Ann Rheum Dis 62(5):388–393
17. Blank M, Shoenfeld Y (2004) Beta-2-glycoprotein-I, infections, antiphospholipid syndrome and therapeutic considerations. Clin Immunol 112(2):190–199
18. Hunt JE et al (1992) A phospholipid-beta 2-glycoprotein I complex is an antigen for anticardiolipin antibodies occurring in autoimmune disease but not with infection. Lupus 1(2):75–81
19. Uthman IW, Gharavi AE (2002) Viral infections and antiphospholipid antibodies. Semin Arthritis Rheum 31(4):256–263
20. Ramos-Casals M et al (2004) Clinical features related to antiphospholipid syndrome in patients with chronic viral infections (hepatitis C virus/HIV infection): description of 82 cases. Clin Infect Dis 38(7):1009–1016
21. Cervera R et al (2004) Antiphospholipid syndrome associated with infections: clinical and microbiological characteristics of 100 patients. Ann Rheum Dis 63(10):1312–1317
22. Rojas-Rodriguez J et al (2000) Catastrophic antiphospholipid syndrome: clinical description and triggering factors in 8 patients. J Rheumatol 27(1):238–240
23. Font C et al (2011) Solid cancer, antiphospholipid antibodies, and venous thromboembolism. Autoimmun Rev 10(4):222–227
24. Yoon KH et al (2003) High prevalence of antiphospholipid antibodies in Asian cancer patients with thrombosis. Lupus 12(2):112–116
25. Miesbach W, Scharrer I, Asherson R (2006) Thrombotic manifestations of the antiphospholipid syndrome in patients with malignancies. Clin Rheumatol 25(6):840–844
26. Armas JB et al (2000) Anticardiolipin and antinuclear antibodies in cancer patients–a case control study. Clin Exp Rheumatol 18(2):227–232
27. Turna H et al (2009) Is there any effect of tumor burden on hemostatic parameters in cancer patients? A case-control study of hemostatic abnormalities and anticardiolipin antibodies in solid tumors. Clin Appl Thromb Hemost 15(4):454–457
28. Schved JF et al (1994) A prospective epidemiological study on the occurrence of antiphospholipid antibody: the Montpellier Antiphospholipid (MAP) Study. Haemostasis 24(3):175–182
29. Ozguroglu M et al (1999) Serum cardiolipin antibodies in cancer patients with thromboembolic events. Clin Appl Thromb Hemost 5(3):181–184
30. Pusterla S et al (2004) Antiphospholipid antibodies in lymphoma: prevalence and clinical significance. Hematol J 5(4):341–346
31. Zuckerman E et al (1995) Increased thromboembolic incidence in anti-cardiolipin-positive patients with malignancy. Br J Cancer 72(2):447–451
32. Bazzan M et al (2009) Presence of low titre of antiphospholipid antibodies in cancer patients: a prospective study. Intern Emerg Med 4(6):491–495
33. de Meis E, Monteiro RQ, Levy RA (2009) Lung adenocarcinoma and antiphospholipid antibodies. Autoimmun Rev 8(6):529–532
34. Biggioggero M, Meroni PL (2010) The geoepidemiology of the antiphospholipid antibody syndrome. Autoimmun Rev 9(5):A299–A304
35. Mahaum N, Prete PE (2011) Antiphospholipid antibodies in malignancy: are these pathogenic or epiphenomena? J Clin Rheumatol 17(8):429–431

36. Atzeni F et al (2005) Autoimmunity and anti-TNF-alpha agents. Ann N Y Acad Sci 1051: 559–569
37. Ferraccioli G et al (2002) Anticardiolipin antibodies in rheumatoid patients treated with etanercept or conventional combination therapy: direct and indirect evidence for a possible association with infections. Ann Rheum Dis 61(4):358–361
38. Bobbio-Pallavicini F et al (2004) Autoantibody profile in rheumatoid arthritis during long-term infliximab treatment. Arthritis Res Ther 6(3):R264–R272
39. Hemmati I, Kur J (2013) Adalimumab-associated antiphospholipid syndrome: a case report and review of the literature. Clin Rheumatol 32(7):1095–1098
40. Vereckei E et al (2010) Anti-TNF-alpha-induced anti-phospholipid syndrome manifested as necrotizing vasculitis. Scand J Rheumatol 39(2):175–177
41. Hughes GR (1983) Thrombosis, abortion, cerebral disease, and the lupus anticoagulant. Br Med J (Clin Res Ed) 287(6399):1088–1089
42. Avcin T et al (2008) Pediatric antiphospholipid syndrome: clinical and immunologic features of 121 patients in an international registry. Pediatrics 122(5):e1100–e1107
43. Petri M (2000) Epidemiology of the antiphospholipid antibody syndrome. J Autoimmun 15(2):145–151
44. Alarcon-Segovia D et al (1992) Preliminary classification criteria for the antiphospholipid syndrome within systemic lupus erythematosus. Semin Arthritis Rheum 21(5):275–286
45. Gomez-Puerta JA et al (2005) Long-term follow-up in 128 patients with primary antiphospholipid syndrome: do they develop lupus? Medicine (Baltimore) 84(4):225–230
46. Freire PV et al (2014) Distinct antibody profile: a clue to primary antiphospholipid syndrome evolving into systemic lupus erythematosus? Clin Rheumatol 33(3):349–353
47. Tarr T et al (2007) Primary antiphospholipid syndrome as the forerunner of systemic lupus erythematosus. Lupus 16(5):324–328
48. Cervera R et al (2002) Antiphospholipid syndrome: clinical and immunologic manifestations and patterns of disease expression in a cohort of 1,000 patients. Arthritis Rheum 46(4):1019–1027
49. Gattorno M et al (2003) Outcome of primary antiphospholipid syndrome in childhood. Lupus 12(6):449–453
50. Uthman I, Khamashta M (2005) Ethnic and geographical variation in antiphospholipid (Hughes) syndrome. Ann Rheum Dis 64(12):1671–1676
51. Domenico Sebastiani G, Minisola G, Galeazzi M (2003) HLA class II alleles and genetic predisposition to the antiphospholipid syndrome. Autoimmun Rev 2(6):387–394
52. Freitas MV et al (2004) Is HLA class II susceptibility to primary antiphospholipid syndrome different from susceptibility to secondary antiphospholipid syndrome? Lupus 13(2): 125–131
53. Caliz R et al (2001) HLA class II gene polymorphisms in antiphospholipid syndrome: haplotype analysis in 83 Caucasoid patients. Rheumatology (Oxford) 40(1):31–36
54. Tincani A et al (2009) The interplay between the antiphospholipid syndrome and systemic lupus erythematosus. Autoimmunity 42(4):257–259
55. Vianna JL et al (1994) Comparison of the primary and secondary antiphospholipid syndrome: a European Multicenter Study of 114 patients. Am J Med 96(1):3–9
56. Soltesz P et al (2003) Evaluation of clinical and laboratory features of antiphospholipid syndrome: a retrospective study of 637 patients. Lupus 12(4):302–307
57. Danowski A et al (2009) Determinants of risk for venous and arterial thrombosis in primary antiphospholipid syndrome and in antiphospholipid syndrome with systemic lupus erythematosus. J Rheumatol 36(6):1195–1199
58. McClain MT et al (2004) The prevalence, onset, and clinical significance of antiphospholipid antibodies prior to diagnosis of systemic lupus erythematosus. Arthritis Rheum 50(4):1226–1232
59. Wahl DG et al (1997) Risk for venous thrombosis related to antiphospholipid antibodies in systemic lupus erythematosus–a meta-analysis. Lupus 6(5):467–473
60. Somers E, Magder LS, Petri M (2002) Antiphospholipid antibodies and incidence of venous thrombosis in a cohort of patients with systemic lupus erythematosus. J Rheumatol 29(12): 2531–2536

61. Clowse ME et al (2006) Early risk factors for pregnancy loss in lupus. Obstet Gynecol 107(2 Pt 1):293–299
62. Cervera R et al (2009) Morbidity and mortality in the antiphospholipid syndrome during a 5-year period: a multicentre prospective study of 1000 patients. Ann Rheum Dis 68(9):1428–1432
63. van Vollenhoven RF et al (2014) Treat-to-target in systemic lupus erythematosus: recommendations from an international task force. Ann Rheum Dis 73(6):958–967
64. Khamashta MA et al (1995) The management of thrombosis in the antiphospholipid-antibody syndrome. N Engl J Med 332(15):993–997
65. Crowther MA et al (2003) A comparison of two intensities of warfarin for the prevention of recurrent thrombosis in patients with the antiphospholipid antibody syndrome. N Engl J Med 349(12):1133–1138
66. Finazzi G et al (2005) A randomized clinical trial of high-intensity warfarin vs. conventional antithrombotic therapy for the prevention of recurrent thrombosis in patients with the antiphospholipid syndrome (WAPS). J Thromb Haemost 3(5):848–853
67. Lim W, Crowther MA, Eikelboom JW (2006) Management of antiphospholipid antibody syndrome: a systematic review. JAMA 295(9):1050–1057
68. Ruiz-Irastorza G, Hunt BJ, Khamashta MA (2007) A systematic review of secondary thromboprophylaxis in patients with antiphospholipid antibodies. Arthritis Rheum 57(8):1487–1495
69. Kleinknecht D et al (1989) Recurrent thrombosis and renal vascular disease in patients with a lupus anticoagulant. Nephrol Dial Transplant 4(10):854–858
70. Leaker B et al (1991) Insidious loss of renal function in patients with anticardiolipin antibodies and absence of overt nephritis. Br J Rheumatol 30(6):422–425
71. Isenberg DA, Griffiths M, Neild GH (1995) Woman with livedo reticularis, renal failure, and benign urinary sediment. Nephrol Dial Transplant 10(2):295–297
72. Hanly JG et al (1999) A prospective analysis of cognitive function and anticardiolipin antibodies in systemic lupus erythematosus. Arthritis Rheum 42(4):728–734
73. Hanly JG et al (2010) Prospective analysis of neuropsychiatric events in an international disease inception cohort of patients with systemic lupus erythematosus. Ann Rheum Dis 69(3):529–535
74. Merkel PA et al (1996) The prevalence and clinical associations of anticardiolipin antibodies in a large inception cohort of patients with connective tissue diseases. Am J Med 101(6):576–583
75. Sanna G et al (2005) Antiphospholipid antibodies in patients with scleroderma: prevalence and clinical significance. Ann Rheum Dis 64(12):1795–1796

The Catastrophic Antiphospholipid Syndrome 20

Ignasi Rodríguez-Pintó, Gerard Espinosa, and Ricard Cervera

20.1 Introduction

The addition of the word "catastrophic" to the term antiphospholipid syndrome (APS) was proposed 20 years ago by Ronald Asherson when he published an editorial in The Journal of Rheumatology describing a group of patients who develop multiple thrombosis in a short period of time and with a much worse prognosis than that attributed to patients with classic APS [1]. Since then, many cases have been published reporting patients with this devastating variant of the APS.

The catastrophic APS (CAPS) is a rare disease that affects around 1 % (0.4–1.6 %) of patients with APS [2] but is associated with a high rate of mortality [3]. The majority of the knowledge on this disease has been provided by studying the cases included in the CAPS Registry. This is a database in a web-based format that includes all patients published or reported directly to the CAPS Registry Project Group with this condition. This registry was created in 2000 by the European Forum on Antiphospholipid Antibodies, a group of experts devoted to perform international collaborative studies on antiphospholipid antibodies (aPLs) [4]. The results are freely available in its web site (https://ontocrf.costaisa.com/en/web/caps). The CAPS Registry includes nowadays more than 500 cases from almost 200 published papers and 100 cases directly reported to the CAPS Registry Project Group.

According to the CAPS Registry, this syndrome affects mainly women with a female to male ratio of 3:1 and involves patients in their fourth decade of life, although cases in newborns and elderly patients have been reported [5]. CAPS is the first manifestation of APS in 56.4 % of patients, and most of them do not present any associated autoimmune disease. In the remaining patients, systemic lupus

I. Rodríguez-Pintó • G. Espinosa • R. Cervera (✉)
Department of Autoimmune Diseases, Hospital Clinic, Villarroel 170, Barcelona, Catalonia 08036, Spain
e-mail: ignasirodriguezpinto@gmail.com; gespino@clinic.cat; RCERVERA@clinic.cat

© Springer International Publishing Switzerland 2015

P.L. Meroni (ed.), *Antiphospholipid Antibody Syndrome: From Bench to Bedside*, Rare Diseases of the Immune System, DOI 10.1007/978-3-319-11044-8_20

erythematosus (SLE) is the autoimmune disease more frequently associated with CAPS, followed by rheumatoid arthritis, dermatomyositis, Behçet disease, or Crohns' disease [5].

20.2 Pathophysiology

The pathological mechanisms involving CAPS are not yet clearly understood [6]. The rarity of this syndrome hindered any effort to perform mechanistic studies, and CAPS is considered to have a multifactorial etiology, including a genetic background and environmental factors. In this sense, an association has been found between several polymorphisms of HLA class II genes and the development of aPLs. However, its role in APS pathogenesis and, especially, in CAPS has not been elucidated.

The role of aPLs in endothelial cell (EC) activation as a pathogenic mechanism of thrombosis in APS was first proposed by Meroni et al. [7]. Rashi et al. [8] later suggested that anti-β2-glycoprotein I (GPI) antibodies might mediate the activation of EC leading to an alteration in the endothelial phenotype and a switch to a procoagulant microenvironment.

Several explanations of these events have been proposed. Asherson and Shoenfeld [9] postulated the molecular mimicry hypothesis, suggesting that some peptides derived from β2-GPI recognized by aPLs might share some amino acid sequences with those found in several microorganisms. The aPLs were found to activate EC and monocytes when they are bound to β2-GPI. The activation of EC and monocytes upregulates the production of tissue factor leading to a procoagulant state [10].

However, no more than 15 % of general population patients with aPLs develop thrombosis [6]. Indeed, β2-GPI does not bind to unstimulated endothelium in vivo [11]. This observation lead to propose the "two-hit" hypothesis to explain the only occasionally clinical observation of thrombotic events in spite of the persistent presence of aPLs in these patients [12]. In this hypothesis, a "first hit" would induce a thrombophilic state but clotting would take place only in the presence of a "second hit." This "second hit" would be another thrombophilic condition that increases the risk for clot formation. The presence of an environmental trigger as a "second hit" has been reported in more than half of cases with CAPS [5]. The most frequent precipitating factor reported are infections, especially in the pediatric age [3, 13]. In this regard, both human monoclonal IgM and polyclonal IgG anti-β2-GPI antibodies were found to induce an endothelial signal similar to that induced through toll-like receptor 4 (TLR-4) activation. The TLR are a type of pattern recognition receptors. These are transmembrane receptors that recognize molecules that are broadly shared by pathogens but different from host molecules, collectively referred as pathogen-associated molecular patterns [14]. TLR4 is known to be essential for innate immune response to components of bacteria, mycobacteria, yeast, and virus [15]. It is expressed in the innate immune system cells surface and EC [16] and is known to be the main receptor in lipopolysaccharide (LPS) signal transduction [17]. Ligand binding to TLR4 triggers the MyD88-dependent pathway finally leading to

NF-κB and AP-1 [8] activation and resulting in transcription of inflammatory genes [18]. On the other hand, virtually all patients with sepsis have coagulation abnormalities [19]. These abnormalities range from subtle activation of coagulation only detectable by sensitive techniques through somewhat subclinical stronger coagulation activation evident by a small decrease in platelet count and prolongation of global clotting times to fulminant disseminated intravascular coagulation, characterized by widespread microthrombosis and profuse bleeding [20]. At the same time, proinflammatory cytokines are important in inducing a procoagulant effect by inducing tissue factor expression on mononuclear cells and EC, probably playing their role in increasing the risk for new thrombosis.

In 1998, Kitchens [21] proposed that intravascular coagulation itself could increase the risk to develop another thrombosis. In this theory, the blood clot would promote thrombin formation and fibrinolysis would become impaired by an increase of plasminogen activator inhibitor (PAI) type I. This would determine the consumption of natural anticoagulant proteins, such as protein C and antithrombin.

However, it is still unclear why some patients with aPLs develop thrombosis affecting large vessels, while others develop this catastrophic situation with simultaneous multiple vascular occlusions that affects predominantly small vessels. In CAPS, probably all these factors are interplaying in a procoagulant milieu that leads to this multiorgan thrombosis in small vessels observed in clinical practice. Some clinical manifestations are not directly related to the blood flow occlusion but to the cytokine overexpression in the ischemic necrotic tissue, leading to the so-called cytokine storm. This, probably, at the same time closes the circle that leads to this devastating situation.

20.3 Precipitating Factors

As previously explained, in the two-hit hypothesis, the presence of a second thrombophilic state has been proposed to explain the observation of thrombosis in patients with circulating aPLs. Different triggers have been reported in as much as 2/3 of CAPS cases. The most common precipitating factors described are infections, followed by neoplasms, surgical procedures, and anticoagulation withdrawal or low international normalized ratio (INR) [3, 5, 22].

Different infectious agents are associated with CAPS. Among them, the most frequent reported are bacteria such as *Escherichia coli, Shigella sp., Salmonella, Streptococcus, Staphylococcus aureus, Klebsiella*, and herpes virus, affecting mainly the lungs and kidneys. Most of them are gram-negative bacteria, and, thus, these infectious agents might act co-signaling with aPLs the TLR signal that leads to the prothrombotic state and, finally, to CAPS.

Not surprisingly, neoplasms are the second most frequent precipitating factor in CAPS. Hematological malignancies are the oncological diseases more frequently associated with CAPS and, among them, Hodgkin's lymphoma. However, CAPS has been reported to be associated with carcinomas and sarcomas [23]. Malignancies have been linked to the development of circulating aPLs [24], and the increased risk of cancer patients to develop thrombosis is well known since last century when Trousseau described the development of thrombophlebitis in these patients [25]. Several reasons have been proposed to explain the increased risk of thrombosis in cancer patients. For instance, blood flow stasis due to vascular invasion, immobilization, upregulation of thrombophilic substances by both tumor and endothelial cells, chemotherapy, and central venous devices have been proposed as conditions that might explain the increased frequency of thrombosis in these patients.

Surgery and trauma are found often associated with the development of CAPS in patients with APS. The increased postoperative risk of thrombosis after major general surgery or multiple trauma has been extensively documented [26, 27]. The inflammatory response to the surgery wound is thought to explain the increased risk described in these patients. Interestingly, pre-surgery measurement such as plasma exchange have been proposed in order to decrease aPL levels and, thus, reduce the thrombotic risk [22].

Other precipitating factors such as anticoagulation withdrawn, pregnancy, and postpartum period have been reported to be linked to a CAPS episode, but in lower frequency.

20.4 Clinical Manifestations

The development of multiple microvascular thrombotic occlusions with microangiopathic anemia and thrombocytopenia is a characteristic finding of patients with CAPS. As a systemic disease, CAPS can affect any organ or system. Clinical manifestations have been classically classified into those attributed to thrombosis itself and those attributable to the cytokine storm [28]. However, sometimes it is difficult to differentiate if a clinical manifestation is attributable to one or the other cause and many times both pathways may work together.

CAPS patients present frequently with renal failure and variable degrees of hypertension, although hypotension does not exclude the diagnosis. Some patients present with proteinuria and sometimes with hematuria [3, 5, 22, 29].

Pulmonary manifestations are reported in 2/3 of cases, classically characterized by acute respiratory distress syndrome (ARDS) attributed typically to the cytokines storm. Pulmonary emboli are associated with dyspnea, and, sometimes, the clinical picture is associated with pulmonary hemorrhage [3, 22, 29, 30].

Almost half of patients with CAPS present with consciousness deterioration manifested as encephalopathy. Many times, it is not clear if this manifestation could be ascribed to general hypoperfusion because of microthrombosis, to generalized shock, or to intracranial large vessel thrombosis. Nevertheless, some patients present with classical neurological deficits with motor or sensitive symptoms and an established stroke. Less often is the report of seizures, and, when present, many times they are associated with other manifestations [3, 22, 29].

Heart failure due to myocardium infarction, angina, or cardiac valvulopathy (Libman-Sacks endocarditis) is described in 50 % of cases, sometimes with cardiogenic shock as part of multiorganic failure, with hypotension, tachycardia, and oliguria. The main valves affected are the mitral and the aortic valves. This condition is mainly reported as valvular insufficiency, and, sometimes, it leads to the requirement of valvular replacement. Intracavitary thrombosis has been seldom reported in patients with CAPS.

Skin complications in a form of livedo reticularis are very often reported; however, few of these cases develop skin necrosis with ulcers and digital ischemia [5, 22, 29].

Other organs affected are the peripheral vessels, the intestine, the spleen, the adrenal glands, the pancreas, the retina, and the bone marrow. Anecdotally, testicular/ovarian infarction, necrosis of the prostate, and acalculous cholecystitis have been reported [5, 22, 29].

20.5 Diagnosis

The differential diagnosis of patients with multiple thrombosis is not easy. Indeed, many times, several thrombophilic situations interplay together, leading to thrombosis in multiple sites throughout the organism.

Most cases of CAPS present as microangiopathic storm rather than large-vessel occlusion, although cases with large-vessel involvement have been reported. The presence of multiple occlusions should always rise the suspicion of a thrombophilic state. However, when this thrombosis presents in large vessels, the search for classical well-known risk factors for thrombosis should be performed. Typical risk factors for thrombosis include malignancy, surgery, obesity, immobility, pregnancy and oral contraception, and hereditary and acquired thrombophilias (i.e., aPLs, antithrombin, protein C and protein S deficiency, factor V Leiden and prothrombin G20210A mutations, and increased levels of several coagulation factors such as factor VIII, IV, or XI). Nevertheless, the microangiopathic storm that is common in CAPS leads to a deferent differential diagnosis that includes diseases characteristically associated with microangiopathy. Classically, the differential diagnosis of patients with CAPS includes severe infections, with or without disseminated intravascular coagulation (DIC), noninfectious-related DIC, thrombotic thrombocytopenic purpura (TTP) or hemolytic uremic syndrome, heparin-induced thrombocytopenia, HELLP (hemolysis, elevated liver enzymes, low platelet count) syndrome, and scleroderma renal crisis.

Even when the presence of aPLs in patients with multiple thrombosis gives habitually the clue for the differential diagnosis of patients with this microangiopathic picture, the presence of aPLs is not pathognomonic of CAPS and have been reported in several other situations. However, when aPLs are found in other settings, they are almost always reported at lower levels [22, 31], but the clinical situation should always guide decision making.

Systemic severe infections may recall the clinical picture of CAPS, and sometimes both situations take place together: the first acting as a trigger of the second.

There is evidence that the activation of inflammation and coagulation in the context of severe sepsis can lead to thrombosis [32], and, at the same time, infections have proved to be able to lead to the development of aPLs [24]. However, although transient aPLs positivity at low levels can be found in severe infections, they have no clinical significance. Thus, the presence of high levels of aPLs should be taken as a highly specific finding for CAPS helping in the differential diagnosis between these two clinical situations [22].

DIC is not a disease entity itself but a complication of several disorders. The most commons disorders associated with DIC are infections, severe trauma, malignancy, and obstetric complications [33, 34]. DIC is characterized clinically by thrombosis and bleeding with coagulation factor consumption leading to coagulation times prolongation and fibrinogen consumption [35]. However, clinical and laboratory features of DIC have been observed in patients with CAPS [36]. Thus, it may not be possible to differentiate between these two clinical situations, and both situations might take place together.

Nevertheless, TTP represents the most difficult differential diagnosis of patients with CAPS. Renal and neurological clinical manifestations with anemia, thrombocytopenia, and the presence of schistocytes in peripheral blood smear can be found in both TTP and CAPS. However, even when the specificity of the ADAMTS-13 activity has been long debated in the literature [37], the presence of low levels of ADAMTS-13 activity might give the clue for the diagnosis of a TTP, while high levels of aPL should favor the diagnosis of CAPS.

Heparin-induced thrombocytopenia (HIT) is a rare but sometimes severe complication of heparin treatment that occurs 4–10 days after the initiation of a therapy with heparin. The severe form (type II) is a disorder characterized by the formation of autoantibodies against the heparin-platelet factor 4 (PF4) complex that binds to platelets leading to cell aggregation and activation [38]. The history of heparin administration and the presence of PF4 antibodies may let physicians to distinguish between these clinical situations [22].

HELLP syndrome is an endothelium disease that affects small vessels of hepatic circulation. It normally takes place at the end of the pregnancy, and sometimes it has been considered an expression of CAPS. However, the small number of patients with CAPS in the obstetric period makes it difficult to differentiate this clinical situation from the CAPS, and probably both clinical situations might favor each other.

Even when scleroderma renal crisis has been proposed as a possible differential diagnosis for patients with CAPS, the presence of classical sclerodermic cutaneous findings, of classical autoantibodies or, at least, the previous history of Raynaud's phenomenon in patients with systemic sclerosis, should differentiate these situations. Nevertheless, although rarely, the development of CAPS in patients with systemic sclerosis has been reported. In these patients, the determination of aPL levels and a renal biopsy are warranted in order to establish the diagnosis.

In this sense, in order to help physicians facing this difficult differential diagnosis, a set of diagnostic criteria for CAPS has been proposed during the 14th

Table 20.1 Diagnostic criteria for CAPS

1. Evidence of involvement of 3 organs, systems, and/or tissues
2. Development of manifestations simultaneously or in less than 1 week
3. Laboratory confirmation of the presence of aPL (LAC and/or aCL and/or anti-2GPI antibodies) in titers higher than 40 UI/l
4. Exclude other diagnosis
Definite CAPS:
All 4 criteria
Probable CAPS:
All 4 criteria, except for involvement of only 2 organs, system, and/or tissues
All 4 criteria, except for the absence of laboratory confirmation at least 12 weeks apart associable to the early death of a patient never tested for aPL before onset of CAPS
1, 2, and 4
1, 3, and 4 and the development of a third event in >1 week but <1 month, despite anticoagulation treatment

International Congress on Antiphospholipid Antibodies (Table 20.1). These criteria take into account the difficulty of performing biopsy in critical care settings, and thus, they do not require the biopsy for the diagnosis although it is highly recommended (Table 20.2).

20.6 Treatment

Due to its bad prognosis, when CAPS is suspected, an aggressive treatment is justified. However, there are no randomized controlled trials to guide the efficacy of the therapies, and data is based on the reported cases and the analysis of the CAPS Registry [39]. Classically, three aspects have been claimed as the basis to treat this situation. First, the so-called supportive general measures; second, the aggressive treatment of any identifiable trigger; and, finally, the specific treatment [39].

The general measures treatment refers to supportive care. It often includes intensive care unit (ICU) admission. Sometimes, intubation is necessary but, mostly, only ICU admission and tight control are necessary. Whenever possible, classical thrombotic risk factors should be avoided, and external pneumatic compression devices might be used when immobility is a concern. When major surgery aim is not taking out necrotic tissue to control the cytokine storm, surgery procedures should be postponed. Additionally, CAPS patients may benefit from glycemic control, stress ulcer prophylaxis, and blood pressure control [39].

Treatment of any precipitating factor is mandatory. When an infection is suspected, an adequately chosen antibiotic treatment should be started, taking into account the infection site, pharmacokinetics, and organism pharmacodynamics. At the same time, amputation and debridation of necrotic tissue might help in controlling the systemic inflammatory response [39–41].

Table 20.2 Differential diagnosis

	CAPS	TTP	HELLP	Sepsis	DIC	HIT
Previous history	Previous APS/SLE/malignancy/pregnancy	Malignancy/non	Pregnancy	Infection	Infection/malignancy	Heparin exposure
Thrombosis	Large/small vessels	Small vessels	Small vessels	Large/small vessels	Small vessels	Large/small vessels
Typical antibodies	aPL	Anti-ADAMS-13	None	None	None	Anti-HP4
Schizocytes	Present	Present	Scanty	Scanty	Scanty	Scanty
Fibrinogen	Normal/high	Normal/high	Normal/high	Normal/low	Normal/low	Normal/high

Abbreviations: *TTP* thrombotic thrombocytopenic purpura, *HELLP* hemolysis, elevated liver enzymes, low platelet count, *DIC* disseminated intravascular coagulation, *HIT* heparin-induced thrombocytopenia, *aPL* antiphospholipid antibodies, *SLE* systemic lupus erythematosus

Since no randomized controlled trials have been conducted in CAPS, the specific treatment of this situation is based on the information provided by the analysis of the CAPS Registry and expert opinion. However, these data permitted the establishment of recommendations and the publication of a treatment algorithm [42].

Heparin is the mainstay of treatment in CAPS patients as it inhibits clot formation and lyses existing clots [22, 28, 30, 39, 43, 44]. Non-fractionated intravenous heparin is often chosen when the patient is in the ICU. Heparin does not only inhibit clot generation but also promotes clot fibrinolysis [45]. Additionally, heparin seems to inhibit aPL binding to their target on the cell surface [46]. Moreover, non-fractionated heparin enables throwback of its effect in case of necessity and it has an antidote. Thus, heparin is always the first line of treatment for thrombosis. Later, non-fractionated heparin can be switched to low molecular weight heparin (LMWH) and finally to oral anticoagulation. Nevertheless, physician should try to keep patients time long enough with heparin to favor clot fibrinolysis.

The combination of corticosteroids with anticoagulant therapy is the standard of care in CAPS treatment.

Many similarities have been observed between the clinical manifestations of patients with CAPS and systemic inflammatory response syndrome (SIRS). Since corticosteroids inhibit the nuclear factor (NF)-κB pathway and aPLs seem to signal NF-κB upregulation, beneficial effects of corticosteroids treatment have been invocated. However, in severe infections and in CAPS, no strong evidence has been found supporting corticosteroid use unless patients develop adrenal insufficiency [47, 48]. Until more studies analyzing the use of corticosteroids can be driven, the consensus treatment guidelines [22] should be followed [44], although there is no clear evidence on the route, dose, and duration of this treatment.

Only recently, the beneficial effects of intravenous immunoglobulins (IVIG) in primary APS have been proved. IVIG proved to decrease aPL titers and therefore, the thrombotic risk of these patients [49, 50]. However, IVIG and plasma exchanges were found few years ago to be a useful complementary tool for the treatment of patients with CAPS [51]. Their high economic cost and low availability may limit their use in patients with CAPS [52]. In this sense, an algorithm for the treatment of CAPS was published in order to guide physician facing these patients and establish treatment priorities [53]. This algorithm proposed to start specific treatment by handling independently each one of the main pathologic pathways. The authors recommended starting on anticoagulation and steroids as soon as the catastrophic situation is suspected. The former is given in order to stop the thrombophilic state and promote clot lysis and the later to downregulate the cytokine storm thought to be the one responsible for SIRS. When the patient is thought to be in a life-threatening condition, the authors suggested adding treatment with IVIG and/or plasma exchanges [53]. In case of active lupus manifestations, treatment with cyclophosphamide should be considered due to the better prognosis of these when they are treated with this drug. Cyclophosphamide is a nitrogen mustard-alkylating agent that binds to deoxyribonucleic acid in immune cells leading to cell death. Cyclophosphamide, probably, promotes the proliferation of T cells, suppression of helper Th1 activity, and enhances Th2 response (Fig. 20.1) [54].

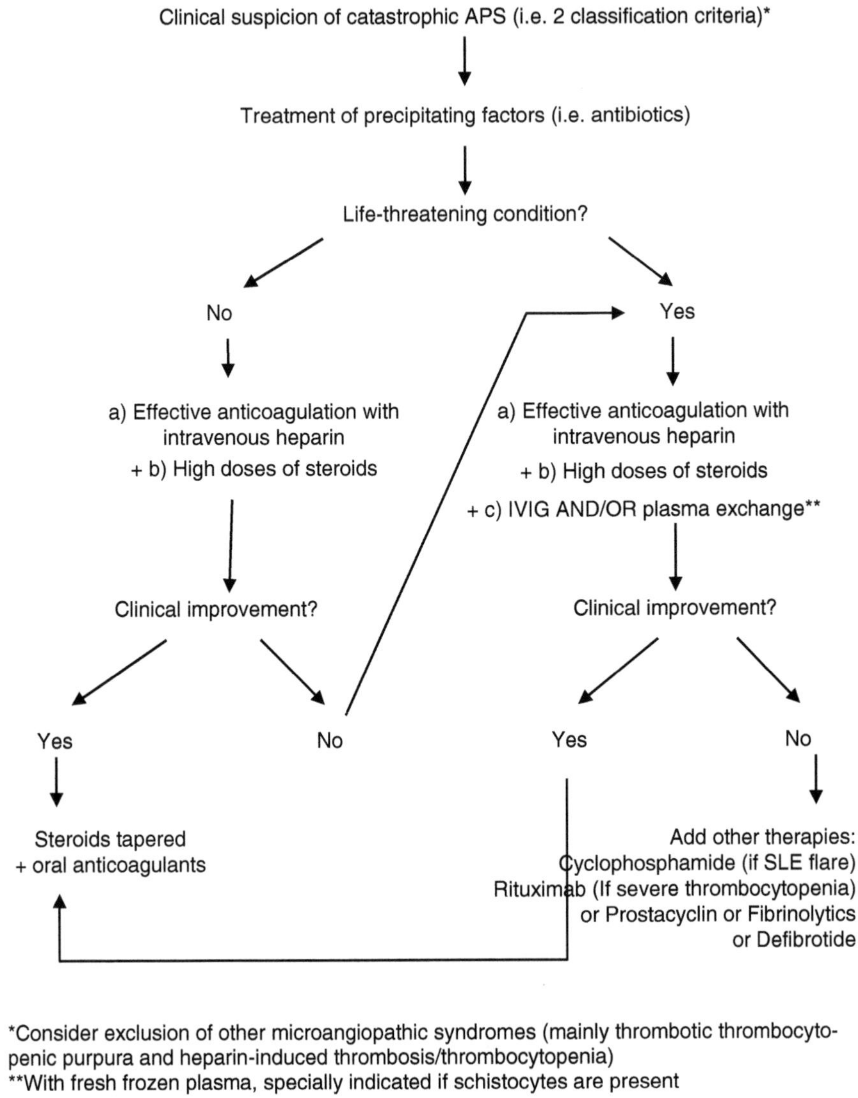

Fig. 20.1 Treatment algorithm of catastrophic APS. Abbreviations: *IVIG* intravenous immunoglobulins, *SLE* systemic lupus erythematosus

Rituximab is a chimeric monoclonal antibody against CD20, a surface protein expressed on the cytoplasmic membrane of B cells. Rituximab is approved for the treatment of B-cell non-Hodgkin lymphoma and rheumatoid arthritis [55]. However, it has been used extensively for the treatment of several other autoimmune diseases [56–58]. Although two randomized controlled trials failed to demonstrate its effectiveness in SLE, it seems to be safe for the treatment of APS. Rituximab has been proposed as a second-line therapy when facing refractory CAPS cases with a relapsing course [59]. The analysis of 18 cases from the CAPS Registry showed that 80 % of them recovered from the CAPS episode in front of the 20 % who did not [22, 59]. Nevertheless, the small number of patients treated with rituximab makes difficult to propose definitive conclusions, but in light of these good results, rituximab has been also proposed as first-line therapy.

20.7 Prognostic

Despite aggressive treatment, mortality in patients with CAPS continues to be high [48]. It accounts for almost 30 % of cases according to the CAPS Registry data [3, 48, 60]. This disease normally have monophasic course, and most patients surviving a CAPS remain symptom free with anticoagulation, although some develop further APS-related events [61]. However, although rare, cases with a recurrent course have been reported. Of note, they present high prevalence of microangiopathic hemolytic anemia laboratory features [51, 62].

References

1. Asherson RA (1992) The catastrophic antiphospholipid syndrome. J Rheumatol 19:508–512
2. Cervera R, Piette J-C, Font J, Khamashta MA, Shoenfeld Y, Camps MT et al (2002) Antiphospholipid syndrome: clinical and immunologic manifestations and patterns of disease expression in a cohort of 1,000 patients. Arthritis Rheum 46:1019–1027
3. Cervera R, Rodríguez-Pintó I, Espinosa G (2014) On behalf of the Task Force on Catastrophic Antiphospholipid Syndrome. Catastrophic antiphospholipid syndrome: task force report summary. Lupus 23:1283–1285
4. Cervera R (2012) CAPS registry. Lupus 21:755–757
5. Cervera R, Bucciarelli S, Plasín MA, Gómez-Puerta JA, Plaza J, Pons-Estel G et al (2009) Catastrophic antiphospholipid syndrome (CAPS): descriptive analysis of a series of 280 patients from the "CAPS Registry". J Autoimmun 32:240–245
6. Ortega-Hernandez O-D, Agmon-Levin N, Blank M, Asherson RA, Shoenfeld Y (2009) The physiopathology of the catastrophic antiphospholipid (Asherson's) syndrome: compelling evidence. J Autoimmun 32:1–6
7. Meroni PL, Raschi E, Camera M, Testoni C, Nicoletti F, Tincani A et al (2000) Endothelial activation by aPL: a potential pathogenetic mechanism for the clinical manifestations of the syndrome. J Autoimmun 15:237–240
8. Raschi E, Testoni C, Bosisio D, Borghi MO, Koike T, Mantovani A et al (2003) Role of the MyD88 transduction signaling pathway in endothelial activation by antiphospholipid antibodies. Blood 101:3495–3500
9. Asherson RA, Shoenfeld Y (2000) The role of infection in the pathogenesis of catastrophic antiphospholipid syndrome–molecular mimicry? J Rheumatol 27:12–14
10. Vega-Ostertag M, Casper K, Swerlick R, Ferrara D, Harris EN, Pierangeli SS (2005) Involvement of p38 MAPK in the up-regulation of tissue factor on endothelial cells by antiphospholipid antibodies. Arthritis Rheum 52:1545–1554
11. Agostinis C, Biffi S, Garrovo C, Durigutto P, Lorenzon A, Bek A et al (2011) In vivo distribution of β2 glycoprotein I under various pathophysiologic conditions. Blood 118:4231–4238

12. Shoenfeld Y, Meroni PL, Toubi E (2009) Antiphospholipid syndrome and systemic lupus erythematosus: are they separate entities or just clinical presentations on the same scale? Curr Opin Rheumatol 21:495–500
13. Berman H, Rodríguez-Pintó I, Cervera R, Gregory S, de Meis E, Rodrigues CEM et al (2014) Pediatric catastrophic antiphospholipid syndrome: descriptive analysis of 45 patients from the "caps registry.". Autoimmun Rev 13:157–162
14. Janeway CA, Medzhitov R (2002) Innate immune recognition. Annu Rev Immunol 20:197–216
15. Kurt-Jones EA, Popova L, Kwinn L, Haynes LM, Jones LP, Tripp RA et al (2000) Pattern recognition receptors TLR4 and CD14 mediate response to respiratory syncytial virus. Nat Immunol 1:398–401
16. Allen KL, Fonseca FV, Betapudi V, Willard B, Zhang J, McCrae KR (2012) A novel pathway for human endothelial cell activation by antiphospholipid/anti-β2 glycoprotein I antibodies. Blood 119:884–893
17. Chow JC, Young DW, Golenbock DT, Christ WJ, Gusovsky F (1999) Toll-like receptor-4 mediates lipopolysaccharide-induced signal transduction. J Biol Chem 274:10689–10692
18. Xie H, Sheng L, Zhou H, Yan J (2014) The role of TLR4 in pathophysiology of antiphospholipid syndrome-associated thrombosis and pregnancy morbidity. Br J Haematol 164:165–176
19. Levi M, Schultz M, van der Poll T (2013) Sepsis and thrombosis. Semin Thromb Hemost 39:559–566
20. Levi M (2008) The coagulant response in sepsis. Clin Chest Med 29:627–642, viii
21. Kitchens CS (1998) Thrombotic storm: when thrombosis begets thrombosis. Am J Med 104: 381–385
22. Cervera R, Rodríguez-Pintó I, Colafrancesco S, Conti F, Valesini G, Rosário C et al (2014) 14th international congress on antiphospholipid antibodies task force report on catastrophic antiphospholipid syndrome. Autoimmun Rev 13:699–707
23. Miesbach W, Asherson RA, Cervera R, Shoenfeld Y, Gomez Puerta J, Bucciarelli S et al (2006) The catastrophic antiphospholipid (Asherson's) syndrome and malignancies. Autoimmun Rev 6:94–97
24. Cervera R, Asherson RA, Acevedo ML, Gómez-Puerta JA, Espinosa G, De La Red G et al (2004) Antiphospholipid syndrome associated with infections: clinical and microbiological characteristics of 100 patients. Ann Rheum Dis 63:1312–1317
25. Trousseau A (1865) Phlegmasia alba dolens. Lectures on clinical medicine, delivered at the Hotel-Dieu, Paris, pp 281–332
26. Anderson FA, Spencer FA (2003) Risk factors for venous thromboembolism. Circulation 107:I9–I16
27. Reed RL, Ericsson CD, Wu A, Miller-Crotchett P, Fischer RP (1992) The pharmacokinetics of prophylactic antibiotics in trauma. J Trauma 32:21–27
28. Rodríguez-pintó I, Espinosa G, Cervera R (2013) Catastrophic antiphospholipid syndrome – 20 years later. Curr Rheumatol Rev 9:73–80
29. Asherson RA, Cervera R, Piette JC, Font J, Lie JT, Burcoglu A et al (1998) Catastrophic antiphospholipid syndrome. Clinical and laboratory features of 50 patients. Medicine (Baltimore) 77:195–207
30. Cervera R, Espinosa G (2012) Update on the catastrophic antiphospholipid syndrome and the "CAPS Registry". Semin Thromb Hemost 38:333–338
31. Gruel Y, Rupin A, Watier H, Vigier S, Bardos P, Leroy J (1992) Anticardiolipin antibodies in heparin-associated thrombocytopenia. Thromb Res 67:601–606
32. Levi M, Keller TT, van Gorp E, ten Cate H (2003) Infection and inflammation and the coagulation system. Cardiovasc Res 60:26–39
33. Spero JA, Lewis JH, Hasiba U (1980) Disseminated intravascular coagulation. Findings in 346 patients. Thromb Haemost 43:28–33
34. Siegal T, Seligsohn U, Aghai E, Modan M (1978) Clinical and laboratory aspects of disseminated intravascular coagulation (DIC): a study of 118 cases. Thromb Haemost 39:122–134

35. Taylor FB Jr, Toh C, Hoots WK, Wada H, Levi M, Scientific and Standardization Committee Communications, *On behalf of the Scientific Subcommittee on Disseminated Intravascular Coagulation (2001) Towards definition, clinical and laboratory criteria, and a scoring system for disseminated intravascular coagulation. Thromb Haemost 86:1327–1330
36. Asherson RA, Espinosa G, Cervera R, Gómez-Puerta JA, Musuruana J, Bucciarelli S et al (2005) Disseminated intravascular coagulation in catastrophic antiphospholipid syndrome: clinical and haematological characteristics of 23 patients. Ann Rheum Dis 64:943–946
37. George JN, Charania RS (2013) Evaluation of patients with microangiopathic hemolytic anemia and thrombocytopenia. Semin Thromb Hemost 39:153–160
38. Arepally GM, Ortel TL (2006) Clinical practice. Heparin-induced thrombocytopenia. N Engl J Med 355:809–817
39. Cervera R (2010) Catastrophic antiphospholipid syndrome (CAPS): update from the "CAPS Registry". Lupus 19:412–418
40. Amital H, Levy Y, Davidson C, Lundberg I, Harju A, Kosach Y et al (2001) Catastrophic antiphospholipid syndrome: remission following leg amputation in 2 cases. Semin Arthritis Rheum 31:127–132
41. Sacks S, Finn J, Sanna G, Khamashta MA, Chowdhury F, Hunt BJ et al (2013) N2010 adult-onset Still's disease complicated by hemophagocytic syndrome and catastrophic antiphospholipid syndrome resulting in four limb amputation. Isr Med Assoc J 15:192–194
42. Asherson RA, Espinosa G, Cervera R, Font J, Reverter JC (2002) Catastrophic antiphospholipid syndrome: proposed guidelines for diagnosis and treatment. J Clin Rheumatol 8:157–165
43. Cervera R, Tektonidou MG, Espinosa G, Cabral AR, González EB, Erkan D et al (2011) Task Force on Catastrophic Antiphospholipid Syndrome (APS) and Non-criteria APS Manifestations (II): thrombocytopenia and skin manifestations. Lupus 20:174–181
44. Erkan D (2006) Therapeutic and prognostic considerations in catastrophic antiphospholipid syndrome. Autoimmun Rev 6:98–103
45. Weitz JI, Hirsh J, Samama MM (2004) New anticoagulant drugs: the Seventh ACCP Conference on antithrombotic and thrombolytic therapy. Chest 126:265S–286S
46. Franklin RD, Kutteh WH (2003) Effects of unfractionated and low molecular weight heparin on antiphospholipid antibody binding in vitro. Obstet Gynecol 101:455–462
47. Manoach S (2008) Corticosteroids for septic shock. N Engl J Med 358:2070; author reply 2070–2071
48. Bucciarelli S, Espinosa G, Cervera R, Erkan D, Gómez-Puerta JA, Ramos-Casals M et al (2006) Mortality in the catastrophic antiphospholipid syndrome: causes of death and prognostic factors in a series of 250 patients. Arthritis Rheum 54:2268–2576
49. Sciascia S, Giachino O, Roccatello D (2012) Prevention of thrombosis relapse in antiphospholipid syndrome patients refractory to conventional therapy using intravenous immunoglobulin. Clin Exp Rheumatol 30:409–413
50. Tenti S, Guidelli GM, Bellisai F, Galeazzi M, Fioravanti A (2013) Long-term treatment of antiphospholipid syndrome with intravenous immunoglobulin in addition to conventional therapy. Clin Exp Rheumatol 31:877–882
51. Bucciarelli S, Erkan D, Espinosa G, Cervera R (2009) Catastrophic antiphospholipid syndrome: treatment, prognosis, and the risk of relapse. Clin Rev Allergy Immunol 36:80–84
52. Erkan D, Espinosa G, Cervera R (2010) Catastrophic antiphospholipid syndrome: updated diagnostic algorithms. Autoimmun Rev 10:74–79
53. Asherson R, Cervera R, de Groot PG, Erkan D, Boffa M-CC, Piette J-CC et al (2003) Catastrophic antiphospholipid syndrome: international consensus statement on classification criteria and treatment guidelines. Lupus 12:530–534
54. Matar P, Rozados VR, Gervasoni SI, Scharovsky GO (2002) Th2/Th1 switch induced by a single low dose of cyclophosphamide in a rat metastatic lymphoma model. Cancer Immunol Immunother 50:588–596

55. Buch MH, Smolen JS, Betteridge N, Breedveld FC, Burmester G, Dörner T et al (2011) Updated consensus statement on the use of rituximab in patients with rheumatoid arthritis. Ann Rheum Dis 70:909–920
56. Ramos-Casals M, Soto MJ, Cuadrado MJ, Khamashta MA (2009) Rituximab in systemic lupus erythematosus: a systematic review of off-label use in 188 cases. Lupus 18:767–776
57. Calich AL, Puéchal X, Pugnet G, London J, Terrier B, Charles P et al (2014) Rituximab for induction and maintenance therapy in granulomatosis with polyangiitis (Wegener's). Results of a single-center cohort study on 66 patients. J Autoimmun 50:135–141
58. Devauchelle-Pensec V, Mariette X, Jousse-Joulin S, Berthelot J-M, Perdriger A, Puéchal X et al (2014) Treatment of primary Sjögren syndrome with rituximab: a randomized trial. Ann Intern Med 160:233–242
59. Berman H, Rodríguez-Pintó I, Cervera R, Morel N, Costedoat-Chalumeau N, Erkan D et al (2013) Rituximab use in the catastrophic antiphospholipid syndrome: descriptive analysis of the CAPS registry patients receiving rituximab. Autoimmun Rev 12:1085–1090
60. Espinosa G, Bucciarelli S, Asherson RA, Cervera R (2008) Morbidity and mortality in the catastrophic antiphospholipid syndrome: pathophysiology, causes of death, and prognostic factors. Semin Thromb Hemost 34:290–294
61. Erkan D, Asherson RA, Espinosa G, Cervera R, Font J, Piette J-C et al (2003) Long term outcome of catastrophic antiphospholipid syndrome survivors. Ann Rheum Dis 62:530–533
62. Espinosa G, Rodríguez-Pintó I, Gomez-Puerta JA, Pons-Estel G, Cervera R (2012) Relapsing catastrophic antiphospholipid syndrome potential role of microangiopathic hemolytic anemia in disease relapses. Semin Arthritis Rheum 42:417–423

Index

© Springer International Publishing Switzerland 2015

P.L. Meroni (ed.), *Antiphospholipid Antibody Syndrome: From Bench to Bedside*, Rare Diseases of the Immune System, DOI 10.1007/978-3-319-11044-8

FSC
www.fsc.org
MIX
Papier aus verantwortungsvollen Quellen
Paper from responsible sources
FSC® C105338

If you have any concerns about our products,
you can contact us on
ProductSafety@springernature.com

In case Publisher is established outside the EU,
the EU authorized representative is:
Springer Nature Customer Service Center GmbH
Europaplatz 3, 69115 Heidelberg, Germany

Printed by Libri Plureos GmbH
in Hamburg, Germany